Foundation Studies for Nursing

Foundation Studies for Nursing

Using Enquiry-Based Learning

Edited by

SUE GRANDIS, GARTH LONG, ALAN GLASPER
and PAM JACKSON

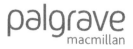

First published 2003 by
PALGRAVE MACMILLAN
Houndmills, Basingstoke, Hampshire RG21 6XS and
175 Fifth Avenue, New York, N.Y. 10010
Companies and representatives throughout the world

PALGRAVE MACMILLAN is the global academic imprint of the Palgrave Macmillan division of St. Martin's Press, LLC and of Palgrave Macmillan Ltd. Macmillan® is a registered trademark in the United States, United Kingdom and other countries. Palgrave is a registered trademark in the European Union and other countries.

ISBN 0–333–77738–7

This book is printed on paper suitable for recycling and made from fully managed and sustained forest sources.

A catalogue record for this book is available from the British Library.

10 9 8 7 6 5 4 3 2 1
12 11 10 09 08 07 06 05 04 03

Typeset by Footnote Graphics Limited, Warminster, Wilts

Printed and bound in Great Britain by Ashford Colour Press Ltd, Gosport.

Contents

3 ■ Insights into Child and Family Health   48

Gill McEwan, Janet Kelsey, Jim Richardson and Alan Glasper

4 ■ Insights into Adolescent Health and Eating Disorders   115

Chris Taylor and Michael Cooper

7 ■ Insights into Learning Disability Nursing 208
Neil Jackson and Tony Gilbert

8 ■ Insights into Community Care 237
Cynthia Akinsanya

12 ■ Insights into Rehabilitation Nursing   379
Stephen O'Connor and Bernard Gibbon

Figures

Tables

Contributors

Cynthia Yolanda Akinsanya, MSc (Surrey), RGN, RM, RFN, PGCEA, DNT, RNT, PWT, Cert Psychology (Lon), Senior Lecturer (Community Health), Anglia Polytechnic University.

Cynthia Akinsanya is a Senior Lecturer in the School of Community Health and Social Studies at Anglia Polytechnic University. She has experience of teaching and research in community health care, with a specific focus on nursing care in the community. Her academic interest involves innovatory principles in learning and teaching approaches in nursing and education. Cynthia has written, published and researched into perspectives in learning and teaching for a number of years.

Alison Cochrane, MA, BA(Hons), RGN, OND, Senior Lecturer (Nursing Older People), University of Central Lancashire.

Alison Cochrane is a Senior Lecturer in Nursing Older People in the Department of Nursing at the University of Central Lancashire. She has experience of teaching the care of older people, with interests in rehabilitation and dementing illness. Her primary academic interest lies in gerontology and she has undertaken research into the sociological/nursing needs of older Asian people and patients' experiences of nutrition on a rehabilitation ward. Prior to her career in education, Alison was a ward sister on an acute assessment and rehabilitation ward for people over the age of 65.

Michael Cooper, MSc, RMN, RNT, Lecturer (Child and Adolescent Mental Health), University of Southampton.

Michael Cooper is a Lecturer in Child and Adolescent Mental Health in the School of Nursing and Midwifery at the University of Southampton. His main academic interest is the therapeutic relationship across a range of nursing settings. He works at present predominantly with children's nurses facing the increasing challenge of mental health issues in the paediatric environment. He has recent clinical experience of a joint appointment, working clinically with adolescents in a CAMH environment. Related clinical work includes providing supervision for practitioners, and also the teaching of communication and counselling skills.

Janet M. Dean, BA(Hons), Dip Nursing, RGN, RNT, Lecturer (Adult Nursing), University of Southampton.

Janet Dean is a Lecturer in Adult Nursing in the School of Nursing and Midwifery at the University of Southampton, where her teaching contribution is primary related to respiratory nursing and the development of nursing skills. Her academic interests include infection control, and she has written and researched hand washing in clinical environments. Janet's clinical background is in acute medical and intensive care nursing. She has a particular interest in respiratory and cardiac nursing and has experience as a lecturer practitioner in acute respiratory care.

Pat Donovan, MA (Ed), MPhil, RGN RM ADM, PGCEA, ILT, Principal Lecturer, (Approved Midwife Teacher) responsible for Quality, University of Central Lancashire.

Pat Donovan is Principal Lecturer in the Department of Midwifery Studies at the University of Central Lancashire. She has experience in developing and teaching on midwifery and neonatal courses at undergraduate and postgraduate level. Her primary academic interest is in professional education, but she is fascinated by, and enjoys teaching, embryology. Pat has also worked abroad and keeps an active interest in overseas work.

Anne Francis, RN, BSc(Hons), Nursing Science ENB Higher Award, PGCE, ENB 264, Dip Nursing, Lecturer Practitioner (Burns and Plastic Surgery), Salisbury NHS Health Care Trust and Bournemouth University.

Anne Francis is Lecturer Practitioner in Burns and Plastic Surgery at the Burns Unit, Salisbury NHS Health Care Trust, and at the Institute of Health and Community Studies, Bournemouth University. She has experience of teaching the ENB 264 burns, plastic and maxillo facial surgery nursing, with a particular focus on wound management within the speciality. Her primary academic interest lies in burns care. Anne worked as the sister on a regional burns unit prior to her career in education, and she has maintained an active clinical role.

Bernard Gibbon, PhD, RMN, RGN, OND, Dip Nursing, Dip ANS, RCNT, RNT, MSc, Head of Department of Nursing, University of Central Lancashire.

Bernard Gibbon is Head of the Department of Nursing at the University of Central Lancashire. Following a clinical career where he worked in both mental health care settings and medical nursing settings, he embarked on a nurse education career. He has a strong interest in clinical nursing practice and engages in nursing research focused on practice issues. He is particularly interested in the care and management of patients requiring post-acute care and rehabilitation, especially stroke rehabilitation, and in multi-professional team working.

Carolyn Gibbon, MA, BA, RN, RCNT, DPSN, Senior Lecturer (Nursing), University of Central Lancashire.

Carolyn Gibbon is a Lecturer in Nursing in the Department of Nursing at the University of Central Lancashire, teaching mainly adult (medical and elderly care) nursing to pre-registration nursing students. Her main interest is in problem-based learning as a teaching and learning methodology. Whilst being a facilitator to students, she also runs workshops for staff in relation to PBL. Recently she was part of a group who successfully won FDTL4 monies to put PBL (triggers with links, e.g. animations) on the Web to assist students, particularly those from diverse backgrounds.

Tony Gilbert, RN, BA(Hons), MSc, PGCEA, PhD, ILTM. Head of Department: Primary Health, Mental Health and Learning Disability, University of Plymouth.

Tony Gilbert is Head of the Department of Primary Health, Mental Health and Learning Disability in the Institute of Health Studies at the University of Plymouth. He has experience as a clinician and teacher in learning disability and has held a number of different appointments across the UK. His present role focuses upon a wide range of population and health issues. Tony has research interests in disability, social policy and sociology, where his work has focused on issues of power, citizenship, trust and managerialism.

Neil Jackson, RN(LD), APN(Cert), RNT, Cert Ed, B Ed, MA, Lecturer (Learning Disability Nursing), University of Southampton.

Neil Jackson is a Lecturer in Learning Disability Nursing in the School of Nursing and Midwifery at the University of Southampton. He has experience of facilitating small learning groups for the past 15 years. He has written on the issue of choice making and he has undertaken research in relation to generic working. His teaching interests are in applied ethics and all aspects of learning disability nursing.

Janet Kelsey, MSc, BSc (Hons), Adv Dip Ed, PGCE, RNT, RSCN, RN, Senior Lecturer (Children's Nursing), University of Plymouth.

Janet Kelsey is a Lecturer in Children's Nursing in the Institute of Health Studies at the University of Plymouth. She has a background of 25 years in paediatric nursing. Her experience includes working in both district general and children's hospitals in various specialities. For the past ten years she has held a variety of roles within nurse education.

Vanessa Lockyer-Stevens, PGCE, Bsc(Hons), RN (Children's Nurse), ENB 100, OND, Clinical Development Coordinator, Princess Margaret Hospital for Children, Western Australia.

Vanessa moved to Perth in Western Australia in 2000, where she currently works as a practice-based Clinical Development Co-ordinator. Her background as Lecturer in Child Health and Critical Care from the UK has enabled her to undertake academic work within several universities from Perth to Broome in north-western West Australia. Her key academic interests lie in paediatric and adult critical care. She is currently researching an aspect of bereavement care, exploring provision for families who may wish to take their child home following sudden death.

Eileen Mann, BSc (Hons), RGN, SCM, PGCE, Consultant Nurse (Pain Management), Poole Hospital NHS Trust and Bournemouth University.

Eileen Mann in a Consultant Nurse in Pain Management who divides her time between Poole Hospital NHS Trust, and the Institute of Health and Community Studies at Bournemouth University. Her teaching experience was gained as a Lecturer Practitioner at Bournemouth University, during which time she co-authored *Pain: Creative Approaches to Effective Management* with Dr Eloise Carr. She still maintains an active clinical role at Poole Hospital NHS Trust where she is involved in integrating practice development, education and research.

Gill McEwing, MSc, Dip Nursing, Cert Ed, RNT, RSCN, RN, Senior Lecturer (Children's Nursing), University of Plymouth.

Gill McEwing is a Senior Lecturer in Children's Nursing in the Institute of Health Studies at the University of Plymouth and has a background of 25 years in paediatric nursing. She has gained experience from working in both district general and specialist children's hospitals both in Britain and abroad. She has been employed in a variety of roles in nurse education for the past 15 years.

Stephen E. O'Connor, PhD, MA, BSc, RN, Cert Ed, Consultant Nurse (Rehabilitation), Winchester and Eastleigh Health Care Trust, and Lecturer (Nursing) University of Southampton.

Stephen O'Connor is a Consultant Nurse in Rehabilitation with the Winchester and Eastleigh Health Care Trust, and a lecturer in Nursing in the School of Nursing and Midwifery at Southampton University. Stephen was one of the first wave of consultant nurses and one of the first in rehabilitation; he has now been in post for two years. His main areas of clinical input are post-acute rehabilitation of the older person and stroke rehabilitation. His primary academic interest has been into the role of the nurse in rehabilitation and has published widely on this subject. He was until recently Chair of the RCN Rehabilitation Forum.

John W. Rawlinson, MN, RGN, RMN, Dip Nursing, Cert Ed, Subject Advisor/ Principal Lecturer (Mental Health), University of Plymouth.

John Rawlinson is Academic Lead for Mental Health in the Institute of Health Studies at the University of Plymouth. Mental Health is the focus and passion of his work. However, despite a community psychiatric nurse background, he increasingly advocates less differentiation between community mental health nursing and other recovery focused mental health work. Course leader for MSc (Mental Health) and BSc (Community Mental Health), his areas of interest include: psychotherapy; psychodrama; personal construct theory; personality disorder; policy; legislation; and service development. Having worked in London, South Africa, Bristol and Cardiff, he moved to Devon in 1996. He is married with grown up children.

Jim Richardson, BA, RGN, RSCN, PGCE, PhD, ILTM, Principal Lecturer (Children's Nursing) School of Care Sciences, University of Glamorgan.

Jim Richardson is a Principal Lecturer in the School of Care Sciences at the University of Glamorgan and has been a children's nurse in a number of settings in Wales and Finland. As a children's nurse educator for the last 12 years, his research and teaching interests have focused on the impact of chronic childhood illness on family life, on cultural aspects of the care of the child and family, and aspects of fatherhood.

Lynda Rogers, MA, BA, RGN, RMN, PGCEA, RNT, Lead Lecturer (Health Psychology and Health Law), University of Southampton.

Lynda Rogers is Lead Lecturer in Health Psychology and Health Law in the School of Nursing and Midwifery University of Southampton. Lynda's areas of teaching reflect her interest within clinical practice. Prior to her career in education she spent many years in clinical practice, both in the acute and community sectors, enabling her to develop her knowledge and experience related to care of the dying person and the family. Her current PhD research relates to curriculum change and the facilitation of students' needs in relationship to loss, grief and bereavement. Lynda is also a volunteer counsellor for a national organisation.

Paula Shobbrook, RGN, BNS, Deputy Director of Nursing, Winchester and Eastleigh Health Care NHS Trust.

Paula Shobbrook is Deputy Director of Nursing based at the Royal Hampshire County Hospital, Winchester. She has experience developing clinical services in primary care, and has worked in community hospital settings and in secondary care, where her area of expertise is respiratory nursing. Paula is studying for an MSc in Nursing and has particular interest in managing and implementing change within the NHS. In her current role Paula leads practice and workforce development for nursing.

Chris Taylor, SRN, RSCN, Dip HE (Community Health and Welfare Studies), ENB 603, Nurse Specialist (Child and Adolescent Mental Health), Child Health Directorate, Southampton General Hospital.

Chris Taylor is a Nurse Specialist in Child and Adolescent Mental Health in Southampton, working in the Paediatric Liaison Team based within an Acute Paediatric Unit. After many years working as a general and paediatric trained nurse, she followed her interest in child and adolescent psychiatry. Her present post enables her to combine her interests in paediatrics and mental health, and her main interests of eating disorders and deliberate self-harm. Chris is currently undertaking an MSc in Family Therapy.

Pauline Turner, B.A. (Hons), M.Phil, RGN, Diploma in Palliative Nursing, Lecturer (Nursing), University of Southampton.

Pauline Turner is Lecturer in Nursing in the School of Nursing and Midwifery at the University of Southampton. She was a member of a community palliative nursing team at Countess Mountbatten House in Southampton for a number of years as well as being part of the education team there. She also has experience of teaching and research in palliative care and has been involved in running interprofessional workshops in palliative care for a number of years. Currently her main responsibilities are in post-qualifying education.

Acknowledgements

This book is dedicated to students of health care who are a great source of inspiration in their thirst for knowledge. Working with students, particularly in learning groups, has been a challenging and stimulating experience and we are grateful to all those students, past and present, we have had the pleasure of teaching.

The editors would also like to express their appreciation to the chapter contributors for their huge commitment to bringing this project to fruition. Thanks also to the many people who have helped us along the way with this project but are too numerous to name individually here, they know who they are and we are grateful to them.

In addition, we are grateful to the following for their kind permission to use copyright material: the University of Southampton School of Nursing and Midwifery for permission to reproduce materials related to enquiry-based learning; The Nursing and Midwifery Council for permission to reproduce the UKCC/NMC Outcomes for entry to the branch programme in Table 1.1; The Royal Cornwall Hospital Trust for permission to reproduce the Nursing Assessment sheet in Table 3.10; Peter Gardiner, medical illustrator, for permission to reproduce the stroke positions on p. 399; the Medical and Elderly Care Directorate, Southampton University Hospital Trust, for permission to reproduce the Nutritional Risk Assessment Tool in Table 10.6.

Every effort has been made to trace the copyright holders but if any have been inadvertently overlooked, the publishers will be pleased to make the necessary arrangements at the earliest opportunity.

Introduction

Sue Grandis, Garth Long, Alan Glasper and Pam Jackson

1

This book is just one of many resources that will help you to acquire the knowledge and skills needed over the first year of your programme in order to meet the required out-comes and to make the transition towards your chosen branch programme.

Exploring the patient's experiences

The scenarios and clinical situations that are visited in each chapter can be explored within the context of any of the four branch programmes so, whichever path you choose to follow, this learning will have direct relevance for you and you will be able to apply it in your own practice setting.

The approach to learning is characterised by:

- Active learning – you will be invited to explore issues and gain further insights through local practice observations.
- Learning individually and in groups – debating issues with colleagues enriches and diversifies your understanding.
- Working through activities and seeking out and responding to questions and dilem-mas, many of which you are encouraged to pose for yourself.

The aim of this book is to help you to embark on the road to becoming a professional nurse practitioner. For this reason the questions and activities that will guide your learn-ing will frequently place you in the role of the qualified nurse, rather than as student or care assistant.

Although some students may wish to leave the programme at the end of the first year and some may choose to work as care assistants, it is not the intention of this book to prepare you for such a role. Therefore, no reference is made to qualifying frameworks such as National Vocational Qualification.

This book will introduce you to a new and refreshing approach to learning nursing. It is a book that uses real client experiences as the focus for learning about nursing; it is therefore more about learning how to think about nursing and how to approach challenging situations than providing all the answers. It is the professional nurse's ability to seek out the answers and provide the best possible care that separates the nurse from non-professional colleagues. Nurses and other health professionals need to be constantly aware of changes, often brought about by research findings, so knowledge is dynamic. Developing the skills to access current information is key to professional practice. It is these skills of enquiry that we hope to promote through your exploration of the chapters in this book.

Learning through enquiry

In taking a client-focused approach we want you to be able to visualise the 'picture on the box' which you will come to recognise as 'nursing', before being tempted to examine each piece of the jigsaw. This, we believe, is fundamental to appreciating the holistic and integrative nature of contemporary health care practice, which crosses professional boundaries in providing best possible patient care. This places learning in context; it gives you the opportunity to experience the excitement and challenge of professional practice from a position of safety, whilst also acknowledging the frustrations that some days can bring. This reality, together with your own experiences drawn from practice, will enable you to seek out and understand the background and detail behind each event.

Being reflective, being inquisitive and solving problems

Using enquiry as the basis of your learning often means starting with something unfamiliar or confusing and then seeking out the information that helps to explain or make sense of this situation or thing. This is a bit like looking for clues to solve a puzzle, something that nurses have to do all the time. Seeking out and making sense of situations that are confusing and dealing with the uncertainties of life are essential skills, equally as important as learning about hard facts.

This is often called being 'reflective' and is often described as a sequence of events known as the reflective cycle. There are several examples which have been developed (Gibbs 1988; Schon 1983).

The following is an adaptation from Gibbs (1988):

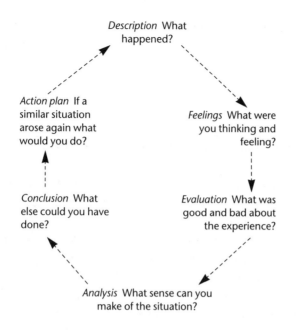

Description What happened?

Action plan If a similar situation arose again what would you do?

Feelings What were you thinking and feeling?

Conclusion What else could you have done?

Evaluation What was good and bad about the experience?

Analysis What sense can you make of the situation?

Figure 1.1   The reflective cycle

There is a further example of the reflective cycle included in Chapter 14, pp. 453–4, 464, which illustrates how it may be used in practice.

It would be helpful to keep these reflective stages in your mind as you explore and make sense of the different scenarios, and the complex world of nursing which unfold in the chapters of this book. Being reflective means getting in touch and keeping in touch with the way you and others practice.

Activity 1.1

Think about a situation that you have recently experienced, perhaps one that did not quite go according to plan. Now work through each of the stages of the reflective cycle exploring your personal experience, looking at what you did and how you might do it differently next time.

Reflection provides a systematic approach to learning and to practising nursing. You will also hear about problem-based approaches to assessing, planning, implementing and evaluating care.

Problem solving can also be seen as a cycle and makes use of some of the principles that have already been introduced in the reflective cycle. In reality you will use both approaches, depending upon the situation you are exploring. For instance, sometimes you will explore a problem and find that there is a definite solution, a right or wrong answer, often proven through past research. On other occasions there is no problem to be solved, just something that appears confusing, that needs to be explored and understood. Such is the world of nursing.

So what is enquiry-based learning?

The approach we are taking in this book is described by us as enquiry-based learning, it will invite you to explore and learn through practice. It will not give you all the answers, but don't worry as it is not intended to.

Enquiry-based learning (EBL) shares similar principles to an approach known as problem-based learning (PBL). It is not necessary for you to be able to distinguish between the two, unless you are particularly interested.

Modern history of the problem-based learning movement began at the medical school at McMaster University in Hamilton, Canada. EBL/PBL found favour as it was perceived by teachers to be an ideal medium for exploring the real world of patient care through which students could learn how to 'solve problems' and think critically. It is, however, important to understand that the term 'problem' encompasses 'enquiry', or the asking of questions about a particular subject which may or may not be directly related to a problem as such, but rather the learning issues to be explored.

This is particularly pertinent in higher education, where the emphasis has moved away from teaching to a more holistic use of the term 'learning'. Hence strategies to enhance learning opportunities, such as the use of EBL/PBL, have been adopted by many disciplines, including nursing. Many traditional boundaries between the health care professions are becoming increasingly blurred in response to changes in health care delivery (Humphris and Masterson 2000) and students are expected to work flexibly across these interprofessional boundaries. This changing workplace environment now requires an innovative approach to health care education, which facilitates greater understanding of the roles of different members of the interdisciplinary health care team. EBL/PBL purports to do this through challenging students to identify the ideas and skills they will need to tackle complexities of health care delivery (Duch et al 2001).

Approaches to learning through EBL/PBL are discussed in more detail at the end of this chapter.

Working with scenarios

Most clients first access health care within the community setting, many attending the local health centre, the occupational health facility at work, or being cared for in their own homes. Some of the scenarios in this book are set within the community, some are also located within a hospital or other residential settings, but all emphasise the importance of providing integrated services, so that wherever people are nursed there is continuity of care.

Central to each chapter is a named individual or a family. They may have health problems, which have resulted from disease, injury or handicap, or have been exacerbated by social circumstances resulting in distress. Each is equally important to the student of nursing. The study of health will enable the nurse to raise health awareness, promote health and, where possible, reduce the likelihood of disease or recurrence of illness. The skills of the nurse are also directed towards those who are already ill, are disabled or having difficulty coping, either in the short or long term. Much is about enabling people to maximise their level of independence, to live fulfilling lives. Nursing is not so much about cure, but providing quality of life, providing comfort and, where needed, supporting the whole family through a period of death and bereavement. This philosophy is reflected in the chapters of this book and the principles are relevant to all branches of nursing.

Practising in a changing world of health care

The ways in which new nurses are prepared for their unique role within health services has changed radically over the last few years. Different health professions now often learn together. There is now more flexible access as well as opportunities to 'step on' and 'step off' courses, as your individual student needs dictate. This book hopes to introduce you to a way of learning that reflects and complements the diversity of this approach. Whether you embark on your studies in a College of Further Education or at University, we intend that this book will act as an effective resource as you begin a career in nursing.

Although the fundamental principles upon which nursing is founded remain unaltered, the ways in which nurses practise, the roles they occupy with others and the public's expectation is constantly changing. In this century more than ever before, nurses will have to adapt their practice to meet the needs of the increasing number of people who are living longer, well into old age. Nurses must find ways of providing the best care possible, yet be constrained by tighter costs and account for their every action.

Whilst research and new technologies will enable more and more dreams to be realised, lives to be saved and health to be optimised, some of the longer established treatments will, as now, be found wanting. We have already entered the arena of the 'super bug'. There are new challenges; old diseases over which we had previous control are increasing again, and the full impact on health from environmental change is yet to be realised. Smoking has increased dramatically amongst young women and we are yet to see a real reduction in the amount of heart disease. Conversely, many people who develop cancer are living much longer after treatment than they previously did.

New ways of working mean that 'e-nursing' is becoming a reality. No wonder public expectation constantly rises as the media proclaims that more and more is possible! At the same time, the expectations and demands of modern living are leading to increased levels of stress, mental illness and suicide in all age groups. New ways of caring for people within the community aim to more effectively support independence. There is the challenge whereby acceptable risks need to be taken, whilst public protection must always be paramount. Nurses have to be able to make such difficult decisions daily. When things go wrong, more people then ever before will know their rights and will have the confidence to seek redress but, because the gap between wealth and poverty continues to widen, the nurse's role in safeguarding the interests of the more vulnerable becomes even more important.

As the boundaries of practice change, nurses will choose to extend their skills into new areas. Some will overlap with the skills of other professionals, and yet all nurses will continue to use those skills which the public recognise and know as 'nursing'. It is this mix of essential skills, knowledge and attitudes interwoven into the fabric of nursing that is central to lifelong professional practice. It is these fundamental principles which will be introduced during the initial period of the course and the way you achieve these will influence the way you will nurse in the future.

Working towards competence

The Nursing and Midwifery Council (NMC), the regulatory body for nursing, sets out a number of common outcomes that all students on a three-year programme, irrespective of where they are studying in the UK, are required to achieve. Meeting these first year outcomes will enable you to proceed to one of four branch programmes: adult; children's; mental health; or learning disability nursing. The NMC Outcomes to be achieved at the end of the first year are set out in Table 1.1.

Table 1.1 NMC Outcomes for entry to the branch programme

Professional and ethical practice

Discuss in an informed manner the implications of professional regulation for nursing practice.

- demonstrate a basic knowledge of professional regulation and self-regulation
- recognise and acknowledge the limitations of one's own abilities
- recognise situations which require referral to a registered practitioner.

Demonstrate an awareness of the NMC code of professional conduct

- commit to the principle that the primary purpose of the registered nurse is to protect and serve society
- accept responsibility for one's own actions and decisions.

Demonstrate an awareness of, and apply ethical principles to, nursing practice

- demonstrate respect for patient and client confidentiality
- identify ethical issues in day-to-day practice.

Demonstrate an awareness of legislation relevant to nursing practice

- identify key issues in relevant legislation relating to mental health, children, data protection, manual handling, and health and safety, etc.

Demonstrate the importance of promoting equity in patient and client care by contributing to nursing care in a fair and anti-discriminatory way

- demonstrate fairness and sensitivity when responding to patients, clients and groups from diverse circumstances
- recognise the needs of patients and clients whose lives are affected by disability, however manifest.

Discuss methods of, barriers to and the boundaries of effective communication and interpersonal relationships

- recognise the effect of one's own values on interactions with patients and clients and their carers, families and friends
- utilise appropriate communication skills with patients and clients
- acknowledge the boundaries of a professional caring relationship.

Demonstrate sensitivity when interacting with and providing information to patients and clients

Contribute to enhancing the health and social well being of patients and clients by understanding how, under the supervision of a registered practitioner, to:

- contribute to the assessment of health needs
- identify opportunities for health promotion
- identify networks of health and social care services.

Table 1.1 (*continued*)

Contribute to the development and documentation of nursing assessments by participating in comprehensive and systematic nursing assessment of the physical, psychological, social and spiritual needs of patients and clients

- be aware of assessment strategies to guide the collection of data for assessing patients and clients and use assessment tools under guidance
- discuss the prioritisation of care needs
- be aware of the need to reassess patients and clients as to their needs for nursing care

Contribute to the planning of nursing care, involving patients and clients and, where possible, their carers, demonstrating an understanding of helping patients and clients to make informed decisions

- identify care needs based on the assessment of patient or client
- participate in the negotiation and agreement of the care plan with the patient or client and with their carer, family or friends, as appropriate, under the supervision of a registered nurse
- inform patients and clients about intended nursing actions, respecting their right to participate in decisions about their care.

Contribute to the implementation of a programme of nursing care, designed and supervised by a registered practitioner

- undertake activities which are consistent with the care plan and within the limits of one's own abilities.

Demonstrate evidence of a developing knowledge base which underpins safe nursing practice

- access and discuss research and other evidence in nursing and related disciplines
- identify examples of the use of evidence in planned nursing interventions.

Demonstrate a range of essential nursing skills, under the supervision of a registered nurse, to meet individuals' needs, which include:

maintaining dignity, privacy and confidentiality, effective communication and observational skills, including listening and taking physiological measurements, safety and health, including moving and handling and infection control, essential first aid and emergency procedures, administration of medicines, emotional, physical and personal care, including meeting the need for comfort, nutrition and personal hygiene.

Contribute to the evaluation of the appropriateness of nursing care delivered

- demonstrate an awareness of the need to assess regularly a patient's or client's response to nursing interventions
- provide for a supervising registered practitioner, evaluative commentary and information on nursing care based on personal observations and actions
- contribute to the documentation of the outcomes of nursing interventions.

Recognise situations in which agreed plans of nursing care no longer appear appropriate and refer these to an appropriate accountable practitioner

- demonstrate the ability to discuss and accept care decisions
- accurately record observations made and communicate these to the relevant members of the health and social care team.

Contribute to the identification of actual and potential risk to patients, clients and their carers, to oneself and to others and participate in measures to promote and ensure health and safety

- understand and implement health and safety principles and policies
- recognise and report situations which are potentially unsafe for patients, clients, oneself and others
- understand and implement health and safety principles and policies.

Demonstrate an understanding of the role of others by participating in inter-professional working practice

- identify the roles of the members of the health and social care team
- work within the health and social care team to maintain and enhance integrated care.

Demonstrate literacy, numeracy and computer skills needed to record, enter, store, retrieve and organise data essential for care delivery

Demonstrate responsibility for one's own learning through the development of a portfolio of practice and recognise when further learning is required

- identify specific learning needs and objectives
- begin to engage with and interpret the evidence base which underpins nursing practice.

Acknowledge the important of seeking supervision to develop safe nursing practice

(Reproduced by kind permission of the Nursing and Midwifery Council 2002)

Getting the most from this book

Because this is a different kind of textbook to many others, not everything will be covered. We have selected aspects which we believe you are most likely to want to explore and which will help you to address each of the NMC Outcomes for entry to the branch programme. These may include a set of particular circumstances, a disease process or set of social issues. This book provides you with the opportunity to identify what you need to learn and to equip yourself with the necessary foundations on which to build your own nursing practice. It will help you explore and experience new ways of learning and to seek out pathways, whilst pointing you towards those resources which will help you to make sense of complex issues. This is enquiry-based learning and we hope you enjoy the challenge, we think you will.

There are a number of steps that characterise the approach to learning that is used in this book. These process steps draw on some of the principles of reflection and problem solving outlined earlier in this introductory chapter. There are several examples of process steps. The steps illustrated here have been adapted from McMaster's handbook for tutors (1996) and Woods (1994).

Enquiry-based learning

The enquiry phase

1 Explore the scenario:
   - Do you understand the context?
   - Are there words that you need to define?
2 What are the main issues?
   Analyse the issues, situation, challenges, problems.
3 Identify what you do not know and need to know (because your lack of knowledge is impeding understanding and action).
4 Decide the exact questions on which you need to work, and prioritise them.
5 Plan your use of resources; for example, plan your time to make the best use of learning opportunities.

The reflective phase

6 Share experiences, new knowledge and learning with others whenever you can create the opportunity. Reflect on the adequacy of the answers to your original questions and identify what remains to be achieved.

When working in a group the seventh stage is:

7 Reflect on the group process (considering what enhances and what inhibits learning within the group learning environment).

Working as an individual you may find it useful to consider your own way of learning and to reflect on your learning strategies, study methods and skills of communication to enable you to create and capitalise on a variety of learning opportunities.

> ### Activity 1.2
>
> Just as you did earlier, try taking a situation or problem and by using the process steps explore ways in which you can find an acceptable way forward, or indeed an answer to your problem.

Getting started

At least a glance at this section may help you to consider effective ways of working with this book so that you can enjoy your learning and make the best use of your study time.

Each chapter has expected learning outcomes; however, as an enquiring student, it is likely that you already have many questions about nursing practice and how this relates to the practice of colleagues from other disciplines. When you start to read each chapter, you may identify with particular clinical or personal experiences which prompt you to question why you thought or reacted in a particular way, so make sure these are noted. You may be exploring some topics for the first time with little or no previous experience, therefore not knowing what you do not know! For many students in health care this can initially raise some anxieties, but you are not alone!

There are prompts for learning in the form of questions and activities at regular points within each chapter. Some of these are best attempted before you read on as they will help you to identify how much you currently know, as well as the level and accuracy of existing knowledge. Sometimes, we don't appreciate what we have previously taken for granted until it is clearly brought to our attention – better in a book than in the clinical environment!

Your very important role as a student is to constantly question, to gain knowledge and to identify the evidence base that underpins accepted nursing practice. Sometimes, this might be based more on 'custom and practice' than evidence and there is a need to seek out the most informed sources, rather than following tradition.

This book helps you to identify the areas of knowledge that you may need to explore and the kinds of questions that you might choose to ask. Developing the confidence to ask questions is a very important part of being a nurse. Nurses need to be able to seek out information from patients and their relatives, often about sensitive or potentially embarrassing topics. Nurses also need to possess assertiveness and interpersonal skills to be able to appropriately question, and sometimes challenge colleagues whether they are from nursing or other disciplines. Clearly, effective communication is immensely important.

Deciding what to focus on

It is also acknowledged that knowledge is constantly changing. This can be a troublesome idea when starting a new career with a vast amount to learn. However, once the overall picture is grasped and the foundations are laid, more complex issues can be tackled. This comes through reading, accessing other resources and also from being an active observer and participant in clinical practice. Soon you will feel more comfortable in questioning accepted practice. As a student you are privileged to experience a wide range of practice environments and you will observe that practices might differ between practitioners. Questioning the rationale for those differences will add to your repertoire of knowledge and skill, rather than accepting that it is just the way that it is done. The manner in which questions are asked are likely to influence the response you receive!

Key points you may like to consider:

- Is this the appropriate time?
- Is this person likely to have the correct information or appropriate experience?
- Do I need permission to ask this person?
- How do I phrase the question; for example, to avoid offence or to ensure the question elicits a relevant answer?

Throughout the book you will be invited to seek the opinions of friends, relatives, patients and others, finding out their views and understanding related to different health issues. By getting into the habit of seeking others' opinions, this will help to develop the skills you will need throughout your professional career. Working in health care is a lifelong learning experience, which requires you to remain open to others' views and opinions.

Most textbooks are studied in isolation. However, it is well established that learning with others can contribute very positively to the learning experience, not only in being more interesting and satisfying, but also in extending ideas. Spending time thinking about practice is useful, but it is likely to be yet more productive if you can engage with others. They may identify aspects which you haven't thought about. Your views may be questioned and this may prompt you to think more laterally – to think the unthinkable!

Your study centre may provide you with opportunities for small group learning and you may have a ready-made group to access. Perhaps you are a member of an email group and could establish a small learning set. You may have friends in other health care educational institutions with similar learning needs.

Each chapter also presents a set of concepts. This list is not definitive. Again, as you approach the topic area in each chapter, you may have your concepts to add to the list. When reviewing the concepts, view them as broadly as possible as this will enhance your understanding. For example, the concept of 'care' will be viewed differently depending on whether you are a patient, client, husband/wife, child, parent, friend, nurse, manager, doctor, physiotherapist, chaplain, undertaker or employer. Accessing the literature will also broaden and deepen your current understanding of each concept. Continually reflect on your personal experience, your current understanding and how new knowledge can change practice. It is through this process that improvements in practice are made.

Some reasons for adopting a model of enquiry-based learning

Since the publication of *Fitness for Practice* (UKCC 1999) many pre-registration nursing curricula have embraced the principles of enquiry-based learning (EBL) as a method of educating students. Enquiry-based learning uses genuine real-life client scenarios, which provide the students with an opportunity to explore a range of issues directly pertaining to client care in a variety of contemporary nursing settings (Long et al 1999). Exploration follows a systematic approach to enquiry, reflection and evaluation and shares many of the principles of problem-based learning (PBL) (Long and Grandis, 2000).

Learning is often undertaken as a group, with individual students taking on specific responsibilities within the group for researching and gathering evidence to bring back to the group. This contributes to the group's overall collective understanding of the issue or problem being explored.

In a recent Canadian study of second year nursing students, Morales-Mann and Kaitell (2001) demonstrated that the factors which most influenced the levels of learning within the group were positive attitudes and group effort. Rhem (1998) believes that the reason why this method is prevailing within higher education institutions is that it orientates students towards strategies of 'meaning making' over simple fact collecting.

In this way the product of the group is greater than the sum of the parts, resulting in higher levels of attainment in which prior learning is valued and built upon. Additionally, this type of co-operative learning brings with it enhanced social skills (Connolly and Seneque 1999) which are highly valued in professions such as nursing.

Perhaps more importantly, the linking of clinical skills (prized by practitioners) and theoretical knowledge (prized by academics) through the medium of EBL/PBL (O'Neil et al 2000; Williams 1999) may bridge the theory–practice gap which has bedevilled the profession for so long. Morales-Mann and Kaitell (2001) have described this type of learning strategy as liberating the academic from the traditional roles associated with teaching.

Acknowledging some challenges

Not all students find the approach easy, indeed some prefer a more structured didactic approach whilst others thrive on the freedom to explore, share and learn in a way that they feel reflects the way in which they will practise as professionals. A study by Glasper (2001) looked at a UK cohort of 15 children's nurses on completion of their three-year pre-registration programme. Using a nominal group technique, he identified five areas which students liked most about EBL and five that they liked least. Students valued the friendships and support generated by working as a group, and believed that EBL enabled them to share experiences, exchange views and gain confidence. They saw EBL as having made the group work 'exceptionally well'. Conversely, students also voiced their frustrations about a lack of structure, having to rely on others to pull their weight and then being provided with poor quality feedback by their peers from what they had researched.

Steele et al (2000) in a comparison of student-led versus tutor-led group work demonstrated a preference for student facilitators. In this study of second year medical students, peer facilitators were given slightly higher ratings than academics, but it was noted by the investigators that peer-facilitated groups often took short cuts in the EBL/PBL process.

Although much of the available literature demonstrates considerable enthusiasm for EBL/PBL as a method of student learning, further research will be required before the efficacy of this type of education can be fully appraised. The outcome of a longitudinal study by Newman (2000) on the efficacy of problem-based learning in post-registration nursing programmes is eagerly awaited.

References

Connolly, C., Seneque, M. (1999) Evaluating problem-based learning in a multilingual student population. *Medical Education* 33 (10), pp. 738–44.

Duch, B. J., Groch, S. E., Allen, D. E. (2001) *The Power of Problem Based Learning: A Practical 'How –To' for Teaching Undergraduate Courses in Any Discipline.* Stirling, VA: Stylus Publishing.

Gibbs, G. (1988) *Learning by Doing: A Guide to Teaching and Learning Methods.* Oxford: Further Education Unit, Oxford Polytechnic (New Oxford Brookes University).

Glasper, E. A., (2001) Child health nurses' perceptions of enquiry-based learning. *British Journal of Nursing* 10 (2), pp. 1343-9.

Humphris, D., Masterson, A. (eds) (2000) *Developing New Clinical Roles: A Guide for Health Professionals.* Edinburgh: Churchill Livingstone.

Long, G., Grandis, S., Glasper, E. A. (1999) Investing in practice: enquiry- and problem-based learning. *British Journal of Nursing* 8 (17), pp. 1171-4.

Long, G., Grandis, S. (2000) Introducing enquiry-based learning into pre-registration nursing programmes. In: Glen, S. and Wilkie, K. (eds). *Problem-Based Learning In Nursing Programmes – A New Model for a New Context.* Macmillan – now Palgrave Macmillan: Basingstoke.

McMaster University (1996) *Tutor Handbook.* Hamilton, Ontario: McMaster University.

Morales-Mann, E. T., Kaitell, C. A. (2001) Problem-based learning in a new Canadian curriculum. *Journal of Advanced Nursing* 33 (1), pp. 13–19.

Newman, M. (2000) Project on the effectiveness of problem based learning (PEPBL): www.hebes.mdx.ac.uk/teaching/research/PEPBL/index.htm.

Nursing and Midwifery Council (2002) *Requirements for Pre-Registration Nursing Programmes*, Section 3 Nursing Competencies. London: NMC, pp. 9–21.

O'Neil, P. A., Morris, J., Baxter, C. M. (2000) Evaluation of an integrated curriculum using problem-based learning in a clinical environment: the Manchester experience. *Medical Education* 34 (3), pp. 222–30.

Rhem, J. (1998) Problem-based learning: an introduction. *NTLF* 8 (1), December. Available at: http://www.ntlf.com/html/pi/9812/pbl_1.htm

Schon, D. A. (1983) *The Reflective Practitioner: How Professionals Think in Actions.* New York: Basic Books.

Steele, D. K., Medder, K. D., Turner, P., (2000) A comparison of learning outcomes and attitudes in student versus faculty-led problem-based learning: an experimental study. *Medical Education* 34 (1), pp. 23–9.

United Kingdom Central Council (1999) *Fitness for Practice* . London: UKCC.

Woods, D. R. (1994) *Problem-Based Learning: How to Gain the Most from PBL.* Hamilton, Ontario: McMaster University.

Insights into Maternal Health

Pat Donovan

Introduction

Midwifery in the United Kingdom is seen as a separate profession to nursing, but maternal health is incorporated within the pre-registration nursing curriculum. Nurses may come into contact with pregnant women in many different ways, from carers and family members to recipients of intensive care. Pregnancy is a normal physiological occurrence and nurses need to be aware of this and to participate in the care that is given. It must be acknowledged, however, that the main care givers during this process are midwives.

Learning outcomes

This chapter will enable the student to:

- Identify the social and health implications of pregnancy and child bearing.
- Recognise common factors which adversely affect the physical, mental and social well-being of patients and clients and take appropriate action.
- Use relevant literature and research to inform the practice of nursing/midwifery.
- Appreciate the influence of social, economic, political and cultural factors in relation to health care.
- Understand the requirements of legislation relevant to the practice of nursing and midwifery.
- Identify physical, social and spiritual needs of the patient or client; and be aware of values and concepts of individual care.
- Aid the midwife in devising a plan of care, contribute to its implementation and evaluation.
- Use appropriate channels of referral for matters not within her/his sphere of practice.

Concepts

- The midwife
- Pregnancy
- Adaptation to parenthood
- Education for parenthood
- The fetus
- Antenatal care
- Teratogenicity
- Empowerment

- Fatherhood
- Childbirth
- Continuity of care
- Autonomy
- Sexuality
- Neonate
- Fertility

Activity 2.1

There may be other concepts which you have already decided that you would like to explore. As you work through the list yet more may arise.

As you work through the chapter refer to a dictionary to check your understanding of technical words and phrases.

Scenario *Introducing Jackie*

To enable appropriate insight into maternal health the scenario will follow one woman throughout her pregnancy and labour to the birth of her baby and early postnatal days.

Jackie thinks that she is pregnant and goes to her Health Centre.

Activity 2.2

What may make Jackie come to the conclusion that she may be pregnant?

Jackie thinks she's pregnant

Jackie has been sexually active and if contraception is not used or fails, then pregnancy can occur. There are physical signs that Jackie may experience due to the high levels of progesterone and oestrogen that are secreted; these are secreted from the corpus luteum, in the ovary during the first 12 weeks of pregnancy, and then from the placenta. One of the first signs noted will be amenorrhoea. This may be obvious, but in women who have an irregular menstrual cycle this may not be the first sign observed or experienced. Other signs may also be present.

> ### Activity 2.3
>
> Consider what other signs you know before reading on.

Possible signs of pregnancy

- Breast changes:
  - A feeling of fullness
  - Tingling
- Bladder irritability which leads to frequency of micturition
- Fetal movements may be felt from 18–20 weeks

Pregnancy testing is also available in the use of kits which can be purchased over the counter, and also performed at pharmacies.

> ### Activity 2.4
>
> In the area where you are living explore the shops where pregnancy kits are for sale, compare their cost with the cost of pharmacy pregnancy testing.

? **What other issues are there about a woman being able to find out for herself if she is pregnant? It may be useful to discuss different viewpoints and experiences with other students.**

Jackie's body will experience major changes and this will affect every physiological system in her body. For a description of this physiology of pregnancy, please refer to a major midwifery text (Bennet and Brown 1999; Sweet 1997). These physiological changes lead to minor discomforts which may affect Jackie's lifestyle. Pregnancy is also a time of major psychological change as Jackie comes to terms with being a mother and having a child who is totally dependent on her. Oakley (1992) argues that the quantity and quality of a person's relationships with significant others positively influences physical health. Therefore, it is important that Jackie receives psychosocial support in this pregnancy, as well as physical support and assessment of fetal and maternal well-being.

Communication is important in caring for women who are pregnant, due to the very intimate nature of sexuality, pregnancy and childbirth.

> ### Activity 2.5
>
> Think about the factors which may influence the psychosocial support for Jackie and for other pregnant women.

> Jackie met with her general practitioner (GP) who agreed to share her care with the consultants at the hospital.

Table 2.1 Jackie's antenatal sheet

LMP: 14/9/X   EDD: 21/6/X   Height: 5'2"   Parity – Gravida: 1   Para: 0   Age: 17

Date	Weeks	Weight	Urine	Blood pressure	Fundal Height	Presentation	Fetal Heart	Oedema	Signature
14/12/X	11	47kg	NAD	90/60				—	Midwife x
17/2/X	22		No spec	110/70				—	GP
19/2/X	22			110/60				—	Consultant
12/3/X	25+		NAD	110/70	28cm	? cephalic	FHH	—	Midwife x
2/4/X	28+		NAD	110/60	30cm	cephalic	FHHR	—	Midwife y
16/4/X	30	53kg	NAD	100/50	32cm	cephalic	FHHR	Nil	GP
7/5/X	33		No spec	130/80	33cm	cephalic	H	Nil	Consultant
3/6/X	37	60kg	NAD	130/75	37cm	cephalic	FHHR	Nil	GP
9/6/X	38	61kg	No spec	130/70	36cm	cephalic	FHH 140 R	Nil	Consultant
19/6/X	39+	59kg	NAD	130/70	39cm	cephalic	H	Nil	Midwife x

In reality this meant that Jackie would see her GP, the midwife who is based at the GP's surgery, and a range of doctors at the hospital. This is not an ideal situation. This multitude of care givers has been challenged (Flint and Poulengeris 1987) and schemes have been set up in order to ensure that pregnant women see fewer people during their pregnancy.

Activity 2.6

A Look at Jackie's antenatal sheet (Table 2.1) to see how many different people gave care to Jackie at this time.
B Can you find out the situation in your local area perhaps by talking to friends or colleagues who have recently had a baby?

The report of the expert Maternity Group (DoH 1993) made recommendations concerning maternity care, one of which was that within five years every woman should know one midwife who ensures continuity of care. Midwives have been changing their way of working and delivering care and are now working in teams or holding their own case load so that continuity of care is possible.

Is there any evidence that Jackie knew what options were available, and have you access to this information in your area?

In order to plan Jackie's care a history is taken by the midwife. This will highlight factors which could affect Jackie's pregnancy and the unborn child. It will also help to highlight specific needs that Jackie may have. This is called the booking interview (see below).

Evidence-based practice

The booking interview
Rosemary Methven (1982) looked at the booking interviews conducted in four maternity hospitals. She looked at the process of the booking interview and the content, and what actually took place at this time. It was a descriptive study and 40 mothers were included. The process of data collection included non-participant observation, satisfaction questionnaires and interviews with the midwives. Her findings were that the antenatal booking interview was obstetric rather than midwifery in orientation, conformed to a medical model of care and was counterproductive to forming a relationship with the pregnant woman. Therefore, the booking interview should be seen as an assessment tool which is available to plan the care in pregnancy. It should be tailored to the needs and wishes of the client and should be perceived as a joint planning venture between the midwife, client and her partner.

The booking interview should occur at a time and place to suit the client. It should take place as soon as possible after the confirmation of the pregnancy. This ensures that advice can be given concerning lifestyle and diet early enough so that it can positively affect the developing embryo.

Jackie's story

Jackie is 19 years old and lives at home with her parents. She has a history of anorexia nervosa and was treated with antidepressants from the age of 15 until she was 17. She smokes 4 cigarettes a day and does not drink alcohol. There is no family history of diabetes, hypertension, multiple pregnancy, genetic or psychiatric illness. This is Jackie's first pregnancy. Her menstrual periods are regular and occur every 28 days and she bleeds for seven days. Her last period was normal and started on 14 September. She had not been on the contraceptive pill, but her boyfriend had used a condom occasionally. Her boyfriend Mark is supportive, and he and his family are also healthy. They plan to move in together during the pregnancy. Jackie works at a local supermarket full-time and Mark is a manager of a computer games shop.

Activity 2.7

Consider what aspects you would want to find out more about to be able to support Jackie confidently during her pregnancy.

Towards a healthy pregnancy

Activity 2.8

Before reading on, list factors about Jackie history which may interfere with her experiencing a fulfilling and safe pregnancy.

Factors that could adversely affect Jackie's pregnancy include the previous anorexia. Weight increases during pregnancy and this could affect Jackie's self-image, therefore she needs practical advice on her diet during the pregnancy with minimal attention overtly given to her weight and the changes in body size and shape. This should be done in a positive manner. Assessing weight gain in pregnancy as an indicator of fetal well-being has been questioned in recent years and now less attention is given to it (Grudzinskas et al 1991). However, nutrition in pregnancy is gaining importance as there is increasing evidence that it may play a major part in programming the physiology and the metabolism of the fetus which could cause disease in the fetus in later life, especially cardiovascular disease (Barker 1992).

Food safety is also important in pregnancy. Any infection that Jackie may acquire during her pregnancy could affect the fetus and the pregnancy. The effect that infection will have is dependent both on the age of the fetus (gestation) and the type of infection. The placenta acts as a partial barrier to many bacteria, but does not prevent the passage of viruses. Some organisms are associated with food and therefore Jackie will be given specific dietary advice (see below).

Dietary advice

- Avoid soft, ripened cheeses such as Brie and Camembert and reheat ready-to-eat poultry and prepared meals until they are hot (DOH 1989; DOH 1992). This is to prevent infection by listeriosis caused by the bacteria Listeria monocytogenes. This has been associated with miscarriages, stillbirths and neonatal deaths (Spedding et al 1995).
- Take extra care when handling poultry, raw meat and eggs. Eggs, meat and poultry should be thoroughly cooked before eating. Raw meat should be kept separate from cooked meats. This is to avoid infection from Salmonella. There is no evidence as yet that Salmonella has a direct effect on the fetus.
- Cook all meat thoroughly and remove soil from vegetables and salads. This is to prevent infection from the parasite Toxoplasma gondii, which causes a flu-like symptom in the mother and a range of symptoms in the fetus which could lead to miscarriage, stillbirth and neonatal death, as well as premature birth and multiple defects. This organism is found in raw meat and cat faeces. Women who keep cats should be advised to wear rubber gloves when disposing of the cat litter tray and all women should be advised to wear rubber gloves when gardening.
- Ensure that only milk that has been heat treated is consumed.

Activity 2.9

You may like to consider how this important information could be given to Jackie so that she accepts and retains it.

The estimation of the expected date of delivery of the baby (EDD) is achieved by adding 7 days to the first day of the last normal menstrual period and then adding 9 months.

This makes Jackie's due date 21 June. Jackie is seen frequently throughout her pregnancy (see Table 2.1) and the growth of the uterus gauged as a measurement of the growth of the fetus.

Developmental levels – from egg to baby

The developing baby goes through three developmental levels:

Pre-embryonic period This is the first three weeks following conception, and includes the fertilised egg embedding into the wall of the uterus.

Embryonic period This is between three and eight weeks following conception (ten weeks following the last menstrual period). This is a time when all the organs develop (organogenesis) and are at risk of damage by infection or drugs. The drug Thalidomide is one of the most well known and caused major limb deformities, abnormalities which are otherwise quite rare.

Fetal period This is between nine weeks (11 weeks from the last menstrual period) and birth. It is a time when all the systems differentiate and mature sufficiently to enable dependent life outside the uterus. The fetus is not a 'man in miniature', and this period is characterised by growth and changes in proportion rather than by the appearance of new features. The length (crown to rump) increases from 3cm to 35cm, and the weight from 4gm to 3000gm. Reflex activities are also practised, such as swallowing and breathing movements as well as general muscle movements which can be felt by the mother and are known as 'Quickening'. This occurs between 16 and 18 weeks in a woman who has been pregnant before (multigravida), and between 18 and 20 weeks in a woman, such as Jackie, who is pregnant for the first time (primigravida).

Activity 2.10

Refer to a physiology or embryology book for more detail.

Before the use of ultrasound scanning this information was used to assess the gestation of the pregnancy if there was doubt about the last menstrual period. During these developmental periods the placenta also develops and secretes the main hormones of pregnancy from the twelfth week of pregnancy until birth. Prior to the twelfth week the main hormones, progesterone and oestrogen, are secreted from the corpus luteum in the ovary.

Antenatal tests

Blood tests are done either at the first visit or at the time of the booking interview. They include tests for:

- Blood group and rhesus factor
- Rubella antibodies
- Haemoglobin and full blood count
- Syphilis (Treponema pallidum haemaglutination assay – TPHA)
- Hepatitis B
- Human immunodeficiency virus – HIV

The midwife should attain informed consent for all these tests and the significance of a positive result should be discussed with women before each test is undertaken. This is especially important for the TPHA, HIV and Hepatitis tests.

 What is the purpose of each of these tests?

Jackie's blood tests

Jackie's results were:

- Blood Group: A Positive
- Haemoglobin: 12.00g/dl
- Rubella: Protective levels detected (immune)
- TPHA: Negative
- Hepatitis B: Negative
- HIV: Negative

Other tests that are performed during the pregnancy relate to the health of the fetus and include an ultrasound scan to detect abnormalities and an alpha fetoprotein test at 18 weeks of pregnancy. If the alpha fetoprotein is raised, it could indicate a fetus with a neural tube defect, such as spina bifida. Other tests can be used to screen for Down's syndrome. This test will show how much the mother is at risk of carrying a baby with Down's syndrome. This test was not offered to Jackie.

 Is this test offered in your area? It may be called the triple test.

Further tests may be performed if there is a high probability that the baby has such defects. These tests include an amniocentesis, when fluid around the baby (the amniotic fluid) is removed and tested and/or a very detailed ultrasound scan is undertaken. See below for evidence regarding ultrasound in pregnancy. If the baby is then diagnosed as having these conditions, a termination of pregnancy is offered. Women have the right to refuse these tests in pregnancy and some might do so on ethical or religious grounds.

 Evidence-based practice

Ultrasound in pregnancy

Ultrasound remains a controversial procedure that the majority of pregnant women undergo during their pregnancy, some up to 12 times. There is no definitive research that has proven the safety of ultrasound in pregnancy, but conversely no evidence exists to prove that it is harmful to the mother or the fetus. It may aid in prenatal bonding when women see their baby on the screen (Welford 1993).

Informed consent is essential for all tests, whether seen as 'routine' or not (see also Chapter 5 on nursing adults, p. 61).

? Why is it so important to have informed consent? Who gives the consent? Does your answer raise any issues?

This informed consent should include:

- An explanation of the test
- Why the test is considered necessary
- The consequences of a positive test for the mother and the fetus
- What action would be taken if the test was positive

There are a number of 'Informed choice' leaflets available for women and their partners in order to give them the most up to date evidence on which to make an informed choice. These leaflets cover:

- Support in labour
- Listening to the baby's heartbeat in labour
- Ultrasound scans
- Alcohol and pregnancy
- Positions in labour and delivery
- Epidurals for pain relief in labour
- Feeding your baby – breast or bottle
- Looking for Down's syndrome and spina bifida in pregnancy
- Breech baby – what are your choices?
- Where will you have your baby – hospital or home?

Activity 2.11

Find out if these leaflets are available in your local area.

Jackie has an appointment at the antenatal clinic to have an ultrasound performed. Mark goes with her.

Activity 2.12

Look at Jackie's antenatal sheet (Table 2.1) to ascertain the frequency of her antenatal visits and the examinations that took place at each visit.

Jackie kept her own notes and she took them to the clinic at each visit and was able to read what was written on them. This has helped Jackie take responsibility for her pregnancy.

Diary extract
Today I went to the clinic and saw my midwife. It's nice to know who I will be seeing when I go. She told me that I was OK and that the baby was growing and she wrote

it on my notes. I asked her what some of the words meant on my notes and she explained things very clearly for me. I like to carry these notes as it means I can see what is written about me.

Table 2.2 Ultrasound report

X NHS Trust

Date	Patient's Name: Jackie X
12/2/XX	**Ultrasound Report**

Measurements:

Biparietal diameter:	54mm = 21 wks + 5 days
Femur length:	38mm = 21 wks + 3 days
Head circumference:	193mm = 21 wks + 5 days
Number of fetuses:	One
Placenta:	Posterior, not low
Normal appearances of:	Head
	Spine
	Chest – four-chamber heart
	Abdomen, stomach, bladder
	Limbs
	Liquor volume

Signature of ultrasonographer: *P. Wilkins*

The Council is in favour of patients and clients being given custody of their own health records in circumstances where it is appropriate. Patient or client held records help to emphasise and make clear the practitioner's responsibility to the patient or client by sharing any information held or assessments made and illustrate the involvement of the patient or client in their own care.
(UKCC 1993)

> Jackie was invited to an education class once she had attended her booking interview.

This class is offered and run by local midwives in the area. It is for all women at the beginning of their pregnancy. General health education is given and the importance of diet and antenatal attendance is stressed. The role of the midwife, general practitioner and obstetrician is also discussed to enable women and their partners to understand why they may be offered different types of care.

 What is the role of an obstetrician?

In what situations is an obstetrician more likely to become involved in care?

The place of birth may be discussed at this class as it is sometimes assumed by their carer that all women wish to deliver in a hospital setting. In many areas there are differing options for place of birth and these may include:

- Home
- A peripheral general practitioner unit (this is away from the main district hospital)
- A central general practitioner unit (a unit within the premises or grounds of a district general hospital)
- A private hospital (not available under the NHS)
- A private maternity unit (not available under the NHS)

? **What options are available in your local area?**

The place of birth may also dictate who would be the main professional carer for the woman in pregnancy and in labour. Normally, at either a home birth or birth in a general practitioner unit, care is given by the midwife and the GP, and the birth is conducted by a midwife who mainly works within the community setting. This is changing in many areas due to the influence of the *Changing Childbirth* report (DoH 1993) as midwives are becoming more flexible and are working in both district hospital and general practitioner unit settings and the community. Private independent midwives also work in some areas and offer antenatal care, during birth at home and then the postnatal period, usually for up to 28 days. In some areas midwifery-led care is also available. This is where a midwife gives total care to a woman at all stages of her pregnancy, labour and the postnatal period. If a problem arises in the pregnancy, the midwife may refer to a doctor or another professional. Women may change their original choice of care once they are aware of all the options that are available to them.

? **How are women in your locality made aware of the possible choices about where the baby is born and who is the main care giver?**

Professional conversation

Lucy Crown, Midwife

The role of the midwife in education for parenthood

'Health counselling and education is a fundamental part of the midwive's role. On both an individual basis and a group basis the midwife is in a prime position to positively influence the health behaviour of new parents and contribute to reducing low birth weight, perinatal morbidity and mortality. Women can also be empowered through the attainment of knowledge and information to enable them to make choices and decisions regarding their care. By familiarising parents with the environment and procedures the midwife can also help to prepare them for labour, and help them to achieve a satisfying experience regardless of the mode of delivery. Through discussion, the fostering of social support systems and the introduction of other members of the primary health care team the midwife can also help parents to face the early challenges of parent education with a degree of confidence.

As a midwife preparing and undertaking antenatal classes I must consider the varying intelligence, ages and personalities of my clients. The expectations and prior knowledge of the group members must be borne in mind.'

Jackie is invited to a set of six classes run by her community midwife where she can learn more about what to expect during the birth and how to prepare for it and the whole aspect of parenthood. This also includes an evening exclusively for prospective fathers and a tour of the hospital where Jackie plans to give birth (see the professional conversation above).

 In your locality are partners invited only for the one evening or can they attend all the classes?

 What might be the implications for including or excluding the partner?

 Activity 2.13

You may like to discuss with colleagues your views about the implications for successful parenting if both prospective parents attend or if the woman attends alone.

The National Childbirth Trust (NCT) also runs classes in many areas with very experienced teachers who have had children.

Activity 2.14

Find your local NCT branch and discover what they offer in the area of antenatal preparation.

Jackie has been reading lots of books about birth and finds talking to Mark's sister Janice very useful, as Janice has a 3-month-old baby who was born in the same hospital where Jackie has planned to give birth. The midwife has also encouraged Jackie to write her wishes for the labour in her notes as she may not be cared for by the team that has given Jackie some of her antenatal care. Jackie finds this very difficult as she does not know what to expect when she starts her labour and how she will cope with the pain. Janice had informed Jackie that she had found the process of labour extremely painful and she had requested 'an epidural' as a method of pain relief.

Jackie is getting extremely worried about this as she does not like needles, and therefore wishes the birth to be as natural as possible without the intervention of invasive procedures. She has written this on her notes and has also discussed this with Mark and her midwife.

Extract from Jackie's Birth Plan

I would like to have my baby naturally and do not want any injections or needles as I do not like needles. I would like to use Entonox if the pain is bad. I agree to have an injection after the baby is born but I do not want to know when it is given. I want my boyfriend to stay with me all the time.

Point of interest – waterbirth

Increasingly, hospitals are offering mothers the choice of water for pain relief and to give birth in. Many hospitals have a specific birthing pool available. If a couple decide on a home birth there are pools available for hire. Each hospital that provides this service has a strict protocol to follow as to who is safe to use the pool and the care to be followed whilst in the pool. Many women have given birth this way with no detrimental effects to themselves or their baby (Beech 1996).

? Is waterbirth available in your area?

Jackie is starting to have regular abdominal pain and has a pink mucous vaginal discharge. The pain has settled down to a regular pattern of every six minutes lasting at least 40 seconds. She has telephoned the hospital where she is going to give birth, and has asked their advice. She has been advised to go to the hospital as she is in labour. She phones Mark who comes home and collects her and takes her to the hospital.

Jackie and Mark are welcomed to the labour ward by midwife Wendy Wilson who is not known to Jackie or Mark. She introduces herself to them and takes them to a delivery room where Jackie is instructed to get undressed and to either put on the nightdress provided or one that she has brought, whichever she will be most comfortable with. Jackie has brought one of Mark's old shirts which she wants to wear in labour, but she knows that it will become quite stained and is prepared to discard it following the birth. Both Jackie and Mark are anxious at this point as Jackie is afraid that she may not be in labour, and that this is a false alarm even though today is her actual due date. She is finding the pain not as bad as Janice had told her and this adds to her feeling that she is not in labour.

The process of labour

How and why labour commences when it does is largely not fully understood (Carson 1997). Pregnancy in the human lasts between 37 and 44 weeks, labour could commence at any time from 37 weeks and women should be prepared from that time on.

Labour can be defined as the onset of regular, painful contractions associated with dilatation of the cervical os. It may be accompanied by:

- A 'show' which is the dislodging from the cervical os of the operculum. This is a mucous plug which has developed during the pregnancy.
- Rupture of the membranes surrounding the baby leading to the amniotic fluid draining through the vagina.

> ### Activity 2.15
>
> Remember to look up the unfamiliar words as you read through. Adding them to your personal glossary may help you to understand and learn them more easily.

Labour is divided into three stages

First Stage

During this time the uterine muscles of the upper part of the uterus contract and retract (become slightly shorter), and the muscles of the lower part of the uterus contract weakly and relax. This enables the upper part of the uterus to pull up the lower part and thus lead to cervical dilatation. Established, active labour commences when the cervical os is 3cm dilated and concludes when it has reached full dilatation. This is 10cm in a full-term pregnancy.

? **How does the midwife know how much the cervix is dilated?**

Second Stage

This commences when the cervical os is fully dilated and concludes following delivery of the baby. It is characterised by fetal descent down the birth canal and the displacement of soft tissue. Due to pressure of the fetal head on the rectum, the mother feels the urge to 'bear down' and this is encouraged once the fetal head is visible at the interoitus.

Third stage

This commences after the baby is born and concludes once the placenta and membranes are delivered. It is usually actively managed, which involves the giving of an oxytocic drug (a drug to contract the uterus) and the use of traction (gentle pulling) on the cord once the uterus has contracted. This shortens the second stage and minimises blood loss. The woman plays a passive role during this stage. If the third stage is managed physiologically, no oxytocic drug is given and the woman plays a more active role in delivering the placenta by 'pushing it out' in a similar manner to the baby. During physiological management the mother is only encouraged to push the placenta out once the midwife has ensured that it has separated from the uterine wall. This will take slightly longer if no oxytocic drug is given.

Responsibilities of the midwife

The clinical actions of the midwife on admission are to assess:

- the progress of the labour
- the mother's condition
- the condition of the unborn baby

The plan of care following admission is dependant on the stage that the labour is at, the condition of both mother and fetus, including the mother's psychological state and how both mother and fetus are coping with the labour, and also the wishes of the mother.

The stage of the labour is ascertained by the history that is given, the onset and present length, strength and frequency of the contractions, abdominal examination and a vaginal examination.

> These findings are discussed with Jackie and Mark and recorded in Jackie's notes:

Activity 2.16

Continue to look up any words or phrases that you are unfamiliar with. Share your findings with a peer. Track down a midwife to answer outstanding questions or to discuss specific issues.

Evidence-based practice

Fetal heart-rate monitoring

The fetal heart can be monitored in labour by the use of the Pinard stethoscope or by electronic means, the Cardiotocograph. The aim of monitoring the fetus during the process of labour is to identify problems which may cause death or morbidity if not corrected. The Cardiotocograph monitors the fetal heartbeat via an abdominal transducer and uses an ultrasonic pulse. Another transducer will also detect the abdominal contractions. Continuous electronic fetal monitoring in labour was introduced into clinical practice in the 1970s and 1980s in the absence of evidence which demonstrated its effectiveness or safety. It is now widely used on over 70 per cent of women in labour (Thacker and Stroup 1998). There appears to be no advantage to using this method of monitoring, and it is associated with a higher incidence of Caesarean sections and operative deliveries (Thacker and Stroup 1998). Continuous electronic monitoring was introduced as it was thought that it would enable clinicians to identify hypoxia of the fetus earlier and more accurately, and thus to intervene promptly, therefore improving outcomes. These hoped for benefits have not been achieved. The use of such routine monitoring influences the roles of the care givers and the focus of the care, with the midwife taking on a more technical role and the obstetrician becoming more involved in the care. The focus becomes the machine and this may also affect the relationship between the woman and her partner. Continuous electronic monitoring also implies a much more passive role for the prospective mother as she is normally confined to a bed or a chair. If lying in a bed, the dorsal position is detrimental to the fetus as this position causes some degree of aorta caval compression, which will lead to diminished uterine and placental blood flow and this can in itself cause problems to the fetus. The National Institute for Clinical Excellence has now issued guidelines for the use of electronic fetal monitoring (NICE 2001).

Table 2.3 Labour notes, extract 1

Date	Labour notes: Jackie X	Signature
21/06/X 12.00 hrs	Admitted from home with a history of contractions, regular since 10 a.m.	
	On admission: Temperature: 36.5 degrees C Pulse: 96 b/m Blood pressure: 110/70mm/Hg Urinalysis : NAD On abdominal palpation: Longitudinal lie Cephalic presentation Right occipito posterior position Head engaged – Fetal heart 135 b/m Coping well with contractions, 1 in every 3 minutes, cardiotocograph (CTG) applied.	Wendy Wilson
21/06/X 13.00 hrs	CTG – good variability with accelerations, early decelerations noted, good recovery to baseline, to continue at present. Vaginal examination to assess progress. Cervix: Fully effaced and soft, Cervical dilation: 6cm, well applied to presenting part Membranes: Intact and bulging Presenting part: Cephalic 1cm above the ischial spines Position: Right occipito posterior position CTG continues. Entonox commenced	Wendy Wilson
13.30 hrs	Reactive CTG, discontinued	Wendy Wilson
14.00 hrs	Coping well with contractions, 1:3 mod/strong on palpation, Fetal heart 135 b/m	Wendy Wilson
14.05 hrs	CTG recommenced	Wendy Wilson

All care given to Jackie is plotted on a partogram which will include the findings of all observations as well as a graph to plot the degree of cervical dilatation and also lists all drugs that are given in labour. Therefore the partogram contains all the details of the fetal and maternal condition as well as the progress of the labour.

Support in labour

Support in labour involves physical contact, such as back rubbing and holding a hand, and emotional support, such as making eye contact and ensuring that the client understands all procedures including results of examinations undertaken and the possible consequences. These will all add to a positive experience of the labour and ensure that the locus of control remains with the client. The partner is in an ideal position to give such support as well as the midwife.

Professional conversation

Eileen, midwife in the delivery suite

Support in labour

'Good rapport between mother and midwife is a pre-requisite for the provision of support in labour. Ideally, this has developed during the antenatal period but, when delivery is taking place in hospital, it is often necessary to strike up a relationship quickly in snatches between contractions. This may be aided by inclusion of the woman's "birthing" partner in discussions and by joint consideration of a written or oral birth plan.

A supportive relationship is not hierarchical and thus it is important that the woman knows my name, and that I am a midwife and how long I will be with her. I need to be sure that I understand her wishes for labour and alert her to any difficulties foreseen or changes that may have to be made. A significant part of providing support is helping the woman to feel that she is in control – even when things are not going as she had hoped. Thus explanation of what I am looking for during observations and monitoring is necessary. Likewise, discussing the findings, their implications (whether or not all is well), consequent options and reasoning is important. This enables the woman and her partner to be part of the decision-making process.

Providing support may mean different things for different people. Eye contact is always important – without it the woman and her partner may not feel that I am being honest with them or that they can trust what I say. Sometimes, in strong labour, eye contact is the only way a woman can hang on to self-control during a contraction. Being supportive requires that I know when to talk or joke, and when to stay silent. Sometimes, it requires that I provide physical support through touch, massage and attending to her comfort. On other occasions, I need to stand back and let the woman focus in on herself or allow her partner to help her (with guidance if necessary). It also requires that an appropriate balance between praise, encouragement and even, on occasions, cajoling be given.'

Support such as this diminishes the need for analgesia and this was seen in Jackie's labour (see Chapter 13 on pain).

Using Entonox

> Jackie commenced using 'Entonox' for pain relief.

Entonox is a 50/50 mix of the gas nitrous oxide and oxygen. It is used in many maternity units and can be used in the home. It is prescribed by the midwife who has been trained in its use. The gas is colourless and odourless, but some women may complain of the smell which is elicited from the black tubing or mask and not from the gas itself. Nitrous oxide is an anaesthetic and therefore Entonox must be self-administered to prevent overdose and loss of consciousness. If Jackie takes too much of the gas, she will drop the mask or tube and thus prevent further administration. The delivery of the gas is triggered by the woman's own effort via the use of a well-fitting mask or a mouth-piece, which is becoming much more popular than the mask. It takes 20 seconds for analgesia to occur and the maximum effect is felt at 45–60 seconds. The mother is therefore instructed to start to take the gas at the commencement of the contraction, which she can feel as a hardening of her uterus. This is felt prior to the perception of the pain. She is instructed to take regular deep breaths and she does not have to let go of the mask or mouth-piece to breathe out as there is a valve system to allow for this. The gas is excreted via the lungs and does not have any known effect on the fetus. It can be used in conjunction with narcotics, but it may not provide adequate analgesia in many cases, especially in women having their first baby. This will be dependant on the woman's expectations, control, place of labour and psychological stress. The use of Entonox is rarely contraindicated due to the presence of 50 per cent oxygen. In earlier times it used to be a mix of nitrous oxide and air, and is still colloquially called 'gas and air'.

During the second stage, a vaginal examination is essential as sometimes when the position of the baby is occipito posterior, that is the baby is facing forwards with his back adjacent to the mother's back, there is a premature urge to push prior to the onset of the second stage of labour. If women attempt to push the baby out prior to full dilatation of the cervix, the supports of the uterus could become damaged and the cervix may become oedematous and this oedema could slow down further dilatation.

> The second stage of labour was diagnosed by the midwife seeing the baby's head at the entrance of the vagina. Jackie had felt the urge to push and the midwife had performed a vaginal examination to assess whether the second stage of labour had commenced.

Evidence-based practice

Amniotomy

Amniotomy or the artificial rupture of the membranes (ARM) has become a controversial issue. The amniotic sac encloses the fetus and protects the fetus from infection ascending up through the birth canal. Once the membranes are ruptured, this protection is eliminated and the baby must be delivered within the following 48 hours. It is thought that rupturing the membranes allows the fetal head to descend on to the cervix, giving better application and greater nerve stimulation leading to more frequent and stronger contractions, and therefore reducing the length of labour. It has also been noted that these shorter labours are also more painful. Once the membranes have been ruptured, the colour of the liquor can be seen. Meconium staining of the liquor may occur in labour if there is some degree of hypoxia, as this may cause the fetus to relax his anal sphincter and empty his bowels. The baby's first stool is a black/green tar-like substance called meconium and this stains the liquor green if passed in the uterus. It is sterile and therefore there is no risk of uterine infection. It must be pointed out that hypoxia can also occur with no meconium staining. Rupturing the membranes also allows free access to the fetal scalp for internal monitoring of the fetal heart as well as biochemical analysis of fetal blood taken from the scalp in cases of fetal hypoxia. Inch (1992) discusses the whole area of the 'cascade of intervention', which is when one intervention leads to another in order to negate the side-effects of the previous procedure. This could all commence with an amniotomy. Amniotomy is also an example of the medical model of care with its desire to control and dominate the physiological process of labour. Routine amniotomy is a part of the policy of many maternity units but, having looked at all the evidence, the WHO (1985) state that this procedure is not scientifically justified.

 What is the Apgar score? (see below when you have thought about it)

Birth

Birth is seen to be the most dangerous journey that a person makes in life. The midwife will observe the condition of the fetus closely and listen to the fetal heart after every contraction during the second stage of labour. The fetus demonstrates well-being by varying his heartbeat by five beats per minute around a baseline of 110 to 150 beats per minute. This demonstrates that he is well oxygenated. If the baby is becoming distressed

Table 2.4 Labour notes, extract 2

Date	Labour notes: Jackie X	Signature
21/06/X 14.40 hrs	Strong urges to push. Vaginal examination to assess progress. Cervix: Fully effaced and soft Cervical dilatation: 9cm, well applied Membranes: Bulging, amniotomy performed, clear liquor Presenting part: Cephalic at the level of the Ischial spines Position: Right occipito lateral Pelvic Outlet: Appears adequate Fetal Heart 138 b/m, using Entonox well with good effect	*Wendy Wilson*
14.45 hrs	CTG recommenced, early decelerations noted after the artificial rupture of the membranes (ARM), baseline fetal heart 120 b/m	*Wendy Wilson*

Table 2.5 Labour notes, extract 3, the third stage of labour

Date	Labour notes: Jackie X	Signature
21/06/X 14.55 hrs	Vertex visible, is pushing	*Wendy Wilson*
15.20 hrs	Turned on to all-fours position, vertex advancing, fetal heart closely observed	*Wendy Wilson*
15.55 hrs	Fetal heart, extended late deceleration noted, perineum infiltrated with 1% lidocaine	*Wendy Wilson*
15.57 hrs	Episiotomy performed for fetal distress	*Wendy Wilson*
16.01 hrs	Normal delivery of a live male infant, Apgar Score 9 at 1 min, good condition at birth	*Wendy Wilson*

 What is the effect of lidocaine?

and perhaps not getting enough oxygen, then there will be alterations in his heart rate, such as decelerations and development of acidosis. This may necessitate speeding up the process of birth. In the second stage of labour an episiotomy will expedite the delivery.

Evidence-based practice

Episiotomy

In the 1980s the episiotomy was the most common surgical procedure performed in hospitals in the United Kingdom. It involves cutting the perineal body in order to deliver the baby. The perineal body is an area of muscle between the rectum and the vagina which, in normal labour, is stretched and flattened to aid delivery of the fetal head. It was thought that an elective, planned episiotomy would prevent damage to the anal sphincter, prevent trauma to the fetal head and prevent damage to the muscles of the pelvic floor. Therefore many maternity units adopted a liberal approach to episiotomy, advocating a routine episiotomy in all women having their first baby. This procedure is not without risks and is associated with haemorrhage, infection and problems of healing which affect women's sexual activity. A large study of over 1000 women was conducted in the early 1980s to explore advantages of a liberal approach to episiotomy and it was discovered that the routine use of such a procedure was not justified (Sleep et al 1984). In many units and for many individual midwives, this procedure has now been reduced to situations where the fetus is felt to be hypoxic and where an episiotomy would reduce the length of the second stage and hasten the delivery of a possibly asphyxiated fetus. This was the indication in Jackie's case. The midwife is also skilled in suturing episiotomies. Episiotomies require consent and it is ideal if the indications for the midwife to perform an episiotomy are discussed with the client before the second stage of labour. This should not preclude the midwife gaining specific consent to perform the procedure if deemed necessary, and discussing the reasoning behind this decision prior to consent being obtained. This consent is usually given verbally.

> **?** How does the weight of Jackie's baby compare with the average birth weight of babies?

The means of assessing the baby's condition soon after birth is via the Apgar score. This gives a total score of two for each of five aspects (see Jackie's labour summary below). Jackie's baby was in a good condition at birth. Birth can be very traumatic for the baby. At birth the baby has to adapt from a liquid environment, where all nutrients and oxygen are available from the maternal circulation via the placenta, to an air environment, where the lungs have to commence being organs of gaseous exchange in order to sustain life. It is vital therefore that the baby is observed closely in the first few hours after birth.

Breathing commences within a few seconds of birth. The fluid that has filled the lungs drains from the nose and mouth at birth due to chest compression within the birth canal. Mechanical mucous extraction is not always necessary. The baby is usually delivered on to the maternal abdomen unless requested otherwise. This skin to skin contact helps

Table 2.6 Labour summary

Spontaneous Onset

Normal Delivery

Duration of first stage: 4 hrs 55 mins

Duration of second stage: 1 hr 6 mins

Duration of third stage: 4 mins

Total duration of labour: 6 hrs 5 mins

Placental delivery

Syntometrine 1ml given with the anterior shoulder

Placenta delivered by controlled cord traction

Condition of placenta

No abnormalities

450g

Complete placenta and membranes

Umbilical cord

No abnormalities, 3 vessels detected, loose around neck, clamped after delivery

Total blood loss

100ml

Perineum

Episiotomy, for fetal distress, sutured

Delivered by midwife: *Wendy WIlson*

Infant's summary

Male

Weight: 3480gm

Head circumference: 34cm

Apgar score at 1 min		Apgar score at 5 mins	
Heart rate:	2	Heart rate:	2
Respiration:	2	Respiration:	2
Muscle tone:	2	Muscle tone:	2
Reflexes:	2	Reflexes:	2
Colour:	1	Colour:	1
Total:	9	Total:	9

Signature of Midwife: *Wendy Wilson*

maintain the baby's temperature. The baby is dried as soon as practicable and left in the arms of his parents.

Survival following birth is also dependent on the relationship built up with the mother who is going to be responsible for the baby. The baby prepares physiologically for birth and at birth appears wide-eyed and alert if no narcotics have been given to the mother in her labour. This is a very sensitive period, and is a time for the parents to explore their child and for the child to get to know its parents. It is the policy, therefore, in many maternity units that after ensuring mother and baby are in a satisfactory condition, parents are given some time alone with their baby. They are also given the means to call for aid if necessary. The relationship developing between parents and their offspring does not start at birth but when the baby is in utero, especially if the parents have seen the baby on 'scan'. Therefore, this time of privacy strengthens this bond. Siblings may also be involved at this time, depending on the place and time of birth, local policy and the wishes of the parents. This period has been seen by some to be important for maternal–infant attachment and has been described as the 'sensitive period'. Other factors also play a role in this attachment. Many mothers and babies are separated at birth due to custom, policy or sickness and this does not appear to have affected the subsequent relationship detrimentally. This 'sensitive period' has yet to be proven or disproved. This early period following the birth is also an ideal time to initiate breast-feeding if this is the choice of the mother.

As the baby is awake and alert, he may be willing to suckle if offered the breast. This is a time when the midwife can offer her help. In a study of ten babies of mothers who had no drugs in labour, the babies commenced spontaneous sucking and rooting movements after 15 minutes (Widstrom et al 1987). Mothers should be encouraged to put the baby to the breast when it shows signs of wanting to feed. Correct positioning of the baby at the breast is vital to successful breast-feeding. If the baby is not positioned accurately, the nipple can be damaged, leading to pain and an unsatisfactory experience for the mother and the baby. Therefore, it is ideal if the midwife observes the baby's first feed to ensure adequate positioning and to give positive feedback to the mother. When helping a mother latch the baby to the breast, the midwife should treat the baby and the mother gently and ask permission to handle the breast if necessary. This is a potentially embarrassing situation for the mother. Feelings of disempowerment, embarrassment and humiliation have been voiced by mothers due to inappropriate and rough handling by midwives (Harper, 1998).

Many factors are known to influence a woman's decision to breast feed her baby. Health professionals are advocates of breast-feeding and parents should be informed of the advantages of breast-feeding (WHO 1989). Some women, however, will choose to artificially feed their baby and therefore the midwife should assist her in that choice.

Activity 2.17

List the advantages and disadvantages of breast- and bottle-feeding.

The Baby Friendly Initiative identified ten practices which help to minimise the number of women choosing to bottle feed or change to bottle-feeding in the first few days of the baby's life. If these ten steps are practised by a hospital, they are awarded the Baby Friendly Initiative award and are then classed as Baby Friendly.

? **Are there any hospitals in your area that are 'Baby Friendly'?**

The midwife will examine the baby soon after birth for signs of abnormality, infection and trauma. Baseline observations of the baby are taken and used in child health follow-up. These include birth weight, head circumference and length.

Babies in the first 28 days of life are termed neonates. They have difficulty in controlling their body temperature as they cannot shiver and therefore the environmental temperature is extremely important. All babies are blue at birth, although within a few minutes they become centrally pink with some peripheral cyanosis. This blue discoloration seen in the hands and feet of neonates is called acrocyanosis and needs no treatment (Fowlie and Forsyth 1994).

Hence, Jackie's baby had an Apgar score of 9 (see Apgar scoring above). Following initial examination of the baby, two labels are attached to him. The mother and baby should never be separated if at all possible. All maternity units should have a policy to ensure that the baby is returned to the correct mother, and a policy to follow should one or both labels become detached. The baby is subsequently examined daily by the midwife and the findings charted in the infant's records.

Table 2.7 Infant's observations

Date	21/6/X	22/6/X	23/6/X	24/6/X
Day	On admission	Day 1	Day 2	Day 3
Eyes	Clear × 2	Clear × 2	Right eye moist	Clear × 2
Mouth	Clean	Clean	Clean	Clean
Axilla	Vernix	Clean	Clean	Clean
Skin	Temp 36.8 Pink with blue extremities	Pink and warm	Pink and warm	Pink and warm
Umbilicus	Clamped – secure	Clamped – secure	Clamped – secure	Clamp removed
Buttocks	Clean	Clean	Clean	Clean
Urine	Has passed urine	Has passed urine	Has passed urine	Has passed urine
Bowels	Not opened	Meconium + + +	Meconium	Changing stool
Labels	× 2 correct	× 2 correct	× 2 correct	× 2 correct
Feeds	Breast-feeding on demand	Breast-feeding well	Breast-feeding well	Breast-feeding well
Weight	3.480 kg	Not weighed	Not weighed	Not weighed
Signature	J. Saunders	E. Blay	J. Saunders	E. Blay
Status	Midwife	Midwife	Midwife	Midwife

? **Why is the baby not weighed every day?**

Postnatal care

The period following childbirth is called the puerperium. It is a time when all the maternal organs return back to their pre-pregnant state and lactation is initiated if the mother wishes to breast feed. This process may take up to eight weeks. The midwife will examine the mother regularly for the first ten days and record the findings in the notes.

Evidence-based practice

Perineal care

Perineal pain is a common discomfort following childbirth irrespective of the type of damage sustained. Sleep et al (1984) found that 23 per cent of women reported some degree of discomfort ten days following a normal delivery. Perineal pain affects the relationship between the mother, her baby and her partner. Bathing does appear to relieve discomfort. Women are advised to add a variety of products to the bath water in order to increase its efficacy, the main products being Savlon bath concentrate and salt. A randomised trial was conducted which included 1800 women, randomly allocated to bathe in salt water, water with Savlon concentrate added, or in water with no additives. No difference was found between the groups in terms of perineal pain at ten days or three months post-delivery. The pattern of wound healing was similar in all groups (Sleep and Grant 1987).

Table 2.8 Jackie's postnatal observations

Date	21/6/X	22/6/X	23/6/X	24/6/X
Day	On admission	Day 1	Day 2	Day 3
Fundal height	Well contracted	Well contracted – above umbilicus	Well contracted and central	Well contracted – below umbilicus
Temperature	36.5	36.6	36.4	36.9
Pulse	80 b/m	76 b/m	78 b/m	80 b/m
B/P	130/75	120/80		
Breasts	Satisfactory	Empty	No problems	Filling
Urine	Has passed urine	No problems	No problems	No problems
Bowels	Bowels not open	Bowels not open	Bowels open	Bowels open
Perineal/abdominal wound	Episiotomy – sutured, no bleeding	Painful and bruised	Painful and oedematous	Bruising less
Lochia	Red – moderate	Red – moderate	Red	Minimal – pink/brown
Legs	No pain/oedema	No pain/oedema	No pain/oedema	No pain/oedema
Signature	J. Saunders	E. Blay	J. Saunders	E. Blay
Status	Midwife	Midwife	Midwife	Midwife

The midwife is also responsible for educating the parents in the care of their baby. In many units this is part of the care plan and is recorded.

Postnatal education

This is a list of such items in Jackie's notes:
Importance of hand-washing
Importance of using the bidet
Importance of daily shower/bath
Postnatal exercises:
  Leaflet given and exercises explained
  Advice on its importance
  Check if performed
Explanation of cold/heat injury
Advice on diet
Advice on rest
Breast care and hygiene (all mothers)
Explanation of demand feeding (where applicable)
Breast-feeding advice:
  No limit to sucking time
  Always start on alternate breasts
  Care of nipples
  Support
Bottle-feeding advice:
  Technique explained
  Advice on amount
Demonstration of making up bottle feeds and sterilisation of equipment
'Top and Tail' of baby
Baby bath
Principles of baby safety whilst in hospital
Mother aware of procedure if:
  Baby's labels are loose
  If one or both labels missing
  If labels are not readable
Advice prior to home:
  Principles of baby safety in the home
  Introduction of the baby to the outside world
  Registration of birth and importance
  Registration of baby with General Practitioner
  Midwife/Health Visitor visits
  Importance of six-week check for mother and baby
  Family planning

Ball (1994) sees that there are three main objectives of postnatal care and these are:

1 Promoting the physical recovery from the effects of pregnancy, labour and delivery of the mother and baby.

2 Establishing sound infant-feeding practices and fostering good maternal–child relationships.

3 Strengthening the mother's confidence in herself and her ability to care for her baby in her own particular social, cultural and family situation.
   (Ball 1994, p. 116)

The adaptation from girlfriend/lover to mother is a very radical change for any woman and is fraught with anxiety. Therefore the midwife must also ensure that Jackie is adapting well to the emotional demands of motherhood, as well as the physical. The first few hours after birth are characterised by physical exhaustion and a range of intense emotional reactions determined by the nature of the birth experience and the condition of the baby. Three main types of emotional disturbance following childbirth are recognised. These are postnatal 'blues', postnatal depression and puerperal psychosis. Postnatal 'blues' affects 70–80 per cent of all mothers and occurs within the first three days following childbirth and is transitory in nature. Postnatal depression affects 10–20 per cent of all mothers and is mainly regarded as a reactive depression, with puerperal psychosis, which is rare, affecting only one per cent of all mothers (Ball 1994). Midwives and Health Visitors are in a prime position to detect postnatal depression and then to give support and refer to the General Practitioner. Partners should also be informed about postnatal depression, as they may be the first to notice it and can inform the General Practitioner or midwife. The consequences of psychiatric illness in the puerperium has been highlighted in the latest confidential enquiry into maternal deaths (RCOG 2001), where it was reported that psychiatric disorders contributed to 12 per cent of maternal deaths in the UK in the period of 1997–99. The family are key providers in the first days following birth, especially the parents of the couple and they may be able to give support to the couple in the care of their new baby. This obviously must be done in a caring and tactful way. Families can help with the household chores, and thus give time for the new parents to learn to care for their baby unhindered by household chores such as laundry and cooking.

The midwife will give continuing care to Jackie and her son at home up to the tenth postnatal day, when the care will be handed over to the Health Visitor. The Health Visitor may be able to put Jackie in touch with postnatal support groups in the area and will discuss with her the immunisation programme that is available for the baby. The National Childbirth Trust (NCT) also runs postnatal groups and has breast-feeding counsellors that are on call if Jackie has a breast-feeding problem.

Professional conversation with a midwife

Marjorie, team midwife

The role of the midwife in the postnatal period

'Continuity of care and carer is an important part of postnatal care. Having already met the women antenatally, you have a relationship with them which will enable you to plan their care knowing their social circumstances and with some knowledge of what they may need. This will change as they identify their specific requirements as time goes on. The aims of postnatal care is to:

● help mothers care for their new babies with confidence
● establish a successful feeding system regardless of the method they have chosen
● monitor normal physiological progress of both the mother and the baby

This entails daily examination and recording of the findings. If there are any problems which require a medical opinion, then the General Practitioner, if the mother is at home; or the Obstetrician, if she is in hospital, will be informed and will visit.

The role of the midwife does not change in the postnatal period, but there is a continuation of the health advisor role through education and the promotion of healthy lifestyles. Midwives also have a role in child protection, both antenatally and postnatally as we visit families in their own homes. Problems such as these are not usually identified just in the postnatal period, but are on-going from before.

There needs to be a good relationship between the midwife and other primary health care workers so that the optimum care can be available to families.

Postnatal depression can affect mothers and needs to be identified as early as possible. Unfortunately, this is not often evident in the time that the midwife visits. However, she will be aware of those mothers who may need help due to this condition because of the background and experiences that each mother has had. This information needs to be communicated to both the General Practitioner and the Health Visitor so that they can continue to monitor the mother's well-being.'

? Who are the other primary care workers that the midwife may have to liaise with?

There are many support groups, pressure groups and voluntary groups that are associated with babies, families and childbirth.

> *Activity 2.18*
>
> Find out what groups are available in your area and what is their role.

Conclusion

This chapter has looked at the care given to a healthy couple during the antenatal period through to the birth of their son, the early postnatal period and the role of the midwife in that care.

Accompanying Jackie on her journey through pregnancy and undertaking the suggested activities will have familiarised you with a wide range of issues to be considered even for a normal pregnancy.

This chapter has demonstrated that the role of the midwife is key to not only ensuring a safe delivery for mother and child but also in empowering the parents to adapt to their new roles. Education and effective communication with continuity of care are important concepts in midwifery.

References

Ball, J. A. (1994) *Reactions to Motherhood: The Role of Postnatal Care.* Cheshire: Books for Midwives Press.

Barker, D. J. P. (ed.) (1992) *Fetal and Infant Origins of Adult Disease.* London: BMJ.

Beech, B. (1996) *Water Birth Unplugged – Proceedings of the First International Water Birth Conference.* Cheshire: Books for Midwives Press.

Bennet, V. R. and Brown, L. K. (eds) (1999) *Myles Textbook for Midwives* (13th Edition) Edinburgh: Churchill Livingstone.

Carson, R. (1997) The mechanisms involved in the initiation of term labour. *Modern Midwife* 7 (7), pp. 12–16.

Department of Health (1988) *Salmonella and Raw Eggs.* London: DoH.

Department of Health (1989) *Listeriosis and Food.* Letter. London: DoH.

Department of Health (1992) *While you are Pregnant: Safe Eating and How to Avoid Infection from Food and Animals.* London: DoH.

Department of Health (1993) *Changing Childbirth.* London: HMSO.

Flint, C., Poulengeris, P. (1987) *The Know Your Midwife Scheme.* London: KYM.

Fowlie, F., Forsyth, S. (1994) Common problems of newborn infants. *Modern Midwife* 14 (12), pp. 16–19.

Grudzinskas, G., Chapman, M., Chard, T. (eds) (1991) *The Embryo: Normal and Abnormal Development and Growth.* London: Springer.

Harper, M. (1998) Latching on. *The Practising Midwife* 1 (7/8), pp. 46–8.

Inch, S. (1992) *Birthrights.* London: Hutchinson.

Methven, R. (1982) The antenatal booking interview: recording an obstetric history or relating with a mother–to-be. *Research and the Midwife.* Conference Proceedings. Manchester: Manchester University Press.

National Institute for Clinical Excellence (2001) *The Use of Electronic Fetal Monitoring.* London: NICE.

Oakley, A., (1992) Measuring the effectiveness of psychosocial interventions in pregnancy. *International Journal of Technology Assessment in Health Care.* 8 (1), pp. 129–38.

Royal College of Obstetricians and Gynaecologists (2001) *Why Mothers Die 1997–1999 – The Confidential Enquiries into Maternal Deaths in the United Kingdom* London: RCOG.

Sleep, J. M., Grant, A., Garcia, J., Elbourne, D., Spencer, J., Chalmers, I. (1984) West Berkshire perineal management trial. *British Medical Journal* 289, pp. 587–90.

Sleep, J. A., Grant, A. (1987) A randomised controlled trial to compare the routine addition of salt or savlon bath concentrate during bathing in the immediate post-partum period. *Research and the Midwife.* Conference Proceedings. Manchester: Manchester University Press.

Spedding ,S., Wilson, J., Wright, S., Jackson, A., (1995) Nutrition for pregnancy and lactation. In: Alexander, J., Levy, V., Roch, S. (eds) *Aspects of Midwifery Practice – A Research-Based Approach.* Basingstoke: Macmillan Press – now Palgrave Macmillan.

Sweet, B. (ed) (1997) *Mayes Midwifery* (12th Edition) London: Ballière Tindall.

Thacker, S. B., Stroup, D. F. (1998) Continuous electronic fetal heart monitoring during Labour. (Cochrane Review) In: *The Cochrane Library*, Issue 2. Oxford: Update Software.

UKCC (United Kingdom Central Council of Nursing, Midwifery and Health Visitors). (1993) Standards for Records and Record Keeping. London: UKCC.

Welford, H. (1993) Scanning for trouble? *Nursing Times* 89 (17), p. 20.

World Health Organisation, UNICEF (1989) *Protecting, Promoting and Supporting Breast-Feeding: The Special Role of Maternity Services: A Joint WHO/UNICEF Statement.* Geneva: WHO.

Widstrom, A. M., Ransjo-Arvidson, A. B., Christensson, H. K., Mattiesen, A. S., Winberg, J., Uvnas-Moberg, K. (1987) Gastric Suction in healthy newborn infants: effects on circulation and developing feeding behaviour. *Acta Paediatric Scandinavica* 76, pp. 566–72.

World Health Organisation (1985) Having a baby in Europe. *Public Health in Europe* 26. Geneva: WHO.

Resources

Further reading

Annotated bibliography

Alexander, J. (1987) *Learning to Care in Midwifery.* London: Hodder & Stoughton.
This is a book written specifically for student nurses in order to inspire them. It covers the whole area of pregnancy, childbirth and postnatal care. It also includes case studies of a teenager, a woman experiencing a pre-term birth and a woman experiencing childbirth after a history of infertility. Each chapter is referenced and concludes with a series of 'test yourself' questions. A very practical and easy to read book even though it is quite old now.

Bennet, V. R. and Brown, L.K. (eds) (1999) *Myles Textbook for Midwives* (13th Edition) Edinburgh: Churchill Livingstone.
This is a standard midwifery text and contains chapters on normal and abnormal midwifery. It is written for midwifery students and includes all aspects of the midwifery curriculum including physiology and social sciences, as well as the history of midwifery.

Hunt, S., Symonds, A. (1995) *The Social Meaning of Midwifery.* Basingstoke: MacMillan Press – now Palgrave Macmillan.
This book is an ethnographic study of two labour wards. It gives a fascinating insight into the maternity services and the roles of midwives and staff within the service. This

book challenges a lot of firmly held assumptions of midwives and midwifery and as such is controversial and potentially threatening.

Inch, S. (1992) *Birthrights*. London: Hutchinson.

An interesting book written for the lay person, but explaining the problems of medicalisation of birth in a clear and distinct manner. A must for anyone in early pregnancy and those who wish to see pregnancy from the perspective of normality.

Niven, C. A. (1992) *Psychological Care for Families: Before, During and After Birth*. Oxford: Butterworth-Heinemann.

A psychological text that covers the areas of pregnancy, birth, the immediate postnatal period, when things go wrong, the early months and problems that may occur. It is easy to read and 95 per cent of the material is based on research findings. The author is a psychologist, nurse and mother.

Royal College of Midwives (2001) *Successful Breastfeeding* (3rd Edition) London: Churchill Livingstone.

This is the third edition of a book that was sent by the Royal College of Midwives to all its members. It is the result of a working group set up to look at the problems of breastfeeding. It is a very extensive handbook that, although small, should be in the possession of any practitioner who is dealing with breast-feeding women. It covers the physiology of breast-feeding as well as the practical issues of the positioning of the baby on the breast and problems that mothers may encounter. There is also a chapter on breast-feeding in special circumstances such as multiple pregnancy and pre-term babies.

Stables, D. (1999) *Physiology in Childbearing with Anatomy and Related Biosciences*. Edinburgh: Ballière Tindall.

This book looks at the childbirth continuum from preconception to the postnatal period and also includes the newborn baby. It covers the physiological processes that take place throughout. You will find this book useful when describing words that are new to you.

@ Web pages

These are changing every day, and offer resources to mothers and midwives. Explore what is on offer on a regular basis. Here are just a few:

www.safemotherhood.org

A site that gives information on the suffering of women worldwide who have not got access to health care during their pregnancy and childbirth.

www.midirs.org

A site for midwives in Britain which includes an enquiry service as well as an up-to-date list of midwifery and maternity organisations. There is also a link and a regular guide to midwifery related web sites.

www.intermid.co.uk

A British site that gives access to peer-reviewed journals.

www.midwifery.com

A site from the USA which gives information for mothers, midwives and aspiring midwives. It covers a range of topics, from gynaecology and contraception to breast-feeding.

www.cemd.org.uk

This is the site where pdf files concerning the confidential enquiry into maternal deaths are available.

www.maternitywise.org

This is a USA site for consumers and professionals and looks at evidence-based care, rights and informed decision making.

www.nelh.nhs.uk/maternity

Informed Choice leaflets can be viewed at this site as well as news, organisations, events and a reference database.

Video

Birth B-Line Productions

An excellent video that shows different births, including a Caesarian section and a birth in water. The mothers contribute and discuss how they felt about their labour and birth. Fascinating watching.

3

Insights into Child and Family Health

Gill McEwing , Janet Kelsey, Jim Richardson and Alan Glasper

Introduction

Children today are regarded as having their own rights, but are acknowledged as vulnerable individuals. This is recognised in contemporary society through robust legislation to protect them. Despite this, the developing child is always at risk in an increasingly dangerous environment and health care settings may present particular risks.

Children's nursing is practised within a philosophy of child-focused and family-centred care in which, whenever possible, the child, parents and carers are equal partners. This partnership enhances self-esteem, enables children to reach their full potential and encourages the development of autonomy in care and decision making (The Quality Assurance Agency for Higher Education 2001). Through these concepts children's nurses strive to improve standards of care through the application of those principles which underpin clinical governance (DoH 1997). This was not always the case and the promotion of family involvement was initiated nationally by the publication of the now famous 'Platt' report published in 1959 (Committee of The Central Health Services 1959). Changes have thus been spurred by the realisation of the harmful effects of admitting children to hospital and a greater identification of their developmental needs, including those of psychosocial care. Attempts to improve the care of children in the UK in a meaningful and altruistic way began much earlier. The work of Thomas Coram in the creation of the London Foundling Hospital in 1739 (Nichols and Wray 1935) is perhaps the starting point of changes to the care of children in society. It was not, however, until the middle of the nineteenth century that hospital inpatient care for children became available. The opening of the Hospital For Sick Children, Great Ormond Street, London, on 14 February 1852 was a major milestone for child health and children's nursing. One of the original aims of the hospital was the education of women in the special duties of children's nursing (Glasper and Charles-Edwards 2002a) and the role of the registered children's nurse since that date has been intimately related to the optimum care of sick children. Although this branch of the nursing profession has a long history which predates that of modern adult nursing, the future of the children's nurse at the pre-registration level remains unclear (Glasper 2002b).

The publication of the public enquiry into the events at Bristol Royal Infirmary has highlighted that challenges remain in delivering care which reflects true partnership with children and their families (DoH 2001). Nightingale herself is attributed as saying, 'it is a real test of a nurse whether she can nurse a sick infant', and Catherine Jane Wood, a former matron in Victorian times of The Hospital For Sick Children, Great Ormond Street, as saying, 'Sick Children require special nursing and sick children's nurses require special training' (Glasper 1995).

Children differ from adults intellectually, emotionally and physically. Childhood is a period of rapid growth and development and children of varying ages from birth to adolescence have very different needs (Bee 2000). Children are particularly vulnerable to the effects of illness and hospitalisation and therefore require specialised and individualised care (Taylor et al 1999).

Learning outcomes

The primary aim of this chapter is to give the reader an introduction to the world of child health nursing through a scenario in which a number of prevailing philosophies and practices will be explored. The scenario relates to an asthmatic child and both cultural and health/illness paradigms will be fully investigated allowing the reader to locate contemporary issues in childhood nursing within a context of family-centred care.

In particular this chapter will enable the student to:

- Use relevant literature and research to inform the practice of nursing.
- Recognise and plan to satisfy the potential care needs of a child with acute asthma.
- Demonstrate knowledge of physiological measurements in children.
- Identify the signs of respiratory distress.
- Discuss the importance of nursing assessment.
- Discuss the effect of hospitalisation on children.
- Describe the importance of play.
- Appreciate the importance of immunisation in children.
- Demonstrate knowledge of basic life support in infants and children.
- Recognise the essential requirements of nutrition in the infant and child.
- Discuss different approaches to the management of care for the sick child.
- Recognise the role of the family in a child's life and well-being and propose strategies to work collaboratively with the child and family.
- Recognise the significance of culture and ethnicity in health care and formulate principles for ensuring that care is delivered in a culturally appropriate way.

Concepts

- Childhood
- The family – structure and function
- Ethnicity, race and culture
- Stereotyping, prejudice and racism
- Social support

- Acute children's nursing and the nurse's role
- Chronic illness in childhood
- Family-centred care
- Nutrition
- Children's rights

Scenario *Introducing Deepak*

Deepak is 8 years old, he has a sister Sanjita aged 5 years and a 3-month-old baby brother, Rachid. Deepak was admitted to hospital at the age of 3 years with an attack of wheezing. By the age of 5 years he had been diagnosed as a severe asthmatic.

Asthma

Asthma is a chronic inflammatory condition of the airways, the cause of which is still not completely understood (Brewin 1997; British Thoracic Society 1990). Asthma is described as, 'airway obstruction that is reversible, airway inflammation, and increased airway responsiveness to a variety of stimuli'.

The asthmatic response includes:

Activity 3.1

Make notes on your current understanding of asthma before reading on.

Activity 3.2

Remember to write down words to check out or cues to pick up on, for example – what 'stimuli'?

Bronchospasm

- Narrowing of the bronchial walls due to contraction of the smooth muscle.
- More severe in the smaller bronchi and bronchioles where there is no cartilage in the walls.

Inflammation

- Causes the airways to become hyper-responsive and narrow easily in reaction to a wide range of stimuli.
- Further narrowing of the airways by the invasion of the mucosa, submucosa and muscle tissue by inflammatory cells.

Inflammatory cells

- These cells are mainly eosinophils, but also contain neutrophils, macrophages and mast cells.
- Contain chemical mediators, including histamine, prostaglandins and leukotrienes, which cause vasodilation and increased capillary permeability.
- This leads to mucous production and oedema.

The lumen of the airways is therefore narrowed by contraction of the smooth muscle, mucosal oedema and the hyper-secretion of mucus (Hunter 1995; Frankes 1997).

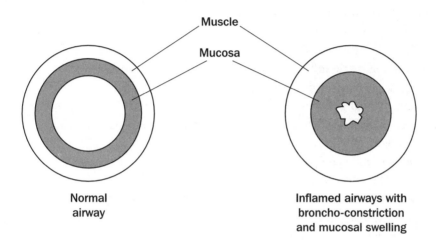

Figure 3.1   Normal and inflamed airways

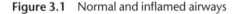

Activity 3.3

List the symptoms that Deepak will experience when he is having an asthmatic attack

There are two phases of the asthmatic response (Thompson and Gustafson 1996):

First phase

- Occurs within minutes of the exposure to the stimuli, reaches a peak in about 30 minutes and subsides after approximately two hours.
- Includes bronchospasm, oedema and mucous secretion.

Second phase

- Occurs about 4–12 hours after the exposure; it reaches a peak after about 4–8 hours, but can last for more than 24 hours.

- Inflammatory reaction, which can lead to damage of lung tissue. Airways are hyper-sensitive to allergic stimulation, which can result in further inflammation and broncho-constriction.

? **Why do you think Deepak was diagnosed as an asthmatic?**

Asthma is the commonest medical condition of childhood (Phelan 1994). It affects approximately 10 per cent of children and the incidence and severity of the disease appears to be increasing (Cross 1999). The changes in prevalence of asthma in children are difficult to deter-

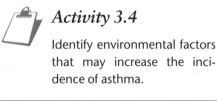

Activity 3.4

Identify environmental factors that may increase the incidence of asthma.

mine owing to changes in diagnostic practice (Magnus and Jaakkola 1997) but, however defined, asthma and wheezing in children has increased dramatically over the past few decades (Kaur et al 1998). This increase is thought to be due to environmental factors (Caldwell 1998).

There are approximately 2000 deaths (adults and children) each year in Britain; 80 per cent of these are thought to be preventable. Asthma is a major cause of morbidity in children. When asthma is not properly controlled, it results in disturbed sleep, absence from school and inability to participate in leisure activities (Welsh Office 1997). Severe childhood asthma can cause disfigurement with chest wall deformities (Cross 1999).

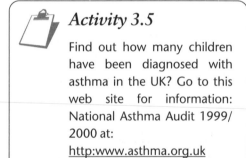

Activity 3.5

Find out how many children have been diagnosed with asthma in the UK? Go to this web site for information: National Asthma Audit 1999/2000 at:

http:www.asthma.org.uk

The course of the disease

- Age of onset varies; it tends to be earlier in boys than girls (Thompson and Gustafson 1996).
- First attack may occur at any age, but approximately 80 per cent of children will have experienced their first symptoms by the age of five years (Valman 1993).
- A better prognosis is associated with an earlier onset, except when the age of onset is less than two years (Thompson and Gustafson 1996).
- Unless the child suffers from severe asthma, generally their condition resolves as they grow older (Thompson and Gustafson 1996).
- Symptoms begin to decline in the teenage years and by the time they reach 30 years 75 per cent of sufferers are symptom free (Jenkins et al 1994).

Key points

- There is no test available to distinguish between acute bronchial infection and asthma.
- Children suffering from persistent recurrent cough or wheeze that responds to treatment with bronchodilator therapy would indicate that the cause might be asthma (Caldwell 1998).
- The child may suddenly develop a cough, which may follow a viral infection. It can be dry or productive, sometimes paroxysmal, and is frequently worse at night.
- The sputum is often thick and rubbery almost like worm casts. This is mainly caused by plasma leakage and the damaged epithelium (Brewin 1997).
- Wheezing is caused by air being forced through the narrowed airways, but if the child's chest is silent this may be due to exhaustion and not a sign of lack of severity of the attack.
- The course of asthma varies from child to child. Most children have discrete episodes of the disease with symptom-free periods in between; however, some children appear to constantly suffer from the symptom (Thompson and Gustafson 1996).
- The degree of symptoms can vary from mild to severe.
- The severity may change depending on the time of year. If the child is sensitive to pollens, then spring and summer could be the time when they experience most episodes of the disease. However, if the child reacts to cold air then the winter months could cause the most concern.

Treatment of asthma will focus on supportive care to ensure that the child receives adequate oxygen and does not tire excessively. Therapy will centre on the use of medication to reverse the physiological changes of asthma in order to ease breathing and return the situation to normal.

> Deepak was very happy at his previous school, but the family have now moved house and Deepak is due to start his new school tomorrow. Deepak is anxious about starting at his new school and was upset when he went to bed. Several hours later his mother realises that Deepak is having some difficulty with his breathing. Deepak uses his inhaler to see if it will improve his breathing.

There are some predisposing factors related to a child developing a hypersensitivity to specific stimuli or triggers.

Activity 3.6

Consider which of the following triggers may have caused Deepak's asthma attack, giving your rationale.

Table 3.1 Predisposing factors

- **Strong genetic factor** (Smith 1995)
- **Family atopy** (Smith 1995)
- **Maternal smoking**
- **Not breast-fed** for first 4 months of life (Oddy et al 1999)

Table 3.2 Indoor triggers

- **Allergy to house-dust mite**
  The allergen is the faeces of the mite. The mite feeds on dead skin cells that can collect on pillows and mattresses (Smith 1995).

  Modern houses with double-glazing tend to lack ventilation and moisture levels allow moulds to grow.

  Partial digestion of skin cells by aspergillus mould encourages the house-dust mite to thrive.
- **Allergy to animal dander** (Caldwell 1998).
- **Tobacco smoke** (Cook and Strachan 1997)
- **Synthetic pillows**
  A study by Strachan and Carey (1995) showed that children with feather pillows suffered less asthmatic response than those using synthetic pillows.

  This suggests that non-feather pillows may pose a greater risk to asthmatics than any allergens associated with feather bedding.

Table 3.3 Outdoor triggers

- **Allergy to pollen**
  The most troublesome time for pollen from flowers and grasses seems to be May/June. It is difficult to stay indoors for these months, but it is recommended that the child avoids being outside in the early evening when the pollen count is at its highest (Smith 1995).
- **Cold weather** (Caldwell 1998).
- **Air pollutants**
- **Industrial chemicals** (Smith 1995)
- **Ozone levels**
  Studies in America and Brazil have shown that air pollution has increased the incidence and severity of asthma, these studies have highlighted the serious effects of ozone on the incidence of childhood asthma and demonstrated clustering of the incidence of the disease around industrialised cities (Camargos et al 1999; Browner 1997).

Table 3.4 Other triggers

- **Viral infections**

  The most common trigger in children is **viral infection**. A study by Johnston et al (1995) showed that upper respiratory infections, mainly rhinoviral infections are associated with 80–85% of reported exacerbations of asthma in a cohort of school age children.

- **Exercise**

  A study carried out by de Bisschop et al (1999) showed that children suffering from exercise induced asthma could significantly reduce post exercise broncho constriction by carrying out a short warm up programme prior to exercise.

- **Food allergies**

  These include food colourings (Tartrazine), nuts, eggs, drinks containing ice or carbon dioxide (Valman 1993).

  Food allergies should be investigated thoroughly before the specific foodstuff is eliminated from the diet.

- **Stress, emotion and laughing**

  It is hard to evaluate the effect psychological factors have on childhood asthma (Valman 1993).

- **Excessive salt**

  There is some research that suggests that a high salt intake may increase bronchial hyperactivity in asthmatics by affecting the smooth muscle of the bronchioles (Medici et al 1993).

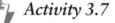

Activity 3.7

Find out what 'atopy' means, and what other allergic conditions are associated with asthma in this syndrome.

Deepak reassures his parents that he has taken his normal medications during the recent move.

All medications should be delivered by inhalation whenever possible. This ensures that the drug acts directly on the bronchioles and therefore has an immediate effect and a lower dose of the drug is required (Rudolf and Levene 1999).

Activity 3.8

Find out what medications are used to treat asthma.

There are two main groups of drugs 'relievers' and 'preventers':

- **Relievers** include beta 2-agonists such as salbutamol and terbutaline and in some cases ipratropium bromide is used.
- The **'preventers'** are the prophylactic drugs such as sodium cromoglycate and steroids (Rudolf and Levene 1999).

Table 3.5 Drugs used to control asthma

Drug group	Effect	Examples	Method
Beta2 agonists	Dilates the smooth muscle of the bronchioles. Reduces the muscle spasm and leads to an increase in the size of the lumen of the airways. Increases movement of the cilia. Decreases chemical mediators.	**SalbuDeepakol** Epinephrine Albuterol Metaproterenol **Terbutaline** Salmeterol long-acting	Inhalation (Can be given intravenously and orally)
Anti-cholinergic bronchodilator	Blocks the vagal stimulus to the bronchi, reduces muscle constriction and mucus production (British Thoracic Society 1997).	Ipratropium bromide	Inhalation
Methylxanthines	Weak bronchodilator. Increases movement of mucous in the airways. Increases the contraction of the diaphragm and respiratory muscles. Inhibits the release of mediators from the inflammatory cells.	Aminophylline Theophylline	Inhalation (Intravenously as life-saving measure)
Corticosteroids	Suppresses the inflammatory process, reduces mucus secretion and mucosal oedema. Reduces hyper-responsiveness of the airways (Hunter 1995).		Inhalation (Prophylactically)
Corticosteroids	Reduces the inflammatory response. Encourages damaged epithelium to heal.		Orally Intravenously Used in acute attacks
Other drugs	Stabilisation of mast cells.	Sodium cromoglycate Cromolyn sodium Nedocromil sodium	Inhalation However, this needs to be taken more frequently and is not so effective in some children (Caldwell 1998).

Deepak's condition worsens. His breathing becomes more rapid and his mother can hear an audible wheeze. The General Practitioner is asked to visit.

 Deepak is very breathless. What signs and symptoms will he present to the GP?

Asthma is one of the respiratory illnesses of childhood that commonly presents as a lower airway obstruction causing respiratory distress (Cropp and Shames 1994). The signs and symptoms of respiratory distress caused by asthma can be differentiated from those of other causes.

The clinical features of severe asthma can be identified as:

- Breathlessness
- Being unable to talk in sentences
- Chest recession
- Peak flow reduced to less than 50 per cent of expected
- Wheezing may or may not be a prominent feature

 What treatment would you expect the GP to administer?

If an acute attack fails to respond to the child's usual treatment, urgent treatment with nebulised salbutamol needs to be given using a compressed air supply or, if available, compressed oxygen (Brewin 1997).

The GP administers nebulised salbutamol, but Deepak is not responding to the treatment and the GP decides to admit him to hospital. The hospital's policy is to admit acute medical admissions directly to the children's ward. The GP reminds Deepak's parents to take all Deepak's medications with them. Deepak's mother accompanies him to hospital with his 3-month-old brother.

 Activity 3.9

Find out from your local hospital if emergency medical admissions are admitted directly to the children's ward, or if they go to Accident and Emergency first and then to the ward following assessment and emergency care. What do you think are the advantages and disadvantages of each approach to admission, for the child and its family?

On arrival to the ward the hospital doctor assesses Deepak. The assessment will include a brief history and examination of Deepak. The aim is to identify if Deepak is at risk of developing a severe exacerbation of his asthma. Deepak is very anxious, as he has not attended this hospital before.

Activity 3.10

Identify what questions the doctor needs to ask in order to ascertain the history and severity of his condition. You may be able to arrange to listen in on the doctor's assessment of such a child.

Table 3.6 Degrees of asthma (Cross 1999)

Mild asthma	Children who do not have continuous symptoms and only experience occasional short attacks.
Moderate asthma	Children who may have continuous mild symptoms and more frequent exacerbations that can last for several days or weeks.
Severe asthma	Children who have continuous symptoms and frequent, severe attacks.

Adverse features in Deepak's history would include:

● Previous episodes of respiratory failure or hypoxic-related seizures due to asthma.
● Deterioration despite the use of oral steroids or frequent inhalation of broncho-dilators at home.
● Recent hospitalisations or emergency-room visits for asthma.
● Dependence on multiple medication, particularly oral steroids.
● Non-compliance/psycho-social problems.

The nurse allocated to Deepak carries out a full nursing assessment.

 What can the nurse learn from looking at and listening to Deepak? What would you expect Deepak's vital signs to be? Consider your responses before reading on.

Table 3.7 Normal respiratory rates

Age (years)	Breaths/min
<1	30–40
2–5	20–30
5–12	15–20
>12	12–16

 Practice tip

Respiratory rates should be measured over a full minute. It should be remembered that young children breath diaphragmatically, and therefore are observed by watching abdominal movement rather than the movement of the chest.

Table 3.8 Normal heart rates

Age (years)	Heart beats/min
<1	110–160
2–5	95–140
5–12	80–120
>12	60–100

Practice tip

An accurate pulse should be measured for a full minute. If measuring the heart rate of children less than two years of age, a stethoscope should be placed over the apex of the heart and the beats counted for a full minute.

Table 3.9 Systolic blood pressure (BP) by age

Age (years)	Systolic BP
<1	70–90
2–5	80–100
5–12	90–110
>12	100–120

Expected systolic BP = 80+(age in years × 2)

Practice tip

The size of the child's limb must be taken into consideration when taking blood pressure. Make sure the width of the BP cuff is about two-thirds the length of the child's upper arm. A cuff that is too large may produce a reading that is too low; a cuff that is too small may give a false high reading (Thomas 1996).

It was previously thought that 37°C was the mean body temperature, however, it is now recognised to be 36.8°C, with a variable fluctuation between individuals of 0.5°C (Mackowiak et al 1992). For example, Anderson et al (1990) describe the normal circadian range of infants' temperatures over the 24-hour period as ranging from 36°C at night, to 37.8°C during active periods in the day.

What are the different methods of assessing the following vital signs: temperature, heart rate, respiratory rate and blood pressure?

 Why are certain methods more appropriate for different groups of children?

For temperature measurement, go to the thermometry page at: http:\\www.graduateresearch.com\thermometry\theory.htm. For further information on assessing children, read Thomas, D., (1996) Assessing children – it's different, *Registered Nurse* 59 (4), pp. 38–45.

To summarise

The ABC criteria for assessment of a patient are useful in any circumstance (Lloyd-Thomas 1990). Physical signs such as wheeze and respiratory rate are poor indicators of the severity of an asthma attack. Contraction of the sternomastoids, chest retraction, pulse rate, peak expiratory flow rate and arterial oxygen saturation are better guides. Cyanosis is a late sign and an indication of a life threatening attack (Advanced Life Support Group 1996).

At this time Deepak has not responded well to the initial treatment of beta2 agonists. He is unable to drink and is finding it increasingly difficult to carry out a conversation with you.

Assessment

Before the nurse can plan the client's care, the client's problems must be defined and identified. Consequently, the assessment phase of planning care begins with the collection of data about the health status of the client and ends with a statement of their problems. The assessment process involves the nurse collecting data. This data can be gathered from a number of sources; primary data is from the client, secondary data is from other sources. It also involves the data being validated; for example, Deepak may say his only health problem is his asthma yet when you talk to him with his parents, they state he has had recurrent ear infections. The data gathered also needs to be recorded in an organised fashion.

There are two different types of data collected:

- Subjective
- Objective

Subjective data includes thoughts, feelings, beliefs and sensations that the client is experiencing. Objective data is that gathered by the use of observation and examination.

Practice tip

It is important to remember that the admission process is the first time that Deepak and his family have met the nursing staff. First impressions can lay the foundation for the future relationship between the nursing staff and Deepak. For this reason, care should be taken to use the opportunity to get to know him. Questions should be asked in language understandable to those being asked. The nurse should be sensitive to the needs of Deepak and time should be given for him and his parents to both answer and ask questions.

Activity 3.11

Consider what other sources may be used to gather information about Deepak. In your current placement find out how information is gathered on assessment, recorded and organised. Detail the objective data that you would need to adequately carry out Deepak's assessment.

There are many different tools available to aid a nursing assessment. Often they are based upon the nursing model which is used to underpin practice. The next section contains a nursing assessment gathered from Deepak and his family.

Activity 3.12

Complete as much as you can of the assessment of Deepak and his family utilising the information you have been given. From your assessment identify the nursing needs of Deepak and his family.

Table 3.10 Nursing assessment sheet

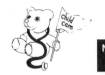

| Nursing Assessment Sheet for 1 to 10 year olds |
| Child Health Directorate |

ROYAL
CORNWALL
HOSPITALS
TRUST

1. Maintaining a Safe Environment

Normally:	Apart from those which are normal for his/her age and stage of development, does your child undertake any hazardous activities?	Yes / No
	If yes, please specify:	
	Does your child have any ongoing health problems?	Yes / No
	If yes, please specify:	
	Is your child fully immunised and vaccinated?	Yes / No

Please indicate: Diphtheria [ ]   Tetanus [ ]
                    Whooping cough [ ]   Polio [ ]   MMR [ ]
                    HIB [ ]   BCG [ ]   Other [ ]

	Is your child allergic to anything: drugs:	Yes / No
	foods:	Yes / No
	other:	Yes / No
	Does your child appreciate danger?	Yes / No
	Does your child respond to commands?	Yes / No
	Would you describe your child as hyperactive?	Yes / No
	Does your child ever have blackouts, convulsions, fits, headaches?	Yes / No
	If yes, please specify:	

On Admission:	Parental medication discussed?	Yes / No
	Has the child had any recent contact with infection?	Yes / No
	If yes, please specify:	
	Is isolation required?	Yes / No
	If yes, please refer to RCH Trust Policy	
	Does the child appear to be in pain?	Yes / No
	If yes, please indicate pain score	
	Identify pain tool used	
	Is the child possibly going for a general anaesthetic?	Yes / No
	If yes, does the parent wish to accompany them?	Yes / No
	Are there any family problems associated with general anaesthetic?	Yes / No
	Other problems:	
	....	
	....	

Child's problem / nursing needs identified (actual or potential):

2. Communication/Fears and Worries

Normally:	Does your child have full language?	Yes / No
	If no, please specify what ability:	
	Is your child able to express his/her feelings/fears?	Yes / No
	Does your child use a 'comforter' of any sort?	Yes / No
	If yes, please specify:	
	Does your child have any problems with:	
	Vision	Yes / No
	Hearing	Yes / No
	Behaviour	Yes / No
	If yes, please specify (e.g. wears glasses, hearing aid, etc.):	
	....	

On Admission:	Has the child ever been in hospital before?	Yes / No
	Indicate the parent's understanding of the reason for admission:	
	....	
	Does the parent feel worried about the admission?	Yes / No
	Please specify worries:	
	Indicate the child's understanding of the reason for admission:	
	....	
	Does the child appear to be worried?	Yes / No
	Please specify child's worries:	
	Other problems:	
	....	

Child's problem / nursing needs identified (actual or potential):

3. Breathing

Normally:	Has your child ever had a breathing problem of any sort?	Yes / No
	If yes, please specify:	
	Does your child take regular medication for his breathing?	Yes / No
	If yes, please specify:	
	Does anyone at home smoke?	Yes / No
On Admission:	Are there signs of respiratory distress?	Yes / No
	If yes, please specify:	
	Is the child's colour clinically normal?	Yes / No
	If no, please specify:	
	Other problems:	
	....	

Child's problem / nursing needs identified (actual or potential):

4. Eating and Drinking

Normally:	Do you restrict your child's diet in any way?	Yes / No
	If yes, please specify:	
	Does your child have a good appetite?	Yes / No
	Does your child have any special likes or dislikes?	Yes / No
	If yes, please specify	
	....	
	What does your child like to drink?	
	Does your child use a cup / feeder / bottle? *(delete as appropriate)*	
	Does your child feed himself?	Yes / No
	If yes, does he/she use a knife / fork / spoon *(delete as appropriate)*	

On Admission:	Is the child eating and drinking normally?	Yes / No
	If no, please specify:	
	Is the child's eating or drinking compromised in any way?	Yes / No
	If yes, please specify:	
	Other problems:	
	....	

Child's problem / nursing needs identified (actual or potential):

5. Elimination

Normally:	Does your child wear nappies day or night?	Yes / No
	If yes, please specify:	
	Is your child clean and dry by day and night?	Yes / No
	If no, please specify:	
	What word does your child use for the toilet?	
	Does your child normally have urinary or bowel problems?	Yes / No
	If yes, please specify:	
	Does your child ever take medicine for bowel or urinary problems?	Yes / No
	If yes, please specify:	

On Admission:	Is the child passing urine normally?	Yes / No
	Are there any problems associated with the urinary tract?	Yes / No
	If yes, please specify:	
	Is the child having normal bowel actions?	Yes / No
	If no, please specify:	
	Other problems:	
	....	

Child's problem / nursing needs identified (actual or potential):

6. Personal Cleansing and Dressing

Normally:	Is your child able to wash and dress independently?	Yes / No
	If no, please specify:	
	Does your child have any soap or lotion allergy?	Yes / No
	If yes, please specify:	
	Does your child use special toiletries?	Yes / No
	If yes, please specify:	
	Can your child clean their own teeth?	Yes / No
	Does he/she visit the dentist regularly?	Yes / No
	How often and when does your child:	
	Bath / Shower?	
	Wash their hair?	
	Clean their teeth?	

On Admission:	Is there a risk of pressure sores?	Yes / No
	Condition of skin	
	Condition of teeth (e.g. loose teeth, braces, etc.)	
	Other problems:	
	....	

Child's problem / nursing needs identified (actual or potential):

7. Temperature Control

Normally:	Is your child prone to high temperatures?	Yes / No
	Has your child ever had a fit associated with high temperature?	Yes / No

On Admission:	Is the child's temperature within the normal range?	Yes / No
	If no, please specify:	
	Has the child had a febrile convulsion prior to admission?	Yes / No
	Other problems (e.g. family history of hyperpyrexia):	
	....	

Child's problem / nursing needs identified (actual or potential):

8. Mobilisation/Milestones

Normally:	Is your child developing normally?	Yes / No
	If no, please specify:	
	Is your child fully mobile?	Yes / No
	If no, please specify:	

On Admission: Is the child partially immobile for any reason?   **Yes / No**

If yes, please specify: ....

....

Other problems: ....

....

....

Child's problem / nursing needs identified (actual or potential):

9. Activities

Normally: Which school does your child attend? ....

Does your child have any schooling difficulties?   **Yes / No**

If yes, please specify: ....

What activities does your child enjoy? ....

....

On Admission: Is the child able to play normally?   **Yes / No**

If no, please specify: ....

Is the child able to attend the hospital school?   **Yes/No/NA**

Hospital school discussed with parents   **Yes/No/NA**

Other problems: ....

....

....

Child's problem / nursing needs identified (actual or potential):

10. Self-Awareness

Normally: Is your child shy or easily embarrassed?   **Yes/No**

(Girls) Has your child started her periods?   **Yes/No**

If yes, when is the next period due? ....

Does your child have any self-image problems?   **Yes/No**

If yes, please specify: ....

On Admission: Other problems: ....

....

....

Child's problem / nursing needs identified (actual or potential):

11. Resting and Sleeping

Normally:	What is your child's normal bedtime?	Yes / No
	Does he/she nap during the day?	Yes / No
	If yes, please specify:	
	Does your child use a pillow?	Yes / No
	Do you want to use your child's own duvet / pillow?	Yes / No
	Does your child have a bedtime routine?	Yes / No
	If yes, please specify:	
	Is your child afraid of the dark?	Yes / No
	Does your child have sleep disturbance/nightmares/sleep walking/ sleep with parents?	Yes / No
	If yes, please specify:	
On Admission:	Is there any reason to suppose that the child may have a disturbed sleep pattern?	Yes / No
	If yes, please specify:	
	Other problems:	
	....	

Child's problem / nursing needs identified (actual or potential):

12. Social Issues

Normally:	Is there a family history of long term illness (e.g. epilepsy, eczema, asthma, diabetes)?	Yes / No
	If yes, please specify:	
	Lives with:	
	Parents' names:	
	Step parents' name(s) (if applicable):	
	Brothers' and Sisters' (names and ages):	
	Name of any other person who regularly looks after your child:	
	Do you have any social or financial problems which may make it difficult for you to stay with / visit your child?	Yes / No
	If yes please specify:	
	Are there any social issues / housing problems that we may be able to help you with?	Yes / No
	If yes, please specify:	
	Do you have a social worker?	Yes / No
	If yes, please state name:	
	Would you like to see a social worker about any of the above?	Yes / No

On Admission:	Can the family / extended family visit easily?	**Yes / No**
	Social Worker required?	**Yes / No**
	Ward visiting discussed?	**Yes / No**
	If no, please specify:	
	Family circumstances / visiting rights:	
	Other problems:	
	....	

Child's problem / nursing needs identified (actual or potential):

13. Cultural/Spiritual Issues

We would like you to know that we respect your family's cultural /religious beliefs

Please indicate your child's culture religion / culture: ....

Is your child baptised?   **Yes / No**

In the case of an emergency would you like us to call a Minister / Elder?   **Yes / No**

If yes, please indicate person to be contacted (or Hospital Chaplain): .....

....

Are there any special religious /cultural observations you would like us to be aware of and respect?

If yes, please specify: ....

| **On Admission:** | Other problems: .... |
| | .... |

Child's problem / nursing needs identified (actual or potential):

14. Care by Parent

This ward operates a 'shared care' system of nursing. We invite you to do as much, or as little, for your child as you feel able.

Please indicate below, how much of your child's care you would like to be involved in but remember that carers need rest too, and we are very willing to take over for you whenever you feel like a break.

Will parent or carer be resident?	**Yes / No**
Basic Care: comfort	**Yes / No**
feeding	**Yes / No**
hygiene	**Yes / No**
Recording temperatures	**Yes / No**
Charting temperatures	**Yes / No**
Charting intake and output	**Yes / No**
Medication	**Yes / No**
Other, please specify:	

On Admission: Does the parent require education on any of the above? **Yes / No**

If yes, please specify: ....

Other problems: ....

....

Child's problem / nursing needs identified (actual or potential):

15. Discharge

Do you foresee any problems with returning home? **Yes / No**

If yes, please specify: ....

On Admission: Are there any reasons to prevent early discharge? **Yes / No**

Discharge plan discussed with parents / family? **Yes / No**

If not, why not?: ....

Discharge plan commenced? **Yes / No**

Provisional discharge date: ....

Other problems: ....

....

Child's problem / nursing needs identified (actual or potential):

Child's / Parent's Valuables

I understand that I am responsible for mine / my child's personal property / valuables during the hospital stay. I have been offered the use of the hospital safe for more valuable possessions and have decided to keep them with me on the ward. I understand that by making this decision, the Royal Cornwall Hospitals Trust is absolved from any liability due to loss or theft.

Parents signature: .... Date: ....

Information which you have shared with us helps build a picture of your child's routine/life. This enables nurses to meet your child's individual requirements / needs during their hospital stay through developing a care plan, and aims to cause as little disruption to usual routine as possible.

If you wish to discuss anything within this document or in the care plans, please ask your named nurse. Thank you for completing the assessment document, please sign box below.

Parent's signature ....

Date ....

Time ....

Assessor's/nurse's signature ....

(Reproduced by kind permission of the Royal Cornwall Hospital Trust)

> **Activity 3.13**
>
> Make a list of the initial priority issues for this family.

You might include such issues as:

Safety It is important to ensure that Deepak is supported, monitored and receives appropriate treatment to improve the situation but also to prevent deterioration.

Information Deepak and his mother need to know both what is happening and why what it is that is being done to support Deepak is important. It is equally important that the nurse is able to establish what the priorities and concerns of Deepak and his mother are. In the light of the fact that Deepak's mother speaks English as a foreign language, particular emphasis should be placed on the effectiveness of information gathering and giving.

> **Activity 3.14**
>
> You may need to ask for the help of an interpreter. Consider what potential problems this may lead to. You will need to consider how the maintenance of Deepak and his mother's confidentiality can be assured.

Comfort It will be helpful to Deepak and his mother if they are treated in a gentle and respectful manner. If the nurse is calm and efficient in her approach to Deepak and his mother's care needs, this may also communicate a reassuring message.

One of the problems you should have identified from the assessment is that Deepak is very anxious about coming into hospital. What causes this anxiety? Much of the research examining the effects of hospitalisation on children has focused on why children react differently to hospital experiences in an attempt to recognise why this occurs. A variety of strategies have been developed by children's nurses to help families cope with the emotional traumas of hospital admission and other related health care interventions. Changes to a child's routine such as hospital admission can expose them to stress and it should be remembered that certain categories of children, for example those with special needs or those for whom English is not the first language, may not be able to adequately articulate their needs (Glasper 2002a).

> **Activity 3.15**
>
> Have you or a member of your family been in hospital as a patient? Think or ask if any of these categories apply and how you felt whilst you were in hospital. Do you think there are any differences between children and adults?

Evidence-based Practice

Features of hospital which may worry children

Visintainer and Wolfer (1975) placed the features of hospital, which may worry children, into five categories:

1 Physical harm or bodily injuries in the form of discomfort, pain, mutilation, or death.
2 Separation from parents and the absence of trusted adults, especially for pre-school children.
3 The strange, the unknown and possibility of surprise.
4 Uncertainty about limits and expected 'acceptable' behaviour.
5 Relative loss of control, autonomy and competence.

Cross (1990) looked at the short-term effects of hospitalisation after the child has been discharged. Of children aged between two and seven years, 54 per cent experienced some difficulties, including nervousness about separation, more demanding behaviour, sleeping difficulties, and difficulty with mother–child relationships. However, McClowry and McLeod (1990) found no changes in behaviour in children between the ages of 8–12 years. There may be many reasons for this difference:

- Older children may be more resilient to the stress of hospitalisation.
- Older children may be disguising their real feelings.
- The measuring tool used in the research may not have been broad enough to encompass this age group.

Other factors may also influence Deepak's anxiety. Cross (1990) found that asthmatic children appeared to have more difficulty with coping than other groups. Crocker (1980) identified that the effect of moving house, birth of a sibling and changing school in addition to being hospitalised may create more stress than the child can handle. An emergency admission means that Deepak has had no preparation for this admission thus potentially increasing his anxiety. It is important to remember that 'routine tests and observations' can be very stressful for the child and family and once again, time should be spent at this stage preparing the children for what is going to happen.

Activity 3.16

Much has been written about different methods of preparation. Read the useful text 'How to prepare', in Taylor et al (1999) *Nursing Children: Psychology, Research and Practice*.

A potential problem for children in hospital is the number of different people involved in their care who they are expected to converse with and who sometimes carry out physical examinations on them.

Activity 3.17

Next time you are on a ward count the number of people one client comes into contact with on your shift.

What system of nursing would help to reduce the number of nurses a child and their family come into contact with?

Children in hospital may meet many new people as a result of their admission and every effort should be made to reduce this added stress.

Play

One method of reducing children's distress is through the use of play as a therapeutic tool. Play was first introduced into paediatric wards in 1963.

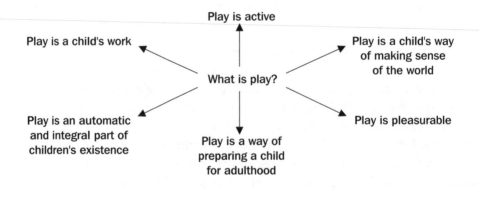

Figure 3.2 What is play?

Play is an activity we all take part in, often without realising it. Normally, play is voluntary and is pleasurable. Rarely does it have extrinsic goals. It is spontaneous and chosen by the player. It can also provide the child with a sense of control (Garvey 1977). Sometimes adults think they have forgotten how to play. However, if you relax and let the children take the lead you will find it easier. Nevertheless, you should be aware that your own expectations and inhibitions might get in the way. Of course, children play for many reasons, some of which are described as to:

- Have fun
- Communicate
- Make sense of and master the environment
- Socialise
- Aid development, this includes:
  - social
  - moral
  - physical
  - cognitive
  - emotional

Play can also be an important child-centred communication tool; sometimes it is seen as a type of language between the child and the carer. By giving up adult-focused language we can gain a child's-eye perspective of their experiences (Webster 2000). Play specialists in areas caring for children work in partnership with parents and other staff, educating them to develop their own play vocabulary. However, they are not the only people who play with children in hospital.

Activity 3.18

Before reading on consider what particular function play can have for a child in hospital.

- Play is an excellent form of communication.
- Play is something that the child normally does in their everyday life, therefore it is familiar.
- Play is usually safe and non-threatening.
- Anyone can be involved.

As part of their emotional development children can learn through play to cope with anxiety producing situations, such as hospitalisation. This is known as therapeutic play and its purpose is to help achieve emotional and physical well being (Sylva 1993). Therapeutic play is different to child-led play in that it is structured by adults and it has extrinsic goals. Play activities are planned to meet the physical and emotional needs of the child in order to decrease the fear and anxiety of hospitalisation. We can use therapeutic play:

- To assess the child's knowledge of a medical condition and treatment.
- To identify and rectify misunderstandings.
- To address issues which cause anxiety or concern.
- To help the child understand what will be expected and what to expect.
- To provide information.

All of these are achieved by sharing information with the child in a developmentally appropriate manner. Therapeutic play employs a variety of techniques to achieve this:

- Projective play, which is described as helping children, can communicate by scaling down their experiences to a manageable size.
- Role-play is that which can help identify any hidden misunderstandings, fears or feelings that the child may have. It allows the child to try on adult roles and one of its aims is to help them as they seek to gain a sense of control.
- Messy play is a great kick against the system and an outlet for the expression of emotion.
- Distraction techniques are acknowledged to help limit anxiety and stress. Their aim is to help the children develop coping strategies in a developmentally appropriate way.
  (Webster 2000)

Some examples of distraction techniques are:

- Blowing bubbles
- Counting
- Hangman (hang the person you are angry with!)
- Puppets
- Imagining
- Breathing
- Relaxation tapes
- Shouting

Visualisation techniques are also used with some children; however, they should only be undertaken by health professionals familiar with the procedure, as particular skills are needed.

Activity 3.19

Have you ever used any of these techniques? Did you recognise what you were doing? Try to write a short reflective account of your feelings at the time. Can you think of any other ways you could maintain Deepak's link with home?

Table 3.11 Play materials for different ages

Play material	Uses	Benefits	Age
Dolls	Role play, discussion, good for checking knowledge	Easy for the child to identify Allows concrete thinking Uses visual and aural memory	2–10 years
Books	Information and good for parents to read to child	Can use again at own pace	2 years onwards
Photo diary	Discussion and detailed explanation	Can make their own Can involve and show to others	6–7 years onwards
Video	Discussion and detailed explanation	Good for those reluctant to play Can use at own pace	6–7 years onwards
Leaflets	Information specific to procedure	Can use again	2 years onwards

Immunisation

During your assessment you should also have asked about Deepak's immunisation record. Immunisation of children is the single most cost-effective form of prevention and a positive health benefit for children. The World Health Organisation (WHO) in its document *Health for All* (1985) clearly aims for the eradication of poliomyelitis, measles, neonatal tetanus, congenital rubella syndrome and diphtheria from Europe by the year 2000.

Activity 3.20

Find out the incidence of these diseases in your area. If you are unsure of the meaning of 'incidence', check in Chapter 12 on rehabilitation.

Protecting children against infectious disease is dependent upon the development of safe and effective vaccines. Once a licence has been granted and the vaccine is in general use, surveillance continues to detect less-common reactions or problems associated with the vaccine. All vaccines can give rise to side-effects, although it is rare that these are severe. However, the complication rate for each disease is greater than that of the vaccine. But no vaccine is 100 per cent effective, although the reasons for this are not fully understood. A proportion of primary vaccine failures may be due to impotent vaccine arising from poor vaccine handling.

- 5–10 per cent of individuals who receive a single dose of live measles vaccine are not protected from the disease (Atkinson and Orenstein 1992).
- A full course of pertussis vaccine confers protection in over 80 per cent of recipients, and in those not fully protected the severity of the disease is reduced (Miller and Fletcher 1976).
- If sufficient individuals in a population are immunised, those who cannot receive vaccine because of medical contraindications and those who did not respond to the vaccine will be protected from disease by herd immunity.
- The level of vaccine coverage required varies for different diseases and is partly dependent on the infectivity of the causative organism.

Immunisation should be postponed for any child who is suffering any acute illness. However, minor infections without fever or systemic upset are not reasons to postpone immunisation. Any vaccine is contraindicated when an individual has had a severe local or general reaction to a preceding dose. Some individuals cannot be given live vaccines because they are unable to make a normal immune response and could suffer disseminated infection. Similarly, inactivated vaccines, while not being dangerous, may be ineffective (DoH 1996).

These include:

- Children undergoing treatment for malignant disease with chemotherapy or generalised radiotherapy, or within six months of terminating treatment.
- Children who have received an organ transplant and are currently on immunosuppressive treatment.
- Children who have received a bone marrow transplant should have their immunity to diphtheria, tetanus, polio, measles, mumps, rubella and Hib checked six months after transplantation and be immunised accordingly.
- Children on high-dose corticosteroids: 2mg/kg/day for at least a week or 1mg/kg/day for one month. Live vaccines should be deferred for at least three months following cessation of treatment. Children on lower dose steroids for prolonged periods need to be assessed individually.
- Live vaccines should not be given within three months of immunoglobulin
- Live vaccines should either be administered simultaneously at different sites or allow a three-week interval.
  (DoH 1996)

A multi-disciplinary team approach to immunisation provision has been found to be particularly beneficial (Peckham et al 1989). This includes opportunistic immunisation of children in contact with health professionals for other reasons and domiciliary services. These additional approaches have proved to be useful in increasing the uptake of vaccinations (Bedford 1997).

Table 3.12 The immunisation schedule

VACCINE			AGE
BCG	*specific high risk*		birth
Diphtheria/tetanus/pertussis		1st dose	2 months
Oral polio	*primary*	2nd dose	3 months
Hib	*course*	3rd dose	4 months
Measles/mumps/rubella (MMR)			12–18 months
Diphtheria tetanus and polio		Booster	4–5 years
MMR		2nd dose	
BCG			10–14 years
(after tuberculin skin test)			
Tetanus/low-dose diphtheria		Booster	15–18 years
Polio			
Hepatitis B			(high risk children)
Pneumococcal			

Activity 3.21

Find out the percentage immunisation uptake for different vaccinations of children in your area. Would you consider asking about Deepak's brother and sister's immunisation status? When do you think this topic should be approached?

Nutrition

Activity 3.22

When you are carrying out your nursing assessment, Deepak's mother asks your advice about how she should feed his 3-month-old brother Rachid. Consider the following and then try to think how you would answer Deepak's mother's question.

During the first year of life growth is rapid and it is essential that the nutritional needs of the infant be met. The infant requires:

- Protein, which is used in infants almost entirely for growth, unlike in adults where it can be used as an energy source or converted to fat. An adequate intake of protein with a balance of amino acids is essential.
- Carbohydrate as the main energy source.

- Fat, which is stored by babies to act as an emergency energy food and used for insulating them from the cold. Fatty acids are also essential to ensure normal growth. Fat reduction should not be considered for children under the age of two years.
- Minerals, although the infant's iron store will last for approximately the first six months it is essential to provide an iron source when mixed feeding is introduced.
- Calcium is needed for the development of the bones and teeth.
- Other trace elements such as copper and zinc must be provided to enable normal development.
- A full range of vitamins is required for normal development.

Weaning is defined by the DoH (1994) as the 'process of expanding the diet to include food and drinks other than breast milk or infant formula'. Thus weaning allows the infant to meet their growing nutritional requirements. The World Health Organisation (WHO) recently changed their recommendation that 'infants should be exclusively breast-fed for the first four to six months of life' to 'exclusive breast-feeding for six months, with introduction of complementary foods and continued breast-feeding there-after'. However, in the United Kingdom we will at present continue to follow the DoH (1994) *Coma* Report recommendations that allows for mothers to choose when to begin introducing solid food when the baby is between 4 and 6 months of age. Not weaning before four months of age does mean waiting until the infant is at least 4 calendar months old, which is 17–18 weeks not 16 weeks.

> ### 📋 *Activity 3.23*
>
> To find out more about the rationale for this decision, read More (2001).

Exclusive breast-feeding for the first four months of life has been associated with significant reduction in the risk of asthma by the age of six years. Public health interventions to promote and increase the duration of breast-feeding may help to reduce the prevalence and severity of childhood asthma (Oddy et al 1999).

The aims of weaning are to:

- Introduce a wide range of tastes and textures
- Take food from a spoon
- Take fluids from a cup
- Provide a more energy dense diet
- Provide iron

Initially weaning should commence by giving one or two teaspoons of food that is a smooth, thick-cream consistency. Half of the breast- or formula-feed should be given first and no salt or sugar added. New flavours are gradually introduced.

The next stage is to introduce food that has soft lumps or is mashed and, by about nine months, minced or finely chopped food can be introduced, ensuring the infant gets lots of different textures so that they can learn to chew.

By 12 months of age children should be getting a good mixed diet with about three meals and two to three healthy snacks in between.

Problems that may be associated with weaning include:

- Failure to thrive
- Risk of choking
- Rejection of solids
- Faddy children
- Constipation
- Diarrhoea
- Obesity
- Dental caries

There are many excellent booklets available from your local health promotion resource centre about the dietary needs of babies and children – you should use these to guide your learning about how to wean infants on to solid food. Another excellent source of information about nutrition is the European Food Information Council at: www.eufic.org/fr/home/fhome.htm.

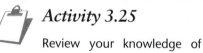

Activity 3.24

Plan a weaning menu for Rachid for one day taking into consideration the family cultural needs. Compare your menu with a colleague.

If Deepak's condition deteriorates he may develop some of the following signs of life threatening asthma:

- Severe chest recession
- Altered consciousness level
- Duskiness or cyanosis
- Marked use of accessory muscles
- Oxygen saturation less than 85 per cent in air
- Peak flow either unrecordable or less than 33 per cent expected
- Silent chest
  (Advanced Life-Support Group 1996)

Should this happen he may require emergency intervention. According to *Advanced Paediatric Life-Support* (1996) 'early diagnosis and aggressive treatment of respiratory or cardiac insufficiency aimed at avoiding cardiac arrest is the key to improving intact survival in seriously ill patients and children. Establishing a clear airway and oxygenation are the most important actions in paediatric resuscitation. These actions are essential prerequisites to other forms of treatment.'

Activity 3.25

Review your knowledge of basic life-support of infants and children

Basic life-support

The epidemiology of paediatric cardiopulmonary arrest is different to that of adults. Cardiac arrest in infants and children is rarely a primary event; it is more likely to be secondary to hypoxia and respiratory acidosis or shock. Respiratory arrest may also arise as a result of neurological dysfunction.

The basic principles of paediatric basic life-support are the same as for adults, but there are some specific differences in technique for different sizes of children which are essential if the optimum support is to be given.

The Resuscitation Council UK (2000) defines an infant as a child under the age of one year, and a child as aged between one and eight years of age. Children over the age of eight years are treated as for a child, but may require different techniques to attain adequate chest compressions.

The major differences in technique for an infant

- To open the airway the head and chin should be tilted to the 'sniffing position'. This is achieved by placing one hand on the forehead and tilting the head back into a neutral position, avoiding excessive neck extension and taking care not to press on the soft issues under the chin. A jaw thrust may be used if cervical spine injury is suspected.
- When delivering rescue breaths, cover the mouth and nose with your mouth, ensuring you have a good seal.
- The brachial pulse is easiest to feel on the inner aspect of the upper arm between the elbow and the shoulder. Gently press with index and middle fingers until you feel the pulse.
- If the pulse rate is less than 60 beats per minute, that is less than one per second, external chest compressions should begin without delay.
- During chest compression the sternum is compressed with two fingers of one hand. Draw an imaginary line between the nipples and place the tips of two fingers one finger's breadth below this line.

The major differences in technique for a child

- To open the airway place one hand on the forehead and tilt the head back into a neutral or slightly extended position. Lift the lower jaw with the tips of two fingers of the other hand. Avoid excessive neck extension and take care not to press on the soft issues under the chin. A jaw thrust may be used if cervical spine injury is suspected.
- To deliver rescue breaths make a mouth-to-mouth seal and pinch the soft part of the child's nose tightly with the thumb and index finger of the hand, maintaining head tilt.

- In children the carotid pulse should be palpated.
- If the pulse is absent, then external chest compressions should begin without delay.
- In children the heel of one hand is used at a compression point two fingers breadth above the xiphisternum. Ensure that the fingers are lifted to prevent pressure being applied over the child's ribs.

In children over the age of approximately eight years, it may be necessary to use the two-handed 'adult' method of chest compression in order to achieve adequate chest compression. In this case the lower half of the sternum is located and the heel of one hand placed there with the other hand on top. Interlock the fingers and raise them off the chest to ensure that pressure is not applied to the child's ribs.

When using this technique, the Resuscitation Council UK (2000) recommends to continue with a rate of 100 times per minute, but the ratio of compressions to breaths for a one-man rescue is 15:2 compared to 5:1 for infants and children.

Basic life-support in infants and children follows the airway, breathing and circulation sequence. They are the same in principle but utilise the different techniques relevant to the child's age as described earlier:

1 Ensure safety of the rescuer and child. It is essential that the rescuer does not become a victim and the child is removed from further danger as quickly as possible. This should precede all further actions.
2 Assess the child's responsiveness. Gently stimulate the child by speaking loudly and asking, are you all right? Shake by the shoulders or pinch gently. Do not shake children with suspected cervical spine injuries. A young child is unlikely to respond in a meaningful way, but may make some sound or open their eyes.
3 If the child responds but is struggling to breathe, leave them in the position in which you find them unless they are in further danger. Children with respiratory distress often position themselves to maintain patency of a partially obstructed airway. Attempts to improve a partially maintained airway, without advanced support being available, is potentially dangerous as total occlusion may occur. Check their condition regularly and get help if needed.

   If the child does not respond, the rescuer should shout for help and then provide basic life-support for one minute before going for assistance. It may be possible to take a small child or infant with you whilst summoning help. Check first to see if there is evidence of trauma. The likelihood of injury may be evident from the child's location or position, for example, a child found at the foot of a tree is more likely to have suffered trauma than a child found in bed. If more than one rescuer is present, then one should go for help whilst the other commences resuscitation.

   After shouting for help, open the child's airway. Use the appropriate technique for the age of the child. Try to do this with the child in the position in which you find him. If this is not possible, then carefully turn the child on to his back and open the airway.

Again if trauma is suspected, then turn the child with head and neck firmly supported. Do not allow the head to twist, roll or tilt. Avoid head tilt if cervical spine injury is suspected.

4 Keep the airway open and check breathing. Look for chest and abdominal movement. Listen at the mouth and nose for breath sounds. Feel for expired air movement on your cheek.

Look, listen and feel for up to 10 seconds before deciding that breathing is absent. If the child is breathing, place them in the recovery position and continue to assess them.

5 If the child is not breathing, carefully check for and remove any obvious airway obstruction, but do not perform a blind finger sweep.

Give up to five rescue breaths. With each breath, the child's chest should move. Take a breath before each rescue breath to optimise the amount of oxygen delivered to the child. Breath slowly and steadily for between 1–1.5 seconds. This minimises the risk of gastric distension, which can reduce the effectiveness of rescue breathing by pushing up the diaphragm and reducing lung volume. If the chest either does not rise or is inadequate, then the airway may be obstructed. Recheck the child's mouth for obvious obstruction. Readjust the airway position. Five attempts should be made to achieve two effective breaths. If you are still unsuccessful, then consider foreign body obstruction and move on to the airway obstruction sequence.

6 Assess the child's circulation. Take no more than 10 seconds to check the pulse using the correct technique for the age of the child. At the same time look for any movement including swallowing or breathing.

If you can detect signs of circulation within the 10 seconds but no breathing, then continue rescue breathing for one minute before going for help. If somebody else has gone for help, continue rescue breathing until the child starts breathing effectively on their own. If at this point the child remains unconscious, then turn them on to their side into the recovery position.

7 If there is no palpable pulse or, in infants, it is less than one beat per second, start chest compressions using an age-appropriate technique and combine the chest compressions with rescue breathing. Remember the ratio of compressions to breaths for infants and children is 5:1, in older children over the age of eight years it is 15:2 for a one-man rescue and 5:1 for a two-man rescue. The recommended rate of compressions is the same for all – 100 times per minute. However, this is the rate and not the number of compressions to be given in a minute, as there will be interruptions for ventilation.

8 Continue to resuscitate until the child demonstrates spontaneous respiration and pulse, or help arrives, or you become exhausted.

Activity 3.26

Once you are confident that you have achieved a good degree of knowledge about basic life-support, you should practise these skills using a resuscitation manikin in the clinical skills laboratory or on a practice placement. It is important that all nurses working with children practise these skills regularly so that they can quickly institute resuscitation procedures on the rare occasions when they are required.

How much of this information do you think you would retain after practising on a manikin?

Activity 3.27

Read the article by H. West (2000) on basic infant life-support. The guidelines for basic life-support in children can be accessed on the internet at: http://www.resus.org.uk/pages/pbls.htm.

Foreign body obstruction sequence

If upper airway obstruction is either witnessed or suspected, then the Resuscitation Council (UK) Guidelines (2000) should be commenced. 'If the child is breathing spontaneously his own efforts to clear the obstruction should be encouraged. Intervention is necessary only if these attempts are clearly ineffective and breathing is inadequate.'

Do not perform blind finger sweeps as this may result in the impaction of a foreign body or cause soft tissue damage. Measures intended to create a sharp increase in pressure in the chest cavity are employed. The sequence is as follows:

- Deliver up to five back blows, holding the infant supported in a prone position with the head lower than the trunk.

If this fails to relieve the obstruction:

- Deliver up to five chest thrusts, holding the infant in a supine position with the head lower than the trunk. Chest thrusts are similar to chest compressions, but sharper and carried out at a rate of approximately 20 per minute.
  Remember to support the head and neck whilst turning the infant.
- Check the mouth and remove any visible foreign bodies.
- Open the airway, reassess breathing.

If the infant is breathing, place in the recovery position and continue to assess breathing. If the infant is not breathing:

- Attempt up to five rescue breaths. Even with a partially obstructed airway you may still achieve effective ventilation.
- If the airway remains obstructed, continue the sequence from the beginning until the infant breathes spontaneously, the airway is cleared or help arrives.

For a child, the above cycle is repeated but substitute abdominal thrusts for chest thrusts on the first cycle and then alternate chest and abdominal thrusts on subsequent cycles. Abdominal thrusts are delivered with the heel of one hand placed in the middle of the upper abdomen with the child in an upright position if they are conscious, but unconscious children should be supported in the supine position.

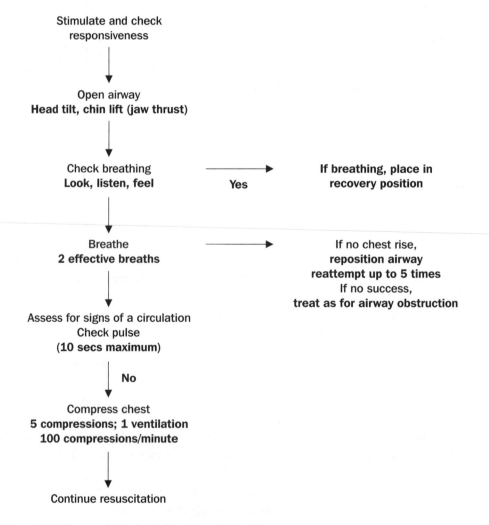

Figure 3.3 The paediatric basic life-support algorithm

> Deepak's condition has not improved and the nurses need to monitor the level of Deepak's respiratory distress.

It is important to realise that although the lung is obviously the primary target of respiratory distress, when respiratory failure follows there may be impairment of other vital organs as a result of decreased arterial blood gases, acidosis and hypercarbia.

The general clinical signs of respiratory distress in children can be described within the systems they affect.

Table 3.13   Clinical signs of respiratory distress

Respiratory

- Tachypnoea
- Altered depth and pattern of breathing
- Intercostal, subcostal and suprasternal inspiratory retractions
- Nasal flaring
- Cyanosis
- Decreased or absent breath sounds
- Expiratory grunting
- Wheeze and or prolonged expiration
- Dyspnoea
- Cough
- Head bobbing
- Stridor
- Seesaw respirations
- Decreased chest expansion
- Decreased breath sounds

Cardiac

- Tachycardia or bradycardia
- Hypertension or hypotension
- Duskiness
- Cyanosis
- Cardiac arrest

General

- Poor skeletal muscle tone
- Fatigue
- Abdominal pain
- Increased sweating
- Altered consciousness level

Cerebral

- Restlessness
- Irritability
- Headache
- Confusion
- Diminished response to parents or pain
- Coma

It can be seen from the above that carefully looking and listening at a child is invaluable in assessing their respiratory status. In addition the measurement of capillary refill, oxygen saturation and peak expiratory flow rate are helpful in making a nursing assessment.

> ### Activity 3.28
>
> For all the systems, check your understanding of the terminology by, for example, checking definitions in a dictionary. Also write key points to explain why breathing difficulties may lead to all these signs and symptoms.

Other systems may also be affected by altered respiratory status, following the ABC criteria (American Academy of Pediatrics 1997) for assessment in conjunction with neurological observations provides a framework for rapid and effective nursing assessment of the child with respiratory problems.

Capillary refill

Capillary refill is a quick and easy method for determining the efficacy of respiratory function. A raised digit is pressed for five seconds and the time taken for blood to return to the area is estimated in seconds. A capillary refill time of greater than two seconds in a child and three seconds in a neonate is a sign of poor oxygenation.

Oxygen saturation

The administration of oxygen may be prescribed to maintain oxygen levels during an asthmatic attack. There are several methods of oxygen administration. The most suitable one will be chosen dependent on the child's age and condition. Oxygen should be humidified whenever possible.

How much oxygen is in the blood depends on:

- Haemoglobin concentration in the blood (Hb g/dl)
- Oxygen saturation of the haemoglobin (Sao_2)
- Partial pressure of oxygen – how much dissolved in the plasma (Pao_2)

Carbon dioxide is transported to the lungs dissolved in the plasma, or as bicarbonate, or carbamino compounds. Carbon dioxide is acidic therefore if the level of carbon dioxide in the plasma rises, the child becomes acidotic.

Analysis of the blood pH and the arterial blood gases provides information of the child's gas exchange and acid-base status:

- Normal partial pressure of oxygen (Pao_2) in the arterial blood is 11–14kPa (Kilo Pascals)
- Lower in neonates Pao_2 = 8–10kPa.
- Normal partial pressure of carbon dioxide ($Paco_2$) in the arterial blood is 4.0–5.5kPa. *(Rudolf and Levene 1999)*

Disturbances in acid-base balance can be caused by respiratory disorders. If respiration is inadequate, the child's blood pH will fall and result in acidosis. Assessment of arterial blood gas values can assist in deciding the best course of treatment.

In asthma the monitoring of arterial blood gases may be necessary:

- If the child shows signs of severe respiratory distress, it will help determine if the child is in respiratory failure and needs respiratory support.
- Controlled ventilation using endotracheal intubation may be necessary for a short period of time, usually 8–12 hours.

Transcutaneous measurement of oxygen saturation is used for continuous oxygen assessment.

Pulse oximetry measures the arterial blood saturation by calculating the percentage of haemoglobin that is saturated with oxygen and, because haemoglobin is photosensitive and has the capacity to absorb different amounts of light, changes in oxygen levels can be rapidly detected. A light emitting sensor and a photodetector are placed in an opposing position around a digit, hand, foot or earlobe. The diode emits red and infrared lights, which pass through the skin to the photodetector. Oxyhaemoglobin absorbs more infrared light than deoxyhaemoglobin. This is detected by the microprocessor, which displays the percentage of oxyhaemoglobin. To enable the sensor to 'pick up' a reading the patient needs to have an adequate pulsatile blood flow to the periphery.

Practice tip

Carrying out pulse oximetry on a site which is already being used for blood pressure monitoring or as access for an arterial catheter will produce inaccurate recordings. Movement of the child has the same effect.

The probe site should be changed every four hours to prevent pressure necrosis or burns from incompatible sensors and oximeters (Murphy et al 1990).

Children like Deepak should have their oxygen saturation recorded on arrival on the ward. Saturations of less than 90 per cent are indicative of a severe attack.

Activity 3.29

Find out normal values for oxygen saturation. If possible measure your own.

Fluid management

From the assessment you should have identified that a child such as Deepak is at risk of dehydration. It is important to ensure the child has a sufficient fluid intake. Oral fluids may be difficult when the child has severe breathing problems. Therefore fluids are administered intravenously to meet normal fluid requirements and to replace additional losses caused by hyperventilation. The amount and type of fluid administered is pre-scribed according to the individual child's size and hydration needs. Measurements of blood gases pH and serum electrolytes will be used to determine the extent of the child's dehydration, acidosis and electrolyte imbalance. The insertion of an intravenous can-nula is a stressful experience for both the child and the parent, therefore age-appropriate preparation for the procedure needs to be given (Campbell and Glasper 1995). The cannula should be inserted into a site that takes into consideration the child's age and level of activity, and should be secured to ensure it remains stable but allows the insertion point to be visible (Moules and Ramsay 1998). An infusion pump is normally used to reduce the risk of circulatory overload. The nurse should, on a regular basis, monitor the rate of the infusion and the infusion site for signs of phlebitis and extra-vasation. There are many risks associated with the administration of intravenous fluids, comprehensive protocols should be available in the ward area and these should be com-plied with to improve safety (Livesley 1993).

> ### Activity 3.30
>
> Find out the recommended intravenous fluid requirements for a child Deepak's age.

Management of care

The Department of Health (1991) suggests that children's wards practise within a philosophy of family-centred care. The main concepts of family-centred care are:

- The unit of care is the family not just the child.
- The individuals that make up the 'family' are decided by each individual family.
- The nursing care and the environment should support and enable the family to care for their child.

The involvement of parents and other family members in the care of the child benefits the child both physically and emotionally (Glasper and Ireland 2000). This is also beneficial to the family as it maintains the family unit, enables them to continue in their parenting role and to develop the knowledge and skills required to care for their sick child (DoH 1991; Audit Commission 1993).

However, there has been some evidence to suggest that parents attempting to care for their sick child in hospital can find it distressing due to the unfamiliar environment and conflict of interests between family members (Callery 1997). Therefore it is important that the nurse works towards what is in the best interests of the child and the family, and that the family decide the level of involvement that is right for them.

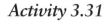

Activity 3.31

It is now generally accepted that a parent or another family member is resident in hospital with a sick child and that they will assist in the care of the child. Discuss the possible advantages and disadvantages of this with the following individuals:

1 Parents
2 Child
3 Nurses
4 Doctors

The children's ward where Deepak has been admitted uses a model of care to enable the nurses to work towards common goals (Moules and Ramsay 1998). The model used on the ward is 'Casey's partnership model of care'; family-centred care is fundamental to this model (Casey 1988).

The philosophy behind Casey's partnership model is that the best people to care for the child is the family. To do this the family may require varying degrees of support and assistance from the health care team. The model also acknowledges that the family can consist of any of its members and anyone else who is emotionally close to the child.

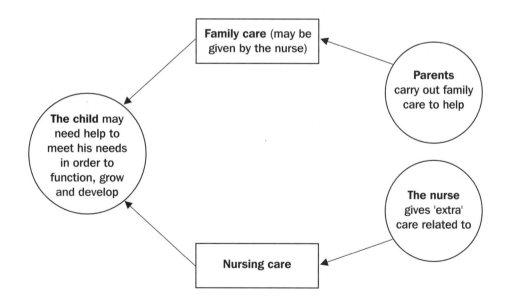

Figure 3.4 Casey's partnership model of nursing
(Casey 1988)

Activity 3.32

Consider the care this family requires. How would you plan to support Deepak and his family to meet his needs? How will you enable Deepak's mother to continue to care for his 3-month-old brother whilst they are in hospital? How would you assist Mr Patel in arranging to take time off work to care for Sanjita?

There has been a lot of criticism of the nursing process approach to care as it imposes rigid constraints on practice, is cumbersome and outdated (Walsh 1997). Critical pathways or integrated care pathways are multi-disciplinary approaches to care that are being developed that provide care that is cost effective, patient focused, multi-disciplinary and collaborative (Herring 1999).

Activity 3.33

A Find out the approach to care used for children with chronic illness on your children's ward. Do you have pre-written care plans or critical pathways? Which approach to care do you consider is most appropriate for Deepak?

B Try to define what might constitute family-centred care.

Professional conversation

Wendy, paediatric ward sister

Issues which characterise family-centred care

'Having been a ward sister for a number of years I really appreciate the recognition of this concept. Of course, many of us feel that we have always recognised that parents or other primary carers satisfy the child's important basic care needs in the normal situation until the child has developed the ability to do this themselves. It's important that we appreciate that parents can usually learn to care for the child's enhanced needs brought about by a change in health status, but that they may need help, support and guidance to learn these skills.

We also have to demonstrate to them that we accept that if parents are to care for their child's needs they may require supportive care themselves. The real challenge for some is the recognition that the nurse's role in this form of care may move from that of care deliverer to that of care facilitator. Most importantly, it is the acceptance that the child is an integral part of the family unit and to improve the child's health involves addressing that family unit as a whole.'

Can you suggest potential advantages and disadvantages to this form of care delivery?

The parent requires the knowledge and skills necessary to care for the child. It is one thing to be responsible for satisfying the child's hygiene needs with a daily bath at home, but it is quite a different situation if the child is on a ward and has an intravenous cannula in his/her hand. Parents may need help to adapt their usual care practices to meet such changed conditions.

Activity 3.34

Make notes on what you think might constitute the supportive care the parent may need while resident on the children's ward and involved in their child's care.

In order to meet the demands of satisfying their child's care needs the parents own care needs need to be attended to. This might include:

- Facilities where the parent can rest and sleep
- Facilities where the parent can wash and change their clothes
- Access to adequate and appropriate food and drink
- The means to communicate with the wider family back home

For many parents, it is equally important that they receive validation that what they are doing is a positive help to their child. It could be argued that these conditions are best achieved by the nurse working side-by-side with the parent and not simply leaving them to get on with their child's care.

Activity 3.35

You will note that in Casey's model 'family' care may be delivery by the nurse. Try to propose reasons for why this may become necessary.

There are many reasons why family care may be delivered by the nurse. For instance:

- The parent may be stressed and tired and the priority is that they are able to rest so that they are able to continue to care for the child.
- The child's situation may require adaptation of the parent's normal care practices. For example, if the child has a plaster cast on a leg, helping the child to bathe or go to the toilet will become more complicated. The parent may need to have this adapted procedure demonstrated and the opportunity to practise its execution while being supported by the nurse.
- The parent may have competing responsibilities. The need to go to work or to care for other children at home may mean that the parent cannot stay in hospital to participate in the child's care. The nurse will then have to explore other methods of ensuring that the parent's participation continues as far as conditions allow.
- On rare occasions, the parent's actions are not in the child's best interests.

Family-centred care occurs in dynamic, ever-changing situations and it is important that continuing assessment of the situation and necessary adjustments to the care approach are undertaken. The cornerstone of collaborative work between parent, child and nurse is effective communication in the form of appraisal and negotiation. The research undertaken by Swallow and Jacoby (2001) illustrates this well. Equally, Darbyshire (1994) was able to show that poor communication precludes collaborative family-centred work.

> **?** In the case of Deepak and his mother, what might be the components of family-centred care?

In the acute phase Mrs Patel might be helped and supported to deliver care which satisfies Deepak's basic needs. She can help Deepak to drink small amounts of fluids, she can help him to wash, she can help to reassure and comfort him. As Mrs Patel's understanding of the tasks of management improve she can begin to take responsibility for monitoring Deepak's condition using observation and peak flow measurement. She can ensure that his medication is administered effectively. In the longer term she can work to ensure the normality of their everyday experience by, for example, minimising the effect of trigger factors which provoke Deepak's asthma. Over time, Deepak and his family will learn to be flexible **and** to adapt these care practices to integrate them into family life and **also in making** the changes necessary to meet new situations.

Action for Sick Children (ASC) (2000), a consumer organisation which represents the views of parents whose children need the services of health care professionals, has summarised the important principles of child health care from their perspective in the *Millennium Charter*. These ideas might be seen as the prerequisites for and the underpinning of family-centred child health care.

> ### Activity 3.36
>
> Having considered the themes introduced in this chapter, can you suggest the principles which should be observed to ensure that family-centred nursing care occurs satisfactorily?

In caring for Deepak's asthma and ensuring his well-being, Deepak and his mother will have to master several tasks.

> ### Activity 3.37
>
> From the knowledge that you have built up about childhood asthma, list what you think are the important knowledge and skills that Deepak and his mother will need to manage this situation.

The millennium charter

- All children shall have equal access to the best clinical care within a network of services that collaborate with each other.
- Health services for children and young people should be provided in a child-centred environment separately from adults so that they are made to feel welcome, safe and secure at all times.
- Parents should be empowered to participate in decisions regarding the treatment and care of their children through a process of clear communication and adequate support.
- Children should be informed and involved to an extent appropriate to their development and understanding.
- Children should be cared for at home with the support and practical assistance of community children's nursing services, unless the care that they require can only be provided in hospital.
- All staff caring for children shall be specifically trained to understand and respond to their clinical, emotional, developmental and cultural needs.
- Every hospital admitting children should provide accommodation for parents, free of charge.
- Parents should be encouraged and supported to participate in the care of their child when they are sick.
- Every child in hospital should have full opportunity for play, recreation and education.
- Adolescents should be recognised as having different needs to those of younger children and adults. Health services should therefore be readily available to meet their particular needs.

(Action for Sick Children 2000)

Your list might include:

- Monitoring Deepak's condition to detect early any signs of deterioration so that action can be taken to deal with this. For example, some children's asthma worsens when they have a viral infection such as a cold. Using an asthma diary might be helpful with this.
- Avoiding factors, which act as triggers. The aim in managing exposure to triggers will be to prevent asthma attacks and to promote normality in the life of the child and family.
- Administering medicine efficiently and effectively. Inhaling medication is not an easy skill to master and the use of inhalers and spacer devices needs to be demonstrated and practised.

> Since moving house, Deepak and his family are separated from their relatives in the UK and the nearest town is very difficult to access by public transport. Although they have recently moved to enable his father to work, the family will still rely on social welfare payments to supplement their basic income. The house they have recently moved to is damp and they know this may prove to be a problem with Deepak's asthma.

From this account, can you identify issues which might pose a challenge for Deepak and his family in their daily lives?

You might suggest:

Social support Who provides Deepak and his family with support, help and encouragement? Who can Deepak's mother discuss her anxieties with? Might Deepak's parents want more social interaction and, if so, who might they ask to baby-sit? This is particularly significant if they cannot be certain, given the unpredictable nature of asthma, when Deepak might have a sudden asthma attack and whether the babysitter might be able to cope appropriately with such a situation. Without social support, Deepak and his family may feel lonely, isolated and uncertain.

Financial Potentially, living on a low income can constitute a chronic stressor for families like Deepak's. Many families who receive social welfare support do not receive the full range of benefits to which they are entitled simply because they are not aware of their entitlement.

Housing Poor living conditions can cause stress, but also the damp state of the house may contribute to Deepak's asthma problems if house-dust mites and fungal spores act as trigger factors in his case.

In order to ascertain whether such factors are indeed issues for this family it will be useful to assess the situation from the family's viewpoint. It is all too easy to make assumptions about people's position. For example that a single parent family suffers from lack of social support and interaction. This may not be the case.

In carrying out an assessment, it may be useful to construct an ecomap to illustrate the family's social position.

The ecomap graphically illustrates relationships within the family and between the family and other individuals such as the wider family, friends and neighbours and with agencies such as the school, the workplace and health care bodies. The ecomap also offers the opportunity to depict information on the nature of these relationships whether they are close, over close or conflictual.

Activity 3.38

You might find it useful to construct an ecomap of your own family or that of a family in your care at the moment. This will allow you to practise the technique and explore its possibilities.

To supplement your understanding of families' experience of caring for an ill child, the papers by Smith and Daughtry (2000) and Neill (2000) offer many insights derived from research work involving such families. You might also find useful views of the child's experience from the work of Sartain et al (2000).

Activity 3.39

Make a list of the observations in these papers which you might want to bear in mind as potential issues when working with families such as Deepak's.

While you read these papers consider, based on the quality and nature of the research they describe, whether you are prepared to accept the findings of these researchers. In other words, is this good quality research that provides results which are valid and reliable? You might find it useful to make notes about the issues you find in the article that convince you that this is good quality research – or not!

It will be important to use such observations critically. Not all families respond in the same ways to difficulties relating to child health. It is unhelpful to assume that difficulties which do not exist are present, but equally unhelpful to fail to recognise difficulties which do. A respect for family individuality and careful information gathering and sharing can help to avoid these pitfalls in planning and delivering care for families such as Deepak's.

Activity 3.40

Suggest which agencies, individuals and professionals might be able to offer help and support to Deepak and his mother if they have any of the potential problems which you have identified.

Among others, your list might include

- Social worker
- Welfare benefits adviser
- Local authority housing officer
- Community groups
- Self-help groups, for example Action Asthma
- Link families with a child with a similar health issue

Mrs Patel came to the UK in the late 1970s with her husband from India. Their families are of Gujurati origin and Gujarati remains their home language. Mrs Patel speaks English but naturally prefers her mother tongue to receive and express complex ideas. Deepak has a native command of both Gujarati and English appropriate to a 8-year-old child.

Given Mrs Patel's Indian background and upbringing, can you propose any cultural issues which it might be helpful to take into account when caring for her and her son?

Attention to cultural issues in health care is called for to avoid discrimination. An awareness of cultural aspects of children's needs should ensure equality. An important appreciation to have when dealing with cultural minority members is that people who are identified as belonging in their beliefs, values and customs are as if members of the majority cultural group. That said, an emphasis on individuality remains the key to working with all consumers of health services. There can be no doubt that people from cultural minority groups have experienced treatment which is different from that delivered to people from the majority cultural group. This difference might be based on ignorance of cultural needs or even on prejudiced attitudes. It might therefore be useful to consider the ramifications of culture as a factor involved in interactions between patients and health care professionals.

It might be profitable to consider the meaning of some of the terms used in trans-cultural nursing practice.

? **Can you define what is meant by the terms 'cultural', 'ethnic' and 'race'?**

Culture has been defined by Helman (2001) as an inherited 'lens' through which a person perceives the world he/she lives in. This can be interpreted as the beliefs and values which guide a person's behaviour or customs, and which allow the person to make sense of the world through explanatory beliefs and ideas about what is right and wrong through those values. These beliefs and values are derived from a person's upbringing and help to identify that person as belonging to a group. Of particular interest to the nurse are those beliefs which a person holds with regard to what health is, how it is preserved and what action should be taken when there is a health problem. Often these beliefs are deeply embedded in our consciousness and can be quite difficult to articulate.

> *Activity 3.41*
>
> Take some time to consider how you explain a minor ailment such as a cold or chill. How do you treat yourself when you have such a problem? How do other members of your family respond when they have the same problem? Your beliefs in this area are affected by culturally determined health beliefs as well as your education.

? **Have you heard the expression, 'feed a cold and starve a fever'? What would you say is the basis for this prescription?**

Suman Fernando (2001) offers an interesting discussion on race, culture and ethnicity. He argues that culture is characterised by behaviour and attitudes which are determined by upbringing and choice, and that these are perceived as changeable through, for example, acculturation. Ethnicity, he proposed, is characterised by a sense of belonging and group identity, both of which are determined by social pressures and psychological need. He makes a case that ethnicity is a partially changeable phenomenon. Finally, Fernando suggests that race is characterised by physical appearance dictated by genetic ancestry and that this is perceived as permanent.

Activity 3.42

Take a few minutes to consider these definitions. Can you think of any grounds on which you might challenge the validity of these ideas?

If Fernando's definition of culture is accepted, then it can be seen that it might be possible to define certain groups in any society as cultural independent of race or ethnicity.

? Could you make a case for the elderly or those in a certain social class or professional group as constituting a cultural group? In what ways might it be useful to use these definitions in this way?

In Mrs Patel's case her culture and ethnicity may have an influence on how she explains Deepak's ill health. This may or may not differ from the Western biomedical explanation for asthma which is the basis of treatment. If Mrs Patel's explanation for Deepak's breathlessness differs from that of his carers, she may find herself bewildered by his treatment. If, for example, she has been brought up to understand that breathlessness can be caused by a dietary imbalance, she may struggle to understand why Deepak is being given medication but no attempt is being made to modify his diet.

? If there is a mismatch between the treatment that Mrs Patel feels her son should receive and that which is actually being given, how might Mrs Patel feel about this?

Consider the situation of the parent who visits a GP with her child, who has an upper respiratory tract infection. She may well expect that her child will be prescribed an antibiotic and might be annoyed if the GP does not agree to do this. The GP knows that this infection is viral in origin, against which the antibiotic would be ineffective.

Moreover, over-prescription of antibiotics when they are not necessary can lead to bacterial resistance to antibiotics. However, the mother may understand that all infections are treatable with antibiotics. The mother's and the GP's perceptions of what should be done differ and, without careful explanation, it is possible that they will not reach common ground. The mother's faith in the GP's advice may be shaken and she may see no usefulness in the GP's suggestion that she give symptomatic care of hydration, rest and anti-pyretic medicine. She may feel it is unnecessary to adhere to this advice.

? Can you propose a strategy for resolving the situation where parent/child and health care professional differ in their understanding of what is an appropriate course of action to deal with a health problem?

You might suggest:

- A careful exploration of what the parent and child understand the problem to be and what they expect should be done to treat the problem. Devoting time to this enquiry can sometimes, from the health care professional's perspective, yield surprising results.
- Offering the parent and child information about the biomedical explanation for the child's problem. Such information may be quite difficult for the parent and child to assimilate and they might require time to think about what they have been told and then have the opportunity to ask questions to clarify some of the issues.

Commonly in health care parents are given explanatory leaflets to supplement the care-related information they have been given.

📋 *Activity 3.43*

List what you think might be the potential benefits and limitations of using the written word for information giving.

Your list might include:

- The parent and child can read the leaflet at their own pace and retain it for later reference.
- These leaflets often contain diagrams which illustrate features of the disorders. For example, the characteristic bronchospasm of asthma can be explained by a drawing.
- The leaflet offers information in one form which may not be understood or may be misunderstood. It will still be important for the nurse to be available to discuss questions which arise from the parent and child's reading of this material.
- Many adults and children have difficulty in reading the sometimes rather sophisticated language contained in explanatory leaflets. This difficulty might be heightened if the parent's native language is not English. In this case, alternative means of information giving such as audio- or videotapes might be explored.

Whatever mode of information giving is employed, it will remain important that the nurse takes time to check on the parent's and child's understanding of the information which has been given.

Other aspects of family life which might be culturally determined include issues such as dietary requirements and preferences, spiritual expression and pastoral care needs, hygiene practices, clothing, language use and child-rearing practices. For all families, it will be important to establish the family's requirements with regard to such daily living practices. Failure to do so may alarm or alienate the parent and child.

Activity 3.44

Working through the assessment framework used in your area, make notes of the factors which might, under the influence of culture, be specific for certain children and families. You might supplement your knowledge in this subject by consulting a textbook such as that by Holland and Hogg (2001) or Culley and Dyson (2001).

Differences between people in cultural or ethnic beliefs have the potential to escalate to form the basis of discrimination, prejudice, or even racism. Many people in cultural and ethnic minority groups have experienced this and will naturally be sensitive and anxious about being exposed to such responses again. It is one of the primary values of the nursing professions that discriminatory attitudes and behaviour are not tolerable, and that all people are approached with respect.

Activity 3.45

Construct a set of theoretical guidelines for nurses working with cultural and ethnic minority families to ensure that anti-discriminatory practice is assured.

Important principles which might be reflected in your guidelines might include:

- Maintaining a respectful attitude towards the beliefs and customs of others so long as these do not lead to harmful effects.
- Remaining committed to achieving an understanding of what parents and children expect of their treatment and why.
- Taking time and patience to explore the parent's and the child's explanation for, and understanding of, the child's health problem.
- Ensuring that the child and family receive a full explanation of the child's problem. This should be in a format which the child and parent can assimilate, negotiating with the child and parent to achieve a consensus about what should be done to alleviate the child's problem and how. Taking the child and parent's resources and preferences into account here could be argued to improve the chances of successful collaboration.

Adopting these strategies have the potential to ensure successful working together not only with those families with particular ethnic backgrounds, but also those with other cultural orientations.

> **Activity 3.46**
>
> Consider whether the operation of these principles in practice might be use-
> ful with other potentially marginalised families in health care. Can you think
> of examples of such families?

Families with subtle differences from the majority norm in their lifestyles and life
expectations might be included here. For example, families made up of two gay or les-
bian parents with children might belong to this group. Taking these principles of working together and translating them into action in planning and delivering child health
care will help to ensure that family-centred care is instituted. Family-centred care has
been evolving in the UK since the 1950s (Smith et al 2002). Nurses working in child
health care have continued to move from making care decisions and delivering that care
to negotiating with families about the child's care needs and who should satisfy these.
The research of Darbyshire (1994) demonstrates that this move is part of a continuing
evolution in care philosophy.

> After Deepak's initial poor response to his treatment, he is now responding well to
> nebulised salbutamol 2-hourly, driven by oxygen. He has also commenced oral
> prednisolone.
>
> During the next 24 hours Deepak's condition continues to improve – he is wheez-
> ing less, his respirations are between 18-22 breaths per minute, his pulse is 90 beats
> per minute at rest, and his oxygen saturation is above 90 per cent. He is able to
> recommence oral fluids and his intravenous infusion is discontinued. The next day,
> he is discharged home. Deepak is a moderate to severe asthmatic, therefore he will
> be advised to follow the national guidelines for chronic asthma management.

Principles of asthma management

The management of asthma is focused on controlling the underlying inflammatory
response using prophylactic therapy, and break-through symptoms being treated with
bronchodilators. It is essential that the child and family are aware that asthma cannot be
cured, the aim is to control the symptoms so that the child can lead a full and active life
(Gregson et al 1993).

National and international guidelines for the management of asthma in children
advise a step approach to drug management (International Paediatric Asthma Consensus Group 1992; British Thoracic Society 1993). Using this protocol, children are
assessed and assigned to a level of treatment related to the severity of their asthma, the
treatment is subsequently adjusted to meet the child's changing needs, and control is
maintained with the lowest possible dosages of drugs. There are five steps in the treatment (Rudolf and Levene 1999):

Table 3.14 Step approach to the drug management of chronic asthma

Step 1   Inhaled beta2 agonists to relieve symptoms, administered no more than 3 times a week.

Step 2   Trial of sodium cromoglycate for six weeks to determine whether there is a prophylactic response. Continue with inhaled beta2 agonists as required.

Step 3   If sodium cromoglycate is unsuccessful, replace with inhaled steroids. Continue with inhaled beta2 agonists as required.

Step 4   Increase dosage of inhaled steroids. Consider long-acting beta2 agonists, or slow-release methylxanthines (orally), or ipratropium bromide.

Step 5   When the maximum dose of inhaled steroids is reached, use low dose oral steroids.

Good inhaler technique is essential for effective treatment and it is important that the most suitable device is chosen for each individual child, trying out a variety of devices may be necessary for the child to be able to find the correct device (Caldwell 1998). The choice of inhaler is affected by the age of the child, prescribed treatment, the child's lifestyle and the child's preference. Over 90 per cent of asthmatics take all the medications they require by inhalation. However, inhaled drugs are not effective during severe asthmatic attacks because the airways are completely obstructed by inflammation and mucus (Jordan and White 2001). Bronchodilators are most effective when delivered as inhaled aerosols, this route of delivery also decreases the amount of the drug entering the systemic circulation and therefore reduces side-effects (Jordan and White 2001).

Activity 3.47

The British Thoracic Society (1997a and 1997b) has published guidelines on asthma management which are also available on their website at: http://www.brit-thoracic.org.uk. Having read these guidelines, satisfy yourself that you understand the forms of therapy used to treat asthma, their modes of administration and actions.

Evidence-based practice

The National Institute of Clinical Excellence (2000) have published a useful review of the use of inhaler systems/devices for children. This can be accessed on their website at: http://www.nice.org.uk. This is also a good example of how the effectiveness of a health care intervention is evaluated.

Which type of inhaler do you think would suit Deepak best?

Inhaler technique

Inhaler devices require different levels of skill and co-ordination to administer effect-ively. The method of administration for inhaled drugs varies with the child's age and ability. Nebulisers are the method of choice for infants and young children. When inhalers are prescribed, the child and family need to be taught how to use the device giving careful instructions, demonstration and then assessing their ability to administer the drug correctly (Gregson et al 1993), as poor technique is one of the main reasons for lack of control of symptoms. All aerosol inhalers must be shaken vigorously before administration. Keeley (1993) maintains that only 2–10 per cent of inhaled drugs actu-ally reach the lungs, the rest is swallowed. However, this percentage can be radically improved by the use of spacer devices. Spacer devices are the best method of delivery for inhaled drugs in young children as they provide a holding chamber from which the child can repeatedly breathe, increasing the opportunity for the child to inhale the drug (Jordan and White 2001). It is important to note that when steroids are inhaled, the child should be encouraged to rinse out their mouth or clean their teeth after adminis-tration to remove any medication left in the mouth (Gregson et al 1993).

Using a spacer with a face mask

For children under the age of 3 years, prescribed metered dose inhalers are best used in conjunction with a spacer and a facemask.

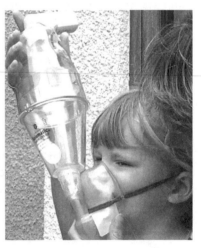

1 Ensure the holes in the face mask are occluded.
2 Attach inverted spacer plus inhaler to the face mask.
3 Place facemask over infant's nose and mouth.
4 Inverting spacer ensures that one-way valve falls open.
5 Activate inhaler.
6 Infant inhales during normal tidal breathing.

Spacer devices

Children over 3 years can usually use spacer devices directly via the mouth-piece. To aid administration the child should stand up to enable full diaphragmatic excursion and look upwards to reduce pharyngeal angle, and therefore minimise depositing the medi-cation in the mouth. Encouraging the child to bite on to the mouth-piece avoids him/her closing the teeth behind it. Another problem can be that the child occludes the mouth-piece with his/her tongue.

Using a spacer device

1 Remove inhaler cap, shake canister and insert into device.
2 Place mouth-piece into child's mouth.
3 Encourage the child to breathe in and out gently (tidal breathing). This will open and close the valve and a clicking noise will be heard.
4 Keeping the device in the same position, depress canister once to release a dose of the drug.
5 The child should continue to tidal breathe for 5 breaths.
6 Remove device from child's mouth.
7 Wait 30 seconds to repeat sequence if second dose is required.

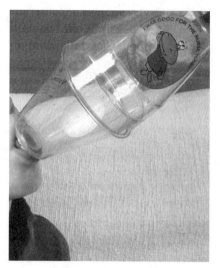

By the age of 5 years children can usually generate enough inspiratory flow to activate dry powder devices and have the skills of co-ordination to use metered dose inhalers.

Metered dose inhaler

1 Shake canister before use.
2 Exhale to functional reserve capacity.
3 Activate inhaler at start of inspiration.
4 Take slow, deep inspiration.
5 Hold breath for 5–10 seconds.
6 Take one puff at a time, break for 30 seconds between puffs.
(Frankes 1997)

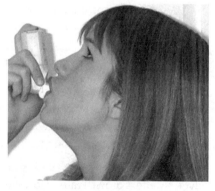

Turbohaler

1 Unscrew and lift off the outer white cover.
2 Hold the turbohaler upright.
3 Twist the grip forwards and backwards as far as you can until you hear the click.
4 Breathe out.
5 Put the mouth-piece between lips and breathe in deeply.
6 Remove inhaler from mouth and hold breath for 10 seconds.
7 Replace white cover on the turbohaler.

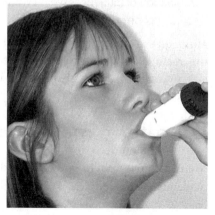

Accuhaler

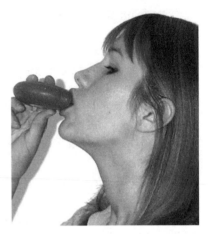

1 Hold outer casing of the accuhaler with one hand whilst pushing the thumb grip away until a click is heard.
2 Hold mouth-piece towards you.
3 Slide lever away until it clicks.
4 Hold inhaler level.
5 Breathe out gently away from the device.
6 Put mouth-piece in mouth and breathe in steadily and deeply.
7 Remove device from the mouth and hold breath for 10 seconds.
8 Close by sliding thumb grip back until it clicks.

> ### Activity 3.48
>
> The step plan is explained to Deepak and his parents, Deepak's mother is worried about the adverse effects of steroids. How could you reassure Deepak and his parents regarding this issue? Look up a recognised pharmacology book to find out the side-effects that Deepak may experience.

Table 3.15   Some of the side-effects of steroids

The most common side-effects of inhaled corticosteroids are oropharyngeal thrush and dysphonia. These are not common and are caused by the drug coming in contact with the oropharynx. They can be reduced by rinsing the mouth after inhalation or using a large volume spacer with the metered dose inhaler (Hunter 1995).

A study by McCowan et al (1998) showed that high doses of inhaled steroids may adversely affect growth rates. However, the reduction in stature may be caused by a combination of influences which would also include the severity of the asthma and the degree of control.

Although use of prophylactic steroids has been demonstrated to be safe and effective in the treatment of childhood asthma (Sharek and Bergman 2000) some parents may feel a little reluctant to give these medicines to their children.

Long-term management of asthma

Many asthmatic children remain undiagnosed, and those that are diagnosed are often inadequately treated (Cross 1999; Caldwell 1998). The greater willingness of doctors to diagnose asthma in children is probably the single most important factor in improving treatment (Phelan 1994). There is no permanent cure for asthma, but appropriate drug regimes abolish symptoms for most asthmatics (Cross 1999).

The British Thoracic Society (1997a and 1997b) produced principles for the management of asthma. These included family and child participation in care, avoiding identified triggers, and using the lowest effective dosages of drugs. They state that the most important aspect of management is that the child and the family understand asthma, the forms of treatment available, and what to do when changes in condition occur. There is a need to educate the child and parents so they understand the difference between preventive and relief treatment, are able to effectively administer inhaled drugs and use a peak flow meter, and are able to monitor symptoms and use a drug usage diary (Caldwell 1998).

Peak flow measurement

Many children are unable to perceive their degree of airway obstruction so, to assist in the monitoring of their condition a peak expiratory flow meter is used. This is a relatively cheap way of making an objective measurement of the rate at which the child can empty his/her lungs in litres per minute. Peak flow meters can be used to monitor the child's asthma at home and to check on diurnal variation or fall, thus anticipating an impending asthma attack and the need for treatment (Brewin 1997). As the airways become more inflamed, more air becomes trapped within them making it difficult to blow out. This results in a reduced peak flow reading. The British Thoracic Society recommends that, where appropriate, every patient with asthma should have their own peak flow meter and should be encouraged to use it to monitor their asthma and the efficacy of inhaled or nebulised medication.

Children can usually learn to use these devices from about 4 years of age. Peak expiratory flow rates (PEFR) vary with age, sex, height and race. A variation of up to 8 per cent of normal values is considered acceptable. PEFR is a good marker of severity of asthma in children who use these meters regularly; however, in children who have not used the meters previously the results should be interpreted with caution.

Mini peak flow meters have been shown to be inaccurate and can overestimate the peak expiratory flow (Sly et al 1994). PEFR should be compared either to the best previous PEFR when well or to the predicted PEFR for height.

The predicted PEFR can be calculated for the height from the formula:

Expected PEFR = (5 × height in centimetres) – 400

Peak flows should be recorded before and 10 minutes after each dose of nebulised salbutamol. The peak flow meter is therefore an important aid in assisting in the management of asthma, but the child's clinical condition must always be taken into account (Caldwell 1998).

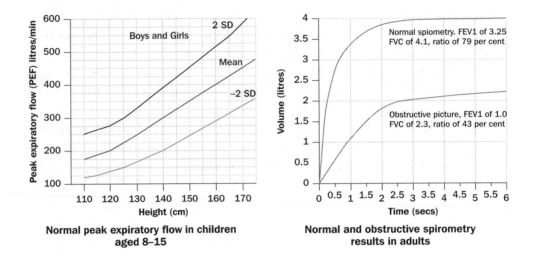

Normal peak expiratory flow in children aged 8–15

Normal and obstructive spirometry results in adults

Figure 3.5 Peak flow chart

Using a peak flow meter

1 Stand
2 Take a full breath in
3 Place the mouth tightly around the mouthpiece
4 Huff out hard and fast
5 Repeat three times
6 Record the highest reading

> *Activity 3.49*
>
> Try to obtain a peak flow meter and record your own peak flow recordings for a period of time. Do your recordings vary, if so can you identify why?

Reducing exposure to triggers

When specific triggers are known, it is recommended that exposure is avoided wherever possible (Smith 1995).

Table 3.16 The eradication of house-dust mites

The bedroom should be well ventilated; there should be no signs of dampness or mould.

The bedding should be laundered frequently to at least 60°C.

The mattress, duvet and pillows can be covered with material that is not porous to house-dust mites.

Ideally, the floor should not be carpeted. If necessary, a minimal pile carpet of synthetic fibre should be used.

The room should be vacuumed regularly with a cleaner that retains dust particles below 5 microns.

In some cases desensitisation to specific triggers is possible.

Table 3.17 Immunotherapy

Allergen specific immunotherapy involves injecting an extract of the allergen under the skin. Research shows that there can be a significant reduction in asthma symptoms and medication following immunotherapy (Abramson et al 1999). Although with some children the therapy is not practical as they find the injections unpleasant, and children often have multiple sensitivities.

It is important to take a positive approach when caring for children with asthma. This, combined with effective prevention, can enable the child to lead a normal life. Parents need to support their children and encourage them to express their feelings about having asthma and develop strategies to cope with these feelings (Caldwell 1998).

One way of ensuring effective high-quality care for the child with asthma has been the multi-disciplinary team approach. The team includes the child, parents, specialist nurse, GP, hospital staff, school teachers and pharmacist (Cross 1999; Gleeson 1996).

Table 3.18 The importance of teachers understanding the needs of the child with asthma

Children spend 40 per cent of their waking life at school (Reynolds 1988), it is important that teachers understand the disease and can support the child with their treatment.

In a study by Bowen (1996) 100 per cent of teachers taught children with asthma, but only 43 per cent felt competent to cope with a child having an asthmatic attack. Therefore the need to educate teachers to form part of the care team is important.

Activity 3.50

Reflect on your knowledge of caring for a child with asthma. Before you completed this chapter would you have been confident dealing with a child having an asthma attack? How much training do you think teachers receive about caring for children in school with asthma? Try to find out from one of your local schools about training offered to teachers (it might be a good idea to speak to the school nurse for this information).

For all chronic childhood illness, adherence with the use of medication might be a problem.

Activity 3.51

Suggest reasons why adherence with the asthma medication regime for asthma might, on occasion, be problematic for the child and family.

Your list might include:

- Methods of administration might be 'fiddly' and difficult. Carter and Dearman (1995, p. 293) suggest which methods of administration might be most useful for different age groups of children.
- The child might be reluctant to be seen to be taking medication, and therefore to be seen to be different from their peers.
- The family might find it difficult to fit the regime of drug administration into their daily life.
- The family may not fully understand the reasons why the drug has been prescribed and may feel dubious about its effects.
- In a disorder such as asthma where the child is often perfectly well between attacks, it may be difficult for the family to appreciate the reason for using a 'preventer' medicine when the child has no symptoms.

Activity 3.52

On re-examining your list of reasons why the family may find adherence with the medication regime problematic, suggest the principal issues which might be addressed in a programme of parent and child education on asthma medication use.

Conclusion

On completion of this chapter you will have become more aware of the special needs of the children and families being cared for by health care professionals. You should be able to utilise this knowledge to enable you to participate in implementing child-friendly, family-centred care in any health care environment. Having considered some of the many key aspects of caring for children, you should recognise the importance of sick children being cared for by appropriately educated and qualified staff who have a greater depth of knowledge and understanding of the differing needs of children and their families.

References

Abramson, M. J., Puy, R. M., Weiner, J. M. (1999) Allergen immunotherapy for asthma. In: *The Cochrane Library*, Issue 3. Oxford: Update Software.

Action for Sick Children (2000) *Millennium Charter for Children's Health Services.* London: ASC.

Advanced Life-Support Group (1996) *Advanced Paediatric Life-Support: The Practical Approach.* London: BMJ.

American Academy of Pediatrics (1997) *Pediatric Advanced Life-Support.* Texas: American Heart Association.

Anderson, E. S., Peterson, S. A., Wailoo, M. P. (1990) Factors influencing body temperature of 3–4 month-old infants at home during the day. *Archives of Disease in Childhood* 65, pp. 1308–10

Anderson, H., Butland, B., Strachan, D. (1994) Trends in the prevalence and severity of childhood asthma. *British Medical Journal* 308, pp. 1600–4.

Atkinson, W. L., Orenstein, W. A. (1992) The resurgence of measles in the United States, 1989-1990. *Annals of Reviews in Medicine* 43, pp. 451–63.

Audit Commission (1993) *Children First: A Study of Hospital Services.* London: HMSO.

Bedford, H. (1997) Childhood immunisation. *Nursing Standard* 11(28), pp. 49–56

Bee, H. (2000) *The Developing Child.* 9th Edition. London: Allyn and Bacon.

Bowen, C. (1996) Educating teachers in children's illnesses: a study. *Nursing Standard* 10(39), pp. 33–6.

Brewin, A. (1997) Comparing asthma and chronic obstructive pulmonary disease (COPD). *Nursing Standard* 12 (4), 15 October, pp. 49–55.

British Thoracic Society (1990) *Guidelines on the Management of Asthma.* London: British Thoracic Society.

British Thoracic Society (1993) Chronic asthma in adults and children. *Thorax* 48 (Supplement), S1–24.

British Thoracic Society (1997a) The British guidelines on asthma management. *Thorax* 52.

British Thoracic Society, The National Asthma Campaign, The Royal College of Physicians of London (1997b) The British guidelines on asthma management: 1995 Review and Position Statement. *Thorax* 1 (Supplement), S1–S21.

Browner, C. (1997) Smog and soot: updating air quality standards. *Public Health Reports* 112 (5), pp. 366–7, Washington DC: US Environmental Protection Agency.

Caldwell, C. (1998) Management of acute asthma in children. *Nursing Standard* 12 (29), 8–14 April, pp. 49–54.

Callery, P. (1997) Using evidence in children's nursing. *Paediatric Nursing* 9 (6), pp. 27–34.

Camargos, P., Castro, R., Feldman, J. (1999) Prevalence of symptoms related to asthma among schoolchildren in Campos Gerais, Brazil. *Pan American Journal of Public Health* 6 (1), 8–15 July.

Campbell, S., Glasper, E. (1995) *Whaley and Wong's Children's Nursing.* Mosby: London.

Carter, B., Dearmun, A. K. (1995) *Child Health Care Nursing: Concepts, Theory and Practice.* Oxford: Blackwell Science.

Casey, A. (1988) A partnership with child and family. *Senior Nurse* 8 (4), pp. 8–9

Casey, A. (1993) Development and use of the partnership model of nursing care. In: Glasper, E. A. and Tucker, A. (eds) *Advances in Child Health Nursing.* London: Scutari Press.

Casey, G. (2001) Oxygen transport and the use of pulse oximetry. *Nursing Standard* 15 (47), pp. 46–53.

Chandler, T. (2000) Oxygen saturation monitoring. *Paediatric Nursing* 12 (8), pp. 37–42.

Committee of the Central Health Services (1959) *The Welfare of Children in Hospital.* London: HMSO.

Cook, D., Strachan, D. (1997) Parental smoking and prevalence of respiratory symptoms and asthma in school aged children. *Thorax* 52, pp. 1081–94.

Crocker, E. (1980) Reactions of children to health care encounters. In: Taylor, J., Muller, D., Wattley, L., and Harris, P. (eds) 1999 N*ursing Children: Psychology, Research and Practice.* 3rd Edition. Cheltenham: Stanley Thornes.

Cropp, G. J., Shames, R. S. (1994) Respiratory and allergic diseases. In: Rudolph, A. M., Kamei, R. K. (eds) *Rudolph's Fundamentals of Pediatrics.* Norwalk, CT: Appleton & Lange.

Cross, C. (1990) Home from hospital. *Nursery World* 90 (3228), pp. 22–3.

Cross, S. (1999) Better care for people with asthma. *Nursing Standard* 13 (46), 4–10 August, pp. 51–4.

Culley, L. Dyson, S. (eds) (2001) *Ethnicity and Nursing Practice.* Basingstoke: Palgrave Macmillan.

Darbyshire, P. (1994) *Living with a Sick Child in Hospital: The Experience of Parents and Nurses.* London: Chapman and Hall.

De Bisschop, C., Guenard, H., Desnot, P., Vergeret, J. (1999) Reduction of exercise-induced asthma in children by short, repeated warm ups. *British Journal of Sports Medicine* 33 (2) April, pp. 100–4.

Department of Health (1991) *Welfare of Children and Young People in Hospital.* London: HMSO.

Department of Health (1994) *Weaning and the Weaning Diet.* Report on Health and Social Subjects 45. London: HMSO.

Department of Health (1996) *Immunisation against Infectious Disease.* London: HMSO.

Department of Health (1997) *The NHS: Modern, Dependable.* London: DoH.

Department of Health (2001) *The Report of the Public Inquiry into Children's Heart Surgery at the Bristol Royal Infirmary, 1984–95: Learning from Bristol.* London: DoH.

Fernando, S. (2001) *Mental Health, Race and Culture.* Basingstoke: Palgrave Macmillan.

Frankes, M. (1997) Asthma in the emergency department. *Journal of Emergency Nursing* 23 (5), October, pp. 429–38

Garvey, C. (1977) *Play.* London: Fontana/Open Books.

Glasper, E. A. (1995) The value of children's nursing in the third millennium. *British Journal of Nursing* 4 (1), pp. 27–30.

Glasper, E. A. Ireland, L. (2000) *Evidence-Based Child Health Care: Challenges for Practice.* Basingstoke: Macmillan – now Palgrave Macmillan.

Glasper, E. A. (2002a) Contemporary issues in the care of sick children and their families. *British Journal of Nursing* 11 (4), pp. 248–56.

Glasper, E. A. (2002b) A review of children's nursing: but does it have a future? *British Journal of Nursing* 11 (7), pp. 492–6.

Glasper, E. A., Charles-Edwards, I. (2002a) The child first and always: the registered children's nurse over 150 years. Part 1. *Paediatric Nursing* 14 (4), pp. 38–42.

Glasper, E. A., Charles-Edwards, I. (2002b) The child first and always: the registered children's nurse over 150 years. Part 2. *Paediatric Nursing* 14 (5), pp. 38–43.

Gleeson, C. (1996) A format for quality. *Nursing Standard* 10 (49), 28 August, pp. 24–-5.

Gregson, R. K., Warner, J. O., Radford, M. (1993) Assessment of the continued supervision and asthma management . . . . *Respiratory Medicine* 89 (7), pp. 487–93.

Hazinski, M. F. (1992) *Nursing Care of the Critically Ill Child.* 2nd Edition. USA: Mosby.

Health Committee (1997) *The Specific Health Needs of Children.* London: The Stationary Office. Cited in Caldwell, C. (1998) Management of acute asthma in children, *Nursing Standard*, 12(29), 8–14 April, pp. 49–54.

Helman, C. G. (2001) *Culture, Health and Illness.* 4th Edition. Oxford: Butterworth Heinemann

Herring, L. (1999) Critical pathways: an efficient way to manage care. *Nursing Standard* 13 (47), 11–17 August, pp. 36–7.

Holland, K., Hogg, C. (2001) *Culture Awareness in Nursing and Health Care.* London: Arnold.

Hubbard, S., Trigg, E. (2001) *Practices in Children's Nursing.* Edinburgh: Churchill Livingstone.

Hunter ,S. (1995) The use of steroids in asthma treatment. *Nursing Standard* 9 (38), 14–20 June, pp. 25–7.

International Paediatric Asthma Consensus Group (1992) Asthma: a follow up statement from an international paediatric consensus group. *Arch Dis Child* 67: pp. 240-8. Cited in Duran-Tauleria, E., Rona, R., Chinn, S. and Burney, P., Influence of ethnic group on asthma treatment in children 1990–1: national cross-sectional study. *British Medical Journal* 313 (1996), 20 July, pp. 148–52.

Jenkins, M. A., Hopper, J. L., Bowes, G., Carlin, B., Flnader, L. B., Giles, G. G. (1994) Factors in childhood as predictors of asthma in adult life *British Medical Journal* 309, pp. 90–3.

Johnston, S., Pattemore, P., Sanderson, G., Smith, S., Lampe, F., Josephs, L., Symington, P., O'Toole, S., Myint, S., Tyrrell, D., Holgate, S. (1995) Community study of role of viral infections in exacerbations of asthma in 9–11-year-old children. *British Medical Journal* 310, 13 May, pp. 1225–9.

Jordan, S., White, J. (2001) Bronchodilators: implications for nursing practice. *Nursing Standard* 15 (27), 21 March, pp. 45–55.

Kaur, B., Anderson, H. R., Austin, J., Burr, M., Harkins, L., Strachan, D., Warner, J. O. (1998) Prevalence of asthma symptoms, diagnosis, and treatment in 12–14-year-old children across Great Britain (international study of asthma and allergies in childhood, ISAAC UK). *British Medical Journal* 316, pp. 118–24.

Keeley, D. (1993) How to achieve better outcome in the treatment of asthma in general practice. *British Medical Journal* 307 (6914), pp. 1261–3.

Livesley, J. (1993) Reducing the risks – management of paediatric intravenous therapy. *Child Health* 1 (2), pp. 68–70.

Lloyd-Thomas, A. R. (1990) ABC of major trauma: primary survey and resuscitation. *British Medical Journal* 301, pp. 334–6.

Mackowiak, P., Wasserman, S., Levine, M. (1992) A critical appraisal of 98.6°F: the upper limit of the normal body temperature. *Journal of the American Medical Association* 286 (12), pp. 1578–80.

Magnus, P., Jaakkola, J. (1997) Secular trend in the occurrence of asthma among children and young adults: critical appraisal of repeated cross sectional surveys. *British Medical Journal* 314, pp. 1795–803.

McClowry, S. G., McLeod, S. M. (1990) The psychological responses of school age children to hospitalization. *Children's Health Care* 19 (3), pp. 155–60.

McCowan, C., Neville, R. G., Thomas, G. E., Crombie, I. K., Ricketts, I. W., Cairns, A. Y., Warner, F. C., Greene, S. A., White, E. (1998) Effect of asthma and its treatment on growth: four-year follow up of cohort of children from general practices in Tayside, Scotland. *British Medical Journal* 316, pp. 668–72.

Medici, T. C., Schmid, A. Z., Hacki, M., Vetter, W. (1993) Are asthmatics salt sensitive? A preliminary controlled study. *Chest: The Cardiopulmonary Journal* 104 (4), October, pp. 1138–43.

Miller, C. L., Fletcher, W. B. (1976) Severity of notified whooping cough. *British Medical Journal* 1, pp. 117–19.

Moules, T., Ramsay, J. (1998) *The Textbook of Children's Nursing.* Cheltenham: Stanley Thornes Publishers.

Murphy, K. G., Secunda, J. A., Rockoff, M. A. (1990) Severe burns from a pulse oximeter. *Aneasthesiology,* 73, pp. 350–1.

National Institute for Clinical Excellence (2000) *Guidance on the Use of Inhaler Systems (Devices) in Children Under the Age of 5 Years with Chronic Asthma.* London: NICE.

Neill, S. (2000) Acute childhood illness at home: the parents' perspective. *Journal of Advanced Nursing* 31 (4), pp. 821–32.

Nichols, R. H., Wray, F. A. (1935) *The History of the Foundling Hospital.* London: Oxford University Press.

Oddy, W. H., Holt, P. G, Sly, P. D., Read, A. W, Landau, L. I., Stanley, F. J., Kendall, G. E.,

Burton, P. R. (1999) Association between breast-feeding and asthma in six-year-old children: findings of a prospective birth cohort study. *British Medical Journal* 319, pp. 815–19.

Peckham, C., Bedford, H., Senturia, Y., Ades, A. (1989) *National Immunisation Study: Factors Influencing Immunisation Uptake in Childhood.* Horsham: Action Research.

Phelan, P. D. (1994) Asthma in children: epidemiology. *British Medical Journal* 308, pp. 1584–5.

Resuscitation Council: http://www.resus.org.uk.

Reynolds, M. A. (1988) How much do school teachers know about asthma? *Paediatric Reviews and Communications* 2, pp. 173–80. Cited in Anderton, J. and Broady, J., Improving schools' asthma policies and procedures. *Nursing Standard* 14 (6), October 1999, pp. 34–8.

Rudolf, M., Levene, M. (1999) *Paediatrics in Child Health* Oxford: Blackwell Science.

Sartain, S. A., Clarke, C. L., Heyman, R. (2000) Hearing the voices of children with chronic illness. *Journal of Advanced Nursing* 32 (4), pp. 913–21.

Sharek, P. J., Bergman, D. A. (2000) Beclometnasone for asthma in children: effects on linear growth. (Cochrane Review) In: the *Cochrane Library.* Issue 1, Oxford: Update Software.

Sly, P., Cahill, P., Willet, K., Burton, P. (1994) Accuracy of mini peak flow meters in indicating changes in lung function in children with asthma. *British Medical Journal* 308, pp. 572–4.

Smith, E. (1995) Guidelines for asthma treatment. *Nursing Standard* 9 (23), 1 March, pp. 3–12.

Smith, L., Daughtrey, H. (2000) Weaving the seamless web of care: an analysis of parents' perceptions of their needs following discharge of their child from hospital. *Journal of Advanced Nursing* 31 (4), pp. 812–20.

Smith, L., Colman, V., Bradshaw, M. (2002) *Family-Centred Care: Concept, Theory and Practice.* Basingstoke: Palgrave Macmillan.

Strachan, D., Carey, I. (1995) Home environment and severe asthma in adolescence: a population based case-control study. *British Medical Journal* 311, pp. 1053–6.

Swallow, V. M., Jacoby, A. (2001) Mothers' evolving relationships with doctors and nurses during the chronic childhood illness trajectory. *Journal of Advanced Nursing* 36 (6), pp. 755–64.

Sylva, K. (1993) Play in hospital: when and why it's effective. *Current Paediatrics* 3, pp. 247–9.

Taylor, J., Muller, D., Wattley, L., Harris, P. (1999) *Nursing Children Psychology, Research & Practice.* 3rd Edition. Cheltenham: Stanley Thornes.

The National Heart, Lung and Blood Institute (1992) International consensus report on the diagnosis and management of asthma. Clinical Exp, allergy, 1–72. Cited in Greyson, R. (1993) Education for control management principles and inhaler techniques for childhood asthma. *Child Health,* June–July.

The Quality Assurance Agency for Higher Education (2001) Subject benchmarks statements: health care programmes – Nursing at: http://www.qaa.ac.uk/crntwork/benchmark/nhsbenchmark/nursing-text.htm. Accessed 21/01/02.

Thomas, D. (1996) Assessing children – it's different. *Registered Nurse* 59 (4), p. 38–45.

Thompson, R., Gustafson, K. (1996) *Adaptation to Chronic Childhood Illness.* Washington, DC: American Psychological Association.

United Kingdom Central Council for Nursing, Midwifery and Health Visiting (1992) *Code of Professional Conduct.* London: UKCC.

Valman, H. (1993) Bronchial asthma. *British Medical Journal* 306, pp. 1676–81.

Visintainer, M. A., Wolfer, J. A. (1975) Psychological preparation for surgical pediatric patients: the effect on children's and parents' stress responses and adjustment. *Pediatrics* 56, pp. 187–202.

Walsh, M. (1997) Will critical pathways replace the nursing process? 11 (52), 17 September, pp. 39–42.

Webster, A. (2000) The facilitating role of the play specialist. *Paediatric Nursing* 12 (7), pp. 24–7.

Welsh Office (1997) *The Health of Children in Wales.* London: Welsh Office.

World Health Organisation. (1985) *Targets for Health for All.* Copenhagen: WHO.

Resources

📖 Further reading

More, J. (2001) Weaning advice in the UK: to change or not to change? *Professional Care of Mother and Child* 11 (5).

Thomas, D., Assessing children – it's different, *Registered Nurse* 59 (4), pp. 38–45.

West, H. (2000) Basic infant life support: retention of knowledge and skill. *Paediatric Nursing* 12 (1), February.

@ Web pages

Basic life-support in children can be accessed on the internet at:
   www.resus.org.uk/pages/pbls/htm.

European Food Information Council at: **www.eufic.org/fr/home/fhome.htm**.

For temperature measurement, go to the thermometry page at:
   www.graduateresearch.com\thermometry\theory.htm.

National Asthma Audit 1999/2000: **www.asthma.org.uk**.

Resuscitation Council: **www.resus.org.uk**.

The British Thoracic Society (1997a and 1997b) **www.brit-thoracic.org.uk**.

The National Institute of Clinical Excellence (2000) at **www.nice.org.uk**.

Insights into Adolescent Health and Eating Disorders

Chris Taylor and Michael Cooper

Introduction

This chapter will explore the issues surrounding eating disorders in adolescence, focusing specifically on anorexia nervosa. Eating disorders will be placed within the context of adolescence and adolescent development. The scenario relates to a young person with an eating disorder and will trace their experiences through various institutional and non-institutional environments looking at the effectiveness of various intervention strategies. Anorexia nervosa will be used to illustrate the complex interplay between the process of adolescence and a major psycho/physiological disorder.

📋 Activity 4.1

Before reading on it may be helpful for you to jot down your current understanding of anorexia nervosa.

Anorexia nervosa is a complex condition with controversial theories of causation. It is characterised by serious loss of weight, which is self-induced by food avoidance, exercise and purging. It is best known as a disorder of adolescent girls and young women, but also occurs in boys and men.

Eating disorders take on a special significance before puberty and in adolescence. In adolescence there is a critical growth period during which the young person physically develops and if missed, the young person is unable to catch up with growth development at a later stage (See Chapter 11 on hydration in relation to 'catch up'). Therefore, when anorexia nervosa occurs during these critical periods, there is a certain urgency for professionals to treat it promptly. One of the primary aims of such interventions will be to help the young person to reach a healthy weight and thereby not miss their critical growth period.

Learning outcomes

This chapter will enable the student to:

- Describe the developmental journey through adolescence.
- Outline the principle theories of the causation of anorexia nervosa.
- Differentiate between anorexia nervosa and other causes of weight loss and anorexia.
- Explore the impact of illness on the adolescent developmental sequence.
- Identify the physiological and psychological implications of extreme low weight.
- Describe nursing interventions required to reach and maintain physiological integrity.
- Understand the patient's desire not to gain weight.
- Be able to recognise and respond therapeutically to the patient's strategies for food avoidance/excess.
- Discuss how the nurse's personal and professional belief systems impact on the giving of care.
- Be able to discuss the nature of a therapeutic relationship with emotionally distressed clients.
- Be able to explore and debate the legal and ethical issues involved in treatment interventions.

Concepts

- Physical and psychological assessment.
- Mental health issues in a paediatric environment.
- Psychological care: managing manipulation, emotional distress, the therapeutic encounter.
- Professional values, social and personal narratives.

- Causation, theoretical issues, personality traits, co-morbidity, family systems.
- Health education: diet, exercise, healthy body weight, body image.
- Moral and legal implications of nursing people with eating disorders.
- Issues around continuing service provision.

Scenario *Introducing Anna*

Anna, aged 12 years, lives with her parents and younger sister in a semi-detached family house which they own. Anna's father James, aged 38 years, has recently changed his job from a milkman to a financial advisor, allowing him to spend more time at home with the family. Anna's mother Jenny, aged 36 years, is a part-time special needs assistant at a local school. Anna has a younger sister Louisa, who is 8 years old.

Genogram and family tree

The challenge of organising information about family members has led to the development of family trees, as a way to record significant information in formats that are accessible and usable for clients and therapists alike.

Family trees or genograms are maps providing a picture of family structure over several generations, with schematic representation of the main stages of the family life cycle. They are a useful adjunct in both assessment and treatment. It gives a concise, graphic summary of the family's current composition.

They can be extended to include dates, marriages, separations, health, occupations, relationships and important points from individuals' past histories.

Activity 4.2

Take time to explore what other assessments, and assessment tools may be used when working with clients and their families.

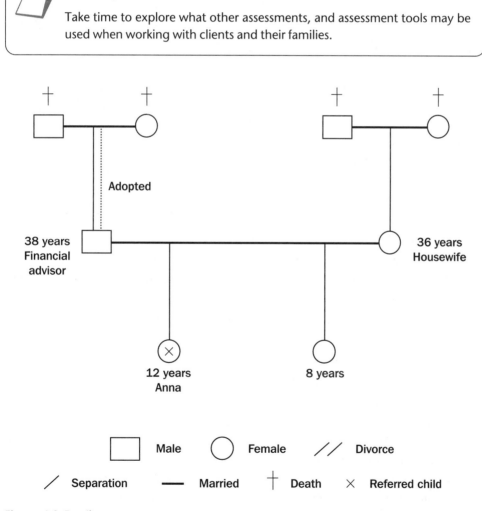

Figure 4.1 Family genogram

The developmental tasks of adolescence

Overview of adolescent development

When talking about adolescence, it is perhaps necessary to sound a note of caution. Developmental theories often describe stages that infer a series of steps to be taken, stages to go through on the road to adulthood. Instead of this linear concept, it would be more helpful to see adolescence as a dynamic process. It is suggested that the concept of adolescence is not as easy to quantify as might first be imagined. Taylor and Muller (1995) use Hauser et al's (1991) definition to illustrate this:

> The adolescent phase of the life cycle refers to a complex terrain of intersecting biological, intra-psychic, and social factors that together contribute to significant transformations in individual development.

These significant transformations have been described both in terms of tasks and stages.

1 Achieving masculine or feminine social roles.
2 Accepting physical build and using the body effectively.
3 Achieving emotional independence from parents and other adults.
4 Preparing for marriage and family life.
5 Preparing for an economic career.
6 Acquiring a set of values and an ethical system as a guide to behaviour and developing an ideology.

Activity 4.3

It might be helpful to spend a little time reflecting on the appropriateness of these developmental task descriptions in the light of the current social and cultural values, and the economic situation.

Erikson (1965) describes the adolescent task/crisis as identity versus confusion. It is perhaps helpful to see the key adolescent task as a search for identity, that is, a separate self, but always in relation to others.

Jacobs (1985) looks at adolescence in three stages (adapted):

1 Early adolescence and sexuality (relates to intimacy).
2 Middle adolescence: authority and independence (relates to individuation).
3 Later adolescence: faith and responsibility (relates to moral development and life values).

The first stage outlined by Jacobs could be linked to changing patterns of intimacy and attachment. The second stage outlined relates to individuation, the process of becoming who we are. This involves renegotiating a self-concept less dependent on our parents' construction of who we are and more reliant on peers and role icons. The final stage relates to developing beliefs and moral values. This is often a time of intense interest in what is right and wrong, fair and unfair, true and not true.

Adolescence can be described as a liminal time when we are neither what we were, involved in childhood, or what we are yet to be, adult. Whilst we may have been impelled on this journey by the physical changes of puberty, many aspects of the terrain are socially defined.

This journey, however it is described, can be impacted upon by illness, whether chronic or transient. Illness itself is a concept that can be both biologically or socially constructed and as such can have a profound effect on the adolescent journey and its outcomes.

>
> ### Activity 4.4
> Reflect on illness and its relationship to your own journey through adolescence. This may be illness that you may have had, or your peers or friends. How did it influence you or your peers?

What are eating disorders? You may like to consider your present perception of this phrase before reading on.

Eating Disorder

The term 'eating disorder' covers a wide spectrum of conditions characterised by psychological and behavioural disturbances associated with weight, food and eating. The term is often used with reference to two specific conditions, anorexia nervosa and bulimia nervosa, and they remain significant health problems in childhood and adolescence.

Eating disorders can be viewed as psychological illnesses in which distress is somatised, or expressed in disordered eating behaviours. Other types of eating disorders occurring in this age range may be related to:

- Food avoidance emotional disorder (FAED)
- Selective eating
- Restrictive eating
- Food refusal
- Dysfunctional dysphagia
- Appetite loss secondary to depression

The prevalence of anorexia nervosa is thought to vary from 0.5 per cent to one per cent among the adolescent population.

Diagnosis of anorexia nervosa

Increasingly, there is an international consensus on the criteria for diagnosing mental and behavioural disorders. There are two major classification systems:

- *The International Classification of Diseases* (ICD-10) (WHO 1994).
- *The Diagnostic and Statistical Manual of Mental Disorders* (DSM-IV-TR) (American Psychiatric Association 1994).

DSM-IV and ICD-10 share many similarities with regard to defining criteria of anorexia nervosa. These pertain to the criteria of weight loss, body image distortion, amenorrhoea and the so-called weight phobia. However, the two systems differ somewhat with respect to the criteria.

Both define weight loss in terms of weight that is 15 per cent below that expected for age and height, but ICD-10 refers to Quatlets Body Mass Index as one way of defining that expectation. Both systems consider the special situation of pre-pubertal patients who fail to meet the expected growth.

ICD–10 has further advantages in that it covers 'self-induced loss of weight', and links body image distortion to the main theme of psychopathology, namely the fear of becoming obese.

Both the syndrome and the spectrum character of eating disorders make it clear that there are atypical cases of anorexia nervosa that do not fulfil the complete sets of criteria listed in the two major systems of classification.

Using the ICD-10 system the following eating disorder diagnoses are possible:

- Anorexia nervosa (F50.0)
- Atypical anorexia nervosa (F50.1)
- Bulimia nervosa (F50.2)
- Atypical bulimia nervosa (F50.3)
- Overeating, with other psychological disturbances (F50.4)
- Vomiting, with other psychological disturbances (F50.5)
- Other eating disorders (F50.8)
- Eating disorder, unspecified (F50.9)

Using the DSM-IV system, there are other possibilities:

- Anorexia nervosa (307.1):
  - restricting type
  - binge eating/purging type
- Bulimia nervosa (307.51):
  - purging type
  - non-purging type
- Eating disorder not otherwise specified (EDNOS) (307.50)

Numerous research studies have focused on the issue of who tends to develop eating disorders. They are more common in women than men but, in children, boys appear to be over-represented when compared to the proportion of males seen in adults with eating disorders.

It has been suggested that eating disorders are more common in social classes 1 and 2, and a number of high-risk groups have been identified including dancers and fashion models. There is increasing evidence that eating disorders are less restricted than previously thought in their occurrence across different cultural and ethnic groups.

The precise aetiology of eating disorders remains obscure, but is probably multi-factorial. Lask and Bryant-Waugh (2000) suggest that an eating disorder does not occur at a particular moment, rather it develops over time with some causative factors being in place since birth, others emerging in early life, and yet others much later.

> ### Activity 4.5
>
> Before reading on consider what factors may contribute to the development of an eating disorder.

The aetiology of eating disorders may be considered under the following headings:

Biological factors   genetic, endocrine, temperament, personality traits.

Sociocultural factors thinness, media, gender, prejudice against obesity.

Familial factors   dysfunctional interaction and communication, abnormal eating, attitudes and behaviour.

Psychological factors stress, adaptation to life events, self-image.

Psychoanalytic perspective

Crisp et al (1992) take the view that anorexia nervosa is an illness of individuals who experience particular difficulty in negotiating their way into the adult world. Crisp suggests that the person with an eating disorder 'solves the crisis' by opting out, with the fear of weight gain expressing a desperate avoidance of normal physical development (regression, growth, sexuality, independence and maturational conflict).

Findings suggest that the course of anorexia nervosa is characterised by high rates of partial recovery and low rates of full recovery, while the course of bulimia nervosa is characterised by higher rates of both partial and full recovery (Herzog et al 1993).

Eating disorders and the nursing role: the nurse's beliefs

Nursing young people with an eating disorder creates particular challenges in the delivery of care.

It is vital that nurses understand the psychological profile of anorexic patients, and know how to overcome difficulties this can create in forming a therapeutic relationship, otherwise anorexic patients may well continue to be seen as 'difficult' patients with a self induced illness, which will prevent therapeutic care.

(*George 1997, p. 902*)

It can be suggested that some of the difficulties experienced in nursing the anorexic young person are related to the nurse's belief system.

Evidence-based practice

Since the seminal work *The Unpopular Patient*, (Stockwell 1972), it has been acknowledged that a nurse's beliefs profoundly influence the care they give. Bodycombe-James (2000) identified a number of research studies over the succeeding years, suggesting a definite pattern to the patient deemed to be unpopular and supporting Stockwell's original work. Her own small study of nurse's attitudes showed that children were described in negative terms if they were unco-operative. Deviant behaviour was also viewed very negatively and made the child unpopular. Her conclusions also suggested that toddlers were generally more popular than adolescents. If the views of the nurses she spoke to were representative of the wider group, then young adolescents with eating disorders are likely to be viewed negatively as a rule. Further

support for this case comes from the work of King and Turner (2000). They identify core values as one of the themes emerging with nurses working with adolescent females with anorexia. These young people challenge nursing core beliefs, leading to emotional turmoil and frustration in the nurse. Resolution occurs through a process of repositioning the young person's situation in relation to core beliefs. These beliefs may have to be expanded or changed to meet the new situation. The change of perspective, in order to promote quality care, can be seen as an element of the therapeutic encounter. Wright (2001) suggested that nurses who believe that the patient with an eating disorder was not responsible for the development of that disorder would be more effective in giving care. Another important belief identified was that the carer has to believe that their intervention can help the patients to achieve a positive outcome. Many nurses can find it hard to believe that

Cooper and Glasper (2001) also emphasise the importance of the nurse's belief system in influencing their therapeutic style. They suggest that the nurse's beliefs are affected by the commonly accepted 'tribal stories'. The unpopular patient identified by Stockwell (1972) would be an example of a tribal story. Such collective beliefs, they suggest, remain unchallenged by the reflective process. The following might be an example of a tribal story:

Sometimes when I am working with the anorexic person I feel that this is all a waste of time. My skills could be better used looking after somebody who has a real illness. We are very busy here. There is not the time to give these people what they need. Anyway, they should be looked after somewhere else. This is not the place for them. They are always manipulative, and they tell lies. I came into nursing to look after children with real illnesses, not these people. Anyway, even if I had time, I would not know what to say. Even if you do speak to her, she won't answer.

Second year student nurse.

 What do you believe about people with anorexia? How might what you believe right now influence the care you may give?

 In order for them to work more effectively with the anorexic patients, how might this example of a nurse's beliefs be challenged?

Having reflected on elements of the nursing role, it is now time to think again about Anna.

Admission and treatment history

Anna, aged 12 years and 6 months, was admitted via a paediatrician, to a busy, acute paediatric medical ward. Her main problem on admission was severe progressive loss of weight. On admission she was 1.52m tall and weighed 27.3kg.

Activity 4.6

Work out her Body Mass Index (BMI) before reading on. For a reminder refer to Chapter 10 on nutrition (Table 10.5).

History and presenting complaints

Anna's BMI is now 11.8. She has always been 'faddy ' about food. At the age of 5 years she complained about the amount of butter on her toast. Over the last year she has progressively cut out foods, including chocolate, meats, fats, dairy products. Daily, she only eats dry toast, one jacket potato without the skin and tuna. She took over cooking six months ago when her mother injured her hand. As her mother's hand improved, food avoidance became more obvious.

Exercise – up until admission to hospital, she attended ten dancing classes per week, participating in six different dancing styles, plus practice and exercise. She admits to a constant, overriding urge to dance or exercise, and difficulty in keeping still. Prior to admission, she was doing 100 sit-ups before breakfast.

Mood low and she has diminished concentration. The only time she smiles is when she is dancing.

Apathy and fatigue – has stopped socialising outside school. She spends her spare time alone in her bedroom, possibly exercising.

Abdominal pain, constipation and headaches. Complains that when she eats, she feels bloated and feels 'like her ribs are going to burst open'.

She is not happy with what she sees when she looks in the mirror. She has a distorted body image and denies knowing her weight. Feels that her tummy and thighs are too fat.

She hates drawing attention to herself. Anna is unhappy with her appearance and her perceived lack of ability. She has difficulty in standing up for herself. She has been exploited by her classmates – doing their homework.
She verbalises how 'horrible 'she is.

Difficulty in dropping off to sleep, and wakes early.

Puberty – had been developing breasts, but this has slowed recently. She has not yet reached menarche.

Activity 4.7

Check out your understanding of 'menarche' and what influences it.

Personality traits

- Always slightly obsessional, and a perfectionist.
- Quiet, unassertive demeanour.
- Spends twice the recommended time on homework, and is still unhappy with her results.
- Has very few close friends, particularly dislikes boys. She chose a secondary school out of her catchment area to avoid contact with boys.
- Is one of the brightest pupils in the school, highest achiever in her year.
- Acknowledges she eats to please others, not herself.

Activity 4.8

Consider how Anna's personality traits compare with those most commonly associated with the anorexic position.

Family history

Father Disrupted attachments. His biological father was killed when he was aged 2 years. His mother was unable to care for him owing to a severe depression. He was subsequently accommodated in a Children's Home until he was 10 years old. He had no further contact with his mother. He was then fostered until aged 18 years, when his foster parents divorced. There has been no further contact. He has a foster sister but has no contact with her. No history of any illnesses.

Mother Has two sisters and a brother. They live locally but have limited contact. Father is alive and well and visits every fortnight, not a close relationship, however. Her own mother died six years ago of lung cancer. Admits to having been very close, and still misses her. She frequently visits the grave.

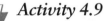

Activity 4.9

Think about how this information may have been collected. What particular skills would a health care professional need to develop to gain such personal and sometimes potentially painful admissions? (See the section on communication in Chapter 14 on palliative care.)

Anna's mother denies ever having an eating problem, but she says she watches what she eats.
Her weight has never been above 51kg.
She has had a recent operation on her hand.

Attachment

Attachment behaviour is defined simply as any form of behaviour that results in a person attaining or retaining proximity to a preferred individual. Attachment is an overall term referring to the state and quality of an individual's attachment. Broadly, attachment can be divided into secure and insecure attachments. Attachment behaviour is triggered by separation or threatened separation from the attachment figure.

Attachment and attachment behaviour are based on an attachment behavioural system, a model of the world in which the self and significant others and their relationships are represented. The ability to form focused, permanent and emotionally meaningful relationships with specific others is one of the most important acquisitions of the infancy period.

The attachment an infant makes to its mother has a powerful influence over its subsequent development. Attachment describes the infant's predisposition to seek proximity to certain people and be more secure in their presence. Ideally, the infant will make a secure attachment, but patterns differ, and in the case of some infants may be characterised by insecurity or ambivalence. The attachment patterns are already established at a year old, and remain constant throughout the life cycle. These early patterns can repeat themselves in later relationships (Bowlby 1969/1980). Disruptions in the first years of life due to inconsistent or inadequate care, or poor parenting skills, may lead to a failure to develop a secure attachment. There is a general assumption that the mother is likely to be the primary care giver in the first years of life, but changing patterns of family life means this is not necessarily the case.

In adolescence the secure attachment shows itself in increasing autonomy and the capacity to evaluate life experiences in a helpful way. Insecure attachments will manifest in a dismissing approach to relationships. Other insecure attachments will be preoccupied, with relationships that are entangled and enmeshed, others will be disorganised (Howe et al 1999). Each of these relational styles will influence the relationship the nurse can make with the young person.

Activity 4.10

1 List factors that may affect attachment.
2 Take time to discover which authors and theories inform the concept of attachment.
3 Consider how Anna and her family members might be described in terms of their attachment behaviours.

As a paediatric nurse, or a nurse who has a working relationship with young families, how can you assist in promoting secure patterns of attachment between parents and their infants?

Family dynamics

There have been long-standing marital problems, recently felt to have been directed towards Anna by her father. Her mother has thought of divorce, but has been threatened that she will have no house or money. It is apparent that there is an alliance between the mother and Anna, and between her father and Anna's sister.

Her father is now 38 years old and is a financial advisor. He has recently changed his occupation from a milkman, having studied at evening classes, and as a consequence is around more. He is described as being authoritative, unsympathetic, detached, and rarely giving praise. He tends to 'fly off the handle', and can go for many weeks without speaking to the family. Anna believes he prefers her younger sister and is jealous of their shared interests in football and television. They have similar personalities.

Anna also feels anorexia is 'her own fault'.

Her mother is 36 years old and works part time as a special needs assistant. She is a youthful, petite woman, who has been referred to as Anna's sister. There is a restrictive but affectionate style of parenting. Her mother finds remaining detached and tolerating her daughter's distress around eating and restricting exercise very difficult. She has an enmeshed relationship with her daughter, and she admits to being very close to her own mother who died six years ago. Both often talk about her and frequently visit her grave together.

Anna's sister is 8 years old and Anna describes her as a 'tomboy and messy'. She is outgoing, independent and makes friends easily. They often argue and fight, although previously they were close. They appear to have no positive feelings for one another.

Anna's developmental history

Uncomplicated pregnancy, birth weight 6lbs 10ozs.
Difficult delivery – face presentation with severe moulding.
Initially spent 24 hours in the Special Care Baby Unit (SCBU).
Her mother described her as a 'whinging baby' who never slept.
Little support from her husband.
Anna required constant attention so that her mother was constantly tired, and felt there was something wrong with the baby.
Anna did not sleep through the night until aged 4 years.
Breast-fed for six months, took to solids well.
She was always a 'faddy' eater and her mother was frequently concerned.
Grew below 50th percentile, but within normal limits.
Anna attended play school from the age of 3 years, with no separation difficulties.
She tended to be quiet with few friends, solitary play.
Infants' school: aged 5 years.
Quiet, hardworking, conscientious.
Few close friends, teased by boys, and found them 'disgusting'.
Measles aged 4 years. No other childhood illnesses or operations.
Coped well when her sister was born, with no sibling rivalry.

Activity 4.11

A What was her birth weight expressed in kilograms?
B Check out your understanding of percentiles. (Refer to Chapter 3 on child and family health.)

An understanding of the developmental and family history might assist the current nursing assessment.

Activity 4.12

Before reading on consider how the above factors may have impinged on Anna. You may like to discuss this with a colleague to share your ideas. You may hold different views which would broaden your views.

There is a possibility that Anna was genetically predisposed to developing a psychiatric problem.

Her father's disrupted attachments may have interfered with his parenting ability.

Having always had a close relationship with her mother, this may have intensified at the time of her grandmother's death, perhaps coinciding with increasing marital disharmony, which has been noticeable since her father's change of occupation.

The combination of tension at home, possible enmeshment with her mother, perceived criticism from her father, sibling rivalry, school pressure, poor peer relations and excessive exercise at the time of early puberty, might have contributed to the onset of an eating disorder now.

Enmeshment The term 'enmeshment' comes from the family systems theory tradition (Von Bertalanffy 1968). It refers to a condition where two or more people weave their lives and identities around one another so tightly that it is difficult for either one of them to function independently. The result is that the behaviour of one family member has an immediate and marked effect on those with whom that person is enmeshed. It is a state without adequate or healthy boundaries (for further descriptions of boundaries, see Minuchin 1974).

The opposite, extreme way of relating, detachment or disengagement, is a condition where the people are so independent in their functioning it is difficult to establish how they are related and function together.

Healthy relationships are thought to occur in the space between enmeshment and detachment.

Activity 4.13

Reflect on how your own family history might influence the assessment process if you were the nurse doing the assessment.

Treatment

Treatment involves a multi-disciplinary approach including medical supervision, nutritional counselling and mental health intervention.

? **How would you describe Anna's current weight of 27.3kg? Refer to the BMI. What is your Body Mass Index?**

Anna's primary nurse, having read the doctor's notes and having made a nursing assessment, creates a care plan.

Activity 4.14

Before reading on think what you would include in the plan. Try to consider the rationale for every nursing action, as if you were explaining it to a more junior colleague, or to Anna or her mother. You may like to use a tool such as the activities of daily living as a checklist (see chapter 12 PB92).

Anna's admission treatment plan

Problem	Nursing action
Excessive activity	Strict bed rest, to remain in a cubicle
	Observe for exercising
	Gentle activities – e.g. puzzles
	Can make telephone calls

Treatment rationale

Excessive exercise can exacerbate physical complications and lead to injury; however, total restriction is unhealthy and unlikely to be successful (Lask and Bryant-Waugh 2000, p. 290).

Problems encountered in practice

Clients feel compelled to exercise and will go to great lengths to increase activity, and also have a constant need to maintain movement. In a busy ward it is difficult to keep up the level of observation and supervision. A further complication of bed rest is to increase the risk of osteoporosis. Therefore strict bed rest should only be used in a limited way, when the advantages outweigh the disadvantages.

Activity 4.15

Identify the challenges or possible risks in imposing such a regime. Consider physical as well as psychological function.

Professional conversation

Jo Green, staff nurse on the unit

The importance of understanding the client

'As a staff nurse in this unit I feel it is important to develop an understanding of the strategies clients might use, and why. Initially, they may have started exercising in pursuit of fitness or for pleasure, but as the activity becomes increasingly compulsive and demanding, it becomes a danger to their health, and often leads to further social isolation. The additional gain that Anna receives from such excessive exercise may be a defence against having to think about worries and fears. Other strategies that I have observed include standing by an open window, and wearing minimal clothing in order to induce shivering thereby increasing energy output. Therefore it is important to establish a realistic regime and provide other diversionary activities as a defence against anxiety.'

Anna's treatment plan

Problem	Nursing action
Low body weight	Monitor by weighing twice weekly, pre-breakfast
	Empty bladder prior to weighing
	Weigh in bra and pants

Treatment rationale

This serves two functions, the first to reassure the patient that they will not be allowed to get fat (Akridge 1989) and the second is to monitor the effectiveness of the treatment programme. The young person's need to control their weight must be relinquished (Lask and Bryant-Waugh 2000, p. 274).

Weight gain can also significantly improve their mental state. An individual diet programme gives a common goal that assists consistency of care. Sometimes a target weight strategy is employed; however, Lask and Bryant-Waugh (2000, p. 274) suggest that a target weight might become an obsessive preoccupation with both the client and staff, increasing potential conflict. They do suggest that there should be a goal in mind.

Problems encountered in practice

This is often viewed as the most difficult area, as it confronts the patient's fears directly. The enforcement of a feeding regime, including naso-gastric feeding if necessary, causes conflict amongst staff. The view might be taken that such enforcement is force-feeding and therefore an infringement of the patient's rights. The legal and ethical issues are introduced in this chapter. Issues around how and when to feed, and the patient's potential dependence on this passive feeding regime, have to be explored.

Discussion of possible solutions

The ethical issues should be discussed with the treatment team. An individual, graded re-feeding plan is negotiated with the dietician.

Activity 4.16

Remember to jot down phrases that may need following up, for example 'individual, graded re-feeding plan'. What does this mean precisely and how is it 'negotiated with the dietician'? What skills does the dietician need in order to work therapeutically with Anna? It may be useful for you to try to negotiate some time to spend with the dietician, being aware that the clients or patients may not always welcome an observer.

Each meal and snack is supervised. The treatment team taking charge at this stage can be seen by the client as helpful. Such a structure could be seen in terms of Winnicott's (1986) concept of 'holding'. It can also be suggested that the staff need 'holding' as well, in order to contain the anxiety generated in the patient, and by the strategy. Consistency among the multi-disciplinary team is essential to avoid the potential of manipulation and division. This would be seen as a function of supervision.

> ### Activity 4.17
>
> Find out in practice what strategies are used to ensure a consistent approach to care is taken.

How do the staff in your practice area support each other? You may like to discuss your findings with various colleagues who work in different practice environments.

It is possible to use other methods for monitoring the effectiveness of the treatment programme, including pelvic ultrasound. This serves the function of helping to determine healthy weight by measuring the size of the ovaries and uterus (Lask and Bryant-Waugh 2000, p. 175).

Anna's treatment plan

Problem	Nursing action
Maintain hygiene	Daily baths, showers and dental care

Treatment rationale

This serves the function of containing the patient's anxiety and encouraging normal healthy daily activities of living and self-care.

Problems encountered in practice

Malnutrition and associated depression can reduce the patient's motivation for self-care. Poor peripheral circulation can cause problems with dry skin, chilblains and occasionally gangrene.

Dental caries can result from acid erosion if there is excessive vomiting.

If there are any self-harming behaviours, for example cutting or scratching, these will need to be addressed.

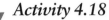 *Activity 4.18*

As a student nurse, consider what your immediate actions might be if you came upon a patient who is self-harming. Where will you find your support to appropriately manage the situation?

Discussion of possible solutions

Encourage and support daily self-care. As weight increases, so will motivation. There is a need to be aware of possible depression.

Anna's treatment plan

Problem	Nursing care
Monitor physical state	4-hourly observations – temperature, pulse, respiration and blood pressure
	Bed rest, or activity as allowed
	Accurate fluid intake/output chart
	Accurate food intake chart
	Quilt and socks to be used

Treatment rationale

Due to Anna's poor physical state, poor peripheral circulation and loss of subcutaneous body fat, frequent observation of her medical state is essential. Postural hypotension on standing could lead to injuries from osteoporosis if she fell. There is a potential for cardiovascular complications and susceptibility to cardiac arhythmias, owing to electrolyte imbalances.

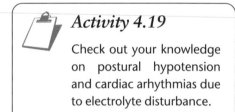 *Activity 4.19*

Check out your knowledge on postural hypotension and cardiac arhythmias due to electrolyte disturbance.

Very emaciated patients can deteriorate suddenly, developing severe infections leading to systemic failure.

? Why is Anna at particular risk of osteoporosis? How might this affect her in later years?

Problems encountered in practice

Resistant to being disturbed as these patients do not see themselves as ill.

Discussion of possible solutions

Management and monitoring of the patient's physical state is a key nursing responsibility. Exact recordings of physical status and dietary intake and output are of special importance.

> ### Activity 4.20
>
> Find out how intake and output for patients with an eating disorder is recorded. Is it different from such recordings in other practice areas? You may find it useful to discuss the challenges of recording such information accurately.

Summation of Anna's treatment

Diet Quarter portions + BD Ensure Plus supplement
Supervision during and half-hour after meals
Meals to include foods from each group – carbohydrate, fats, protein
Can identify three food dislikes, not to be changed once chosen
No low calorie foods/drinks
All changes to be decided by the dietician

> ### Activity 4.21
>
> Consider your ability to assist in choosing appropriate foods from the three groups for balanced meals. Refer to Chapter 10 on nutritional needs to check out your knowledge.

Changes to Anna's treatment plan

One week later the only changes to Anna's treatment plan are:
Some weight loss, 27kgs
Diet – meals increased to half portions
Medication – Lactulose

Two weeks later:
Hygiene – hair can be washed once weekly
Diet – full portions + overnight naso-gastric feeds as there is further weight loss
Parents – able to stay for meals as long as they are able to remain detached and not undermine nursing efforts with feeding

3 weeks later:
Struggling with full portions
Complains of abdominal pain, constipated

Anna is transferred to the adolescent psychiatric unit

Anna is re-admitted six months later.
She had reached her target weight of 43kg prior to discharge.
She was discharged ten days ago. Weight loss 5.5kg.
She is now only eating quarter of an orange, one piece of pasta, and diluted diet coke daily.
Anna feels life is not worth living.

Plan

Restart original plan with quarter-food portions and naso-gastric feeding.

Anna is refusing all oral intake except sips of water. She agreed to drink 100ml water hourly or she would require additional intravenous fluids. Her oral intake improved, and she returned to the psychiatric unit as a day patient six days later.

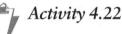 *Activity 4.22*

Think about the risk of hospital acquired infection in Anna's case.

Anna is re-admitted

Anna is re-admitted three months later. Anna was attending as a day patient at the psychiatric unit, but has not eaten or drunk for five days. She collapsed.
  A very difficult admission.

Sixteen days later Anna's weight has increased to 34.4kg. Once her physical state is stable, Anna could be transferred back to the adolescent unit. There is the need to introduce a small oral intake, to reintroduce the concept of feeding.

Twenty-two days later – Anna's weight has increased to 35.2kg.
Day 22 – Anna is transferred back to the psychiatric unit.

Activity 4.23

Anna has made some progress in her treatment and is gaining weight. She is still very distressed at her weight and still has difficulty eating. Think about what could be the risks to her.

 What other agencies might be involved in managing future care?

> **Activity 4.24**
>
> **A** Discuss how anorexia nervosa might be situated within the wider social discourses of both women and men in society.
>
> **B** Explore and debate the legal and ethical issues involved in treatment interventions.

Conclusion

The majority of adolescents with anorexia nervosa will recover or improve sufficiently to obtain a good quality of life. A significant number will go on to develop a severe form of the disorder or develop further serious mental health problems (Crisp et al 1992).

The most commonly observed psychiatric problems, even in those who have recovered from their eating disorder, include depression, anxiety disorders, obsessive compulsive disorder and drug and alcohol misuse (Steinhausen et al 1991). Two-thirds, or even more, of former patients accomplish employment and normal educational careers, but only a minority enter marriage or a stable relationship.

Some authors, for example Herzog et al (1993), claim that a younger age of onset is predictive of a better outcome, and other studies (Bryant-Waugh et al 1996) have shown no significant correlation between age of onset and outcome.

However, eating disorders in all age groups represent the severe end of psychiatric morbidity, having an adverse effect in virtually all areas of life, and not infrequently leading to a premature death. Mortality rates are as high as 22 per cent in some samples, although results are variable (Lucas et al 1976).

There is evidence to show that specialist treatment can result in a better outcome for patients than non-specialist treatment (Crisp et al 1991), but access to specialist units remains problematic and most patients are cared for in primary and secondary care settings. However, contrary findings from Burls et al (2001) suggest that outpatient care had slightly better results in some areas. In terms of the evidence base, it is fair to say that as yet the relative effectiveness of care strategies for the person with anorexia is unclear. The National Research Register also indexes six studies currently under way to examine the effectiveness of inpatient treatment. The earliest is not likely to report until 2004.

Nurses can, however, contribute to improved care for these patients by increasing their awareness and knowledge in this challenging area.

> **Activity 4.25**
>
> Consider how the information that you have gained from this chapter may impact in a range of settings on your care of patients who may experience difficulties with eating.

References

Akridge, K. (1989) Principles and practice: anorexia nervosa. *Journal of Obstetric, Gynaecologic & Neonatal Nursing* 18, pp. 25–30.

American Psychiatric Association (1994) *Diagnostic and Statistical Manual of Mental Disorders* (DSM-IV-TR). Washington, DC: APA.

Bodycombe-James, M. (2000) Paediatric nurses' enjoyment of caring for sick children. In: Glasper, E. A. Ireland, L. (eds) (2000) *Evidenced-Based Child Health Care: Challenges for Practice*. Basingstoke: Palgrave Macmillan.

Bowlby, J. (1969/1980) *Attachment and Loss*. Vol.1. London: Hogarth.

Bryant-Waugh, R. et al (1996). A prospective follow up of children with anorexia nervosa. *Journal of Youth and Adolescence* 25 (4), pp. 431–7.

Burls, A., Gold, L., Meads, C. (2001) How effective is outpatient care compared to inpatient care for the treatment of anorexia nervosa? A systematic review. *European Eating Disorders* Review 9, pp. 229–41.

Cooper, M. A., Glasper, E. A. (2001) Deliberate self-harm in children: the nurse's therapeutic style. *British Journal of Nursing*, 10 (1) pp. 34–40.

Crisp, A. H., Callender, R., JS, Halek, C., Hsu LKG,(1992) Long-term mortality in anorexia nervosa; a twenty-year follow up of the St Georges and Aberdeen cohorts. *British Journal of Psychiatry* 161, pp. 104–7.

Crisp, A. H., Norton, K., Gowers, S. et al (1991) A controlled study of the effect of therapies aimed at adolescent and family psychopathology in anorexia nervosa. *British Journal of Psychiatry* 159, pp. 325–9.

Erikson, E. (1965) *Childhood and Society*. Harmondsworth: Penguin.

George, L. (1997) The psychological characteristics of patients suffering from anorexia nervosa and the nurses role in creating a therapeutic relationship. *Journal of Advanced Nursing* 26, pp. 899–908.

Hauser, S. T., with Powers, S. I., Noam, G. G. (1991) *Adolescents and Their Families: Paths of Ego Development*, New York: Free Press.

Herzog, D. B., Sacks, N. R., Keller, M. B. (1993) Patterns and predictors of recovery in anorexia nervosa and bulimia nervosa. *Journal of The Academy of Child & Adolescent Psychiatry* 32, pp. 835–42.

Howe, D., Brandon, M., Hinings, D., Schofield, G. (1999) *Attachment Theory, Child Maltreatment and Family Support*. Basingstoke: Macmillan Press – now Palgrave Macmillan.

Jacobs, M. (1985) *The Presenting Past: An Introduction to Practical Psychodynamic Counselling*. Milton Keynes: Open University Press, ch. 7.

King, S. J., Turner, S. (2000) Caring for adolescent females with anorexia nervosa: registered nurses perspective. *Journal of Advanced Nursing* 32 (1), pp. 139–47.

Lask, B., Bryant-Waugh, R. (2000) *Anorexia Nervosa and Related Eating Disorders in Childhood and Adolescence*. 2nd Edition. Hove: Psychology Press, pp. 290–2.

Lucas, A., Duncan, J. W., Piens, V. (1976)The Treatment of anorexia nervosa. *American Journal of Psychiarty* 133, pp. 1034–8.

Minuchin, S. (1974) *Families and Family Therapy*. Cambridge, MA: Harvard University Press.

Steinhausen, H. C., Rauss-Mason, C., Seidel, R. (1991) Follow up studies of anorexia nervosa: a review of four decades of outcome research. *Psychological Medicine* 21, pp. 447–54.

Stockwell, F. (1972) *The Unpopular Patient*. London: RCN.

Taylor, J., Muller, D. (1995) *Nursing Adolescents: Research and Psychological Perspectives*. Oxford: Blackwell Science.

Von Bertalanffy, L. (1968) *General Systems Theory: Foundations, Development, Application*. New York: Braziller.

Winnicott, D. (1986) *Holding and Interpretation: Fragment of an Analysis*. London: The Hogarth Press and The Institute of Psychoanalysis.

World Health Organisation (1994) *The International Classification of Diseases* (ICD-10). Copenhagen: WHO.

Wright, S. (2001) Eating disorders: why do nurses choose this field? *Nursing Times* 97 (46), pp. 37–8.

5

Insights into Adult Nursing

Janet Dean and Paula Shobbrook

Nursing adults takes place in a range of settings: in their own homes, in residential care settings as well as within hospitals, both as outpatients and inpatients.

Using an example of a man who is experiencing a chest disorder, this chapter will illustrate the context of nursing adult patients.

Introduction

Many investigative procedures and treatments are now available to patients as 'day cases' and this is generally accepted to be more convenient and less stressful for many people. It also allows for cost effective use of limited resources. Such an approach to patient care, however, provides a particular challenge for nurses, who must be able to establish an effective and supportive relationship with a number of patients in a stressful situation, often in a very limited time. The nurse must ensure that not only does the patient receive excellent care whilst in the unit, but also that their communication skills promote continuity of care once the patient has left the department.

This scenario, related to a man who is to have a bronchoscopy, will explore some of the professional issues raised by the attendance in a day unit of an adult patient for an invasive investigative procedure.

Learning outcomes

This chapter will enable the student to:

- Identify the health risks associated with smoking, and discuss strategies which may help patients to stop smoking.
- Discuss the pathophysiological effects of lung cancer, and identify implications for nursing care.
- Outline the advantages and disadvantages of day case investigative procedures for patients, carers and health care professionals.
- Explore the legal and ethical considerations in adult nursing related to informed consent and information giving.

- Suggest four strategies which may reduce patient anxiety.
- Identify and discuss six key aspects of respiratory assessment.
- Describe the preparation required for a patient undergoing fibreoptic brochoscopy and list potential complications.
- Describe the role of the nurse during bronchoscopy, and the aftercare needed.
- Discuss discharge planning following day case procedures.
- Recognise the importance of interprofessional communication, and suggest ways in which this could be enhanced.

Concepts

- Consent
- Informed consent
- Informed choice
- Trust
- Information giving
- Diagnostic interventions
- Invasive procedures
- Anxiety
- Sedation
- Nurse's role pre-, peri- and post-procedure
- Assessment
- Respiratory assessment
- Monitoring

- Evaluating outcomes
- Nursing judgements
- Patient safety
- Emergency care
- Scope of professional practice
- Health risks
- Malignant
- Benign
- Infection control
- Emergency care
- Day case treatment
- Nursing research

Scenario *Introducing Mr Stevens*

Mr William Stevens is 58 years old, he is divorced and works as a roofer. He lives in a first-floor council-owned flat with his adult daughter who has a 3-month-old baby. He has smoked since the age of 15, preferring to 'roll his own' and continues to do so, although he has recently cut down from four to two ounces of tobacco per week. He drinks alcohol occasionally and does not own a car, using public transport, with his daughter giving him lifts when she can.

Health history

Mr Stevens had been fit and well, apart from occasional upper respiratory tract infections and a 'smoker's cough' in the morning for some years.

Mr Stevens became unwell six weeks ago. He developed a 'flu-like' illness and became lethargic. He also noticed a painless hoarseness of his voice. After a week he visited his GP who prescribed a course of oral antibiotics, to which there was no response. Mr Stevens then developed pain in his chest and back which was made worse by lying down, and unrelieved by taking paracetamol. He returned to his GP and reported the pain. An outpatient chest X-ray was then organised at the local hospital, and Mr Stevens was referred to a medical consultant, specialising in respiratory disease, for assessment of his chest X-ray and clinical condition.

He was seen in the outpatients department two weeks later. The consultant suspected carcinoma of the bronchus and organised an urgent bronchoscopy. Prior to the bronchoscopy, Mr Stevens was asked to attend outpatients again to have blood tests performed and for pulmonary function tests.

After ten days, he was asked to attend the day unit at the local hospital for a fibreoptic bronchoscopy.

Activity 5.1

Visit an outpatients clinic, or talk to a nurse working in the area. How does the nurse's role differ from that of a ward-based nurse?

 What is a bronchoscopy? Consider your response before reading on.

Activity 5.2

You may find it useful to look up or review the anatomy of the respiratory tract.

Flexible fibreoptic bronchoscopy allows direct, detailed examination of the larynx, trachea and bronchi. The procedure is tolerated well by the majority of patients (although particular care should be taken when examining critically ill, hypoxic or asthmatic patients), and does not require a general anaesthetic (Bassett 1997).

A bronchoscopy may be diagnostic or therapeutic. Most are performed to confirm a suspected diagnosis, often of lung cancer as in Mr Steven's case, or of infection (such as tuberculosis). Bronchoscopy can also be useful in identifying other causes of haemoptysis.

Therapeutically, bronchoscopy can be used to remove foreign bodies or excess secretions from the airways, to control bleeding points and to allow direct treatment of tumours (Belli 1999). A doctor with specialist training usually performs the procedure, although some nurses now carry out endoscopic procedures.

Are there any nurse endoscopists practising in your area? What are the professional implications for nurses who choose to extend the scope of their professional practice in this way?

Before the procedure, the patient is starved ('nil by mouth') to reduce the risk of aspiration of stomach contents into the lungs if the patient should vomit.

A written, informed consent is obtained. The patient is then sedated using an intravenous drug, and the mucosa of the nose and throat are sprayed with local anaesthetic agent to reduce discomfort. The bronchoscope is then passed through the nose or mouth, via the vocal cords, into the tracheobronchial tree. Coughing is suppressed with local anaesthetic spray through the bronchoscope as the procedure progresses. Any abnormal tissue seen can be sampled by taking a biopsy, or a brush can protrude from the end of the bronchoscope and sweep off some of the superficial mucosal cells to collect them in a specimen jar. Sputum specimens can also be obtained.

> ### Activity 5.3
>
> Find out in your practice areas how long patients are 'starved' before operative procedures. Find out the rationale if there are differences.

During the procedure the patient's condition is continually monitored by the person performing the procedure and by the assisting nurse. Once the procedure is completed, the patient is encouraged to rest to allow the effects of the sedation to wear off, and he is observed for any sign of complications.

> ### Activity 5.4
>
> Consider what complications may occur following this procedure.

Patients must remain 'nil by mouth' until their swallowing reflex (which is depressed by the local anaesthetic) has returned to normal, usually two to four hours after the procedure. As the effects of sedation may persist for many hours, patients are not allowed to drive home.

Complications are rare, but can include:

- Respiratory distress, hypoxia, bronchospasm
- Pnuemothorax
- Perforation of the trachea
- Aspiration
- Haemorrhage
- Infection
- Cardiac dysrhythmias
- Hypotension
- Drug reactions

> ### Activity 5.5
>
> 1 List the patient monitoring techniques that you already know about. Could they be used to detect such complications?
>
> 2 It is well worth organising a visit to an endoscopy unit to observe some procedures. This will enable you to respond more accurately to patients' questions when preparing them for investigations, and gives you a better idea of what they have been through!
> If this is not possible, watching a video is a good alternative.

? What other endoscopic procedures are performed?

 Practice tip

Many information leaflets have been written to help health professionals prepare patients for investigative procedures. If such leaflets are to prove beneficial to patients, it is important that they are used appropriately:

- Leaflets should be used in addition to verbal information – not instead of.
- Select an appropriate leaflet in the correct language, and ensure that the patient can read it, or that somebody can read it to him.
- Provide the leaflet well before the procedure, to allow time for assimilation of the information.
- Make sure that the patient knows who can answer any questions, and how to contact them.
- It may be useful to highlight or mark crucial information, such as the need to remain 'nil by mouth', or not to drive following procedures, for additional emphasis.

Activity 5.6

Have a careful look at some of the information leaflets available for patients in your practice area. Consider how effective they would be for a variety of patient groups; for example, a person with a learning disability, a person who has a visual impairment, as well as people whose first language is not English.

Lung cancer

Lung cancer is the commonest form of malignant disease in the Western world and 80 to 90 per cent is caused by smoking. Other causes are thought to include passive smoking, exposure to radioactive materials, radon gas and asbestos.

The risk of developing lung cancer is directly related to the duration and intensity of the smoking. The risk of lung cancer in smokers is 15 times that of lifelong non-smokers (NHS Executive 1998), thus a patient like Mr Stevens, a heavy smoker for 43 years, would be at high risk.

Practice tip

Many patients seem reluctant to admit the extent of their smoking habit, and will initially underestimate the amount they smoke when questioned. A non-judgmental approach is essential.

Lung cancer is an umbrella term which includes several different tumours, arising from different cells within the respiratory tract. It is important to identify the exact type of tumour a patient has, as both treatment and prognosis vary from type to type. Occasionally, a lung tumour may be benign (without the capacity to spread to other parts of the body as a malignant tumour can), but this is rare.

Lung tumours can be crudely divided into 'small cell ' and 'non-small cell tumours'.

Small cell tumours are highly malignant. They can divide and spread (metastasise) very rapidly, whereas non-small cell tumours (including adenocarcinomas, squamous cell and large cell tumours) are slower growing (Quinn 1999). However, generally the prognosis for patients with lung cancer is very poor: only 5 per cent of patients will still be alive five years after diagnosis.

One of the difficulties in improving the survival of patients with lung cancer is the lack of an effective screening procedure to detect the disease in the early stages when curative treatment may be possible (Day 1998; Kosco and Held-Warmkessel 2000). Often, as with Mr Stevens, by the time patients seek medical advice the disease is already well established and curative treatment is not possible.

? **What symptoms might occur with this condition which would make a person ask for an appointment with the GP?**

Signs and symptoms which are suggestive of lung cancer include:

- Cough – with or without haemoptysis
- Pain in the chest, neck or back
- Recurrent respiratory infections
- Malaise
- Weight loss
- Dyspnoea

Some patients suffer with hoarseness, which is due to paralysis of one of the vocal cords, rendering normal speech impossible. The paralysis is caused by the tumour damaging the left recurrent laryngeal nerve as it passes through the chest to supply the left vocal cord (Quinn 1999).

A doctor may suspect lung cancer if a patient presents with such signs and symptoms, particularly if the patient is a smoker, or has been exposed to other causative agents.

To confirm the diagnosis a chest X-ray is performed, which will reveal the presence of a tumour, but not its type. To identify the exact nature of the tumour, cells must be obtained from the growth for histological examination, either from biopsy specimens (usually obtained via a bronchoscopy) or from sputum specimens, as tumour cells are shed into sputum. Once the cell type of tumour has been identified, treatment can be offered.

The treatment available for lung cancer depends on several factors including the type and position of the tumour, the extent of any metastatic disease, and the physical condition of the patient. Surgery, radiotherapy and/or chemotherapy can be used, either as potentially curative treatment, or as palliation in an attempt to improve the quality of the patient's remaining life by reducing the severity of symptoms (Claxton 1999, Dest 2000).

Health of the Nation

Lung cancer was one of the target areas identified in the *Health of the Nation* White Paper by the Conservative government in 1992.

The aim was to reduce lung cancer death rates by 30 per cent in men under 75, and by 15 per cent in women under 75 by 2010, and the following preventative measures were advocated:

- Health education on the effects of smoking
- Helping people not to start smoking
- Helping people to stop smoking
- Protecting non-smokers from passive smoking
- Preventing occupational exposure to causative agents

? What were the other target areas identified in the *Health of the Nation*? Consider your responses before checking below.

? Many smokers are aware of the potential health risks associated with smoking, but they continue to smoke – why? You may like to discuss this with friends and colleagues who smoke and consider the range of responses. Compare these with smokers' comment later in the chapter.

Saving Lives: Our Healthier Nation

When the Labour government came to power in 1998, they reviewed the previous Conservative government's health strategies and subsequently produced a White Paper, *Saving Lives: Our Healthier Nation* (DoH 1999a). This is presented as an action plan to tackle poor health. The key agenda is to:

- Improve the health of everyone
- Improve the health of the worst off in particular

The plan is focused on the main causes of early death: cancer, coronary heart disease and stroke, accidents and mental illness. Targets have been established for priority areas – by the year 2010:

- Cancer: to reduce the death rate in people under 75 by at least 20 per cent.
- Coronary heart disease: to reduce the death rate in people under 75 by at least 40 per cent.

- Accidents: to reduce the death rate by at least 20 per cent and serious injury by 10 per cent.
- Mental health: to reduce the death rate from suicide and undetermined injury by at least 20 per cent.

Our Healthier Nation places more emphasis on people taking responsibility for their own health through physical activity, better diet and stopping smoking. It is proposed that this will be supported by:

- NHS Direct – a nurse-led telephone helpline and Internet service providing advice and information on health.
- Health skills programmes for people to help themselves and others.
- Expert Patient programmes to help people manage their own illnesses.

> ### Activity 5.7
>
> This White Paper underpins the political development of the health service today. The executive summary provides an overview of the key points. The White Paper can be found on the Internet at: http://www.onh.gov.uk or visit your library for a copy.

Health risks: smoking

Smoking is a major health risk – 'the largest single preventable cause of death' (Department of Health 1999b) and nurses have an important role in helping patients to give up smoking or not to take up smoking. As well as lung cancer, smoking causes other tumours: cancer of the mouth, nose, larynx, oesophagus, pancreas, bladder, cervix and leukaemia. It also causes emphysema, bronchitis, atherosclerosis, peptic ulcers, infertility and female smokers are at higher risk of osteoporosis, spontaneous abortion and of giving birth to low birth weight babies (Burgess 1994; and also see Chapter 2 on maternal health, p. 20). There is also increasing concern regarding the health effects of passive smoking.

Despite the general knowledge that smoking is 'bad for your health', in 1999 28 per cent of adults, approximately 13 million people, in the United Kingdom were smokers (DoH 1999b). Most smokers are introduced to the habit in their teens. There are many reasons why people begin or continue to smoke, including curiosity, peer pressure, anticipating adulthood, rebelliousness and role modelling. Once established as a behaviour, smoking becomes a habit and addiction to nicotine can result, making it very difficult to stop. Smoking is related to social class, being more prevalent in lower socio-economic classes (as defined by the Registrar General); for example, 21 per cent of men in social class 1 smoke, as compared to 49 per cent of men in social class 5. This clearly has implications for the targeting of health education, screening and health care provision. There is also concern that the downward trend in smoking, which has been evident since the 1960s, is now levelling out and increasing numbers of young people are starting to smoke (DoH 1999b).

The National Health Service Executive (1998) has issued guidance on the commissioning of cancer services, and indicates areas of good practice related to reducing the incidence of smoking. Primary prevention of smoking is felt to be crucial, and strategies include school-based prevention programmes, mass media campaigns, restrictions on cigarette sales to minors, and the banning of cigarette advertising and sponsorship. Increasing taxation to increase the price of tobacco products may also reduce smoking levels; however, given the higher incidence of smoking amongst those of low income, price rises may simply increase financial hardship.

It is vital to remember that giving up smoking is a very difficult process. This is also true for health care professional who smoke, and they should be encouraged and supported to become non-smoking role models (Claxton 1999).

Evidence-based practice

Several smoking cessation interventions have been shown to be effective:

- Brief advice from a health care professional
- Nicotine replacement therapy with advice
- Advice and support to pregnant women

Current evidence suggests that other strategies may be less effective, including:

- Use of anti-depressant and anxiety reducing drugs
- Behavioural therapy such as aversive conditioning
- Acupuncture
- Hypnosis
- Self-help materials such as booklets and pamphlets

(NHS Centre for Review and Dissemination 1998)

Nurses need to be fully informed of the physiological, psychological and social causes and effects of smoking to enable them to function effectively as a health educator, as nurses often interact with smokers in both hospital and community settings. The risk of developing lung cancer does diminish after stopping smoking, becoming apparent after about 5 years. However, the risk of a former smoker remains greater than that of a non-smoker, even 20 to 25 years after stopping (Day 1998).

 Are there any support groups in your area which provide additional help?

Activity 5.8

Consider for a few moments how effective you could be in supporting a patient, friend or relative who wanted to give up smoking.

Professional conversation

Jane Phillips, ward manager

Smoking – too late to stop?

'Mr Stevens has been smoking for many years and would probably find it very difficult to stop, particularly now when he is very anxious regarding his state of health. If he has lung cancer, it could be argued that it is too late for him to stop. The damage to his health is already done, and if it is one of the pleasures in his life, would it not be kinder to allow him to continue to smoke for the limited time he has left?

There are, however, other issues to consider. If Mr Stevens does have lung cancer, the best chance for curative treatment would be surgery, and if it is possible to operate on Mr Stevens, stopping smoking six weeks prior to the operation can make a significant difference in terms of morbidity and mortality. Passive smoking may also be having detrimental effects on the health of Mr Stevens's granddaughter and daughter. It may be "too late" for Mr Stevens, but not for those living with him.'

Smoking Kills

In 1999, the government published a White Paper *Smoking Kills*, which outlines proposed government action aimed at reducing the number of smoking-related deaths in the United Kingdom, and in particular to reduce smoking by children and pregnant women (see Chapter 2 on maternal health, p. 20). These actions include:

- A ban on tobacco advertising.
- Increased support for those wishing to stop via GP services, including a limited supply of nicotine replacement therapy for some.
- Priority attention to pregnant women who smoke.
- Additional funding to reduce cigarette smuggling.
- Enforcement of legislation related to under-age sales and proof-of-age cards to protect young people
(DoH 1999b)

Mr Stevens arrives in the day unit with his daughter at 10 a.m., where a nurse welcomes him. She escorts him into a private room to assess his current situation. As instructed, he has taken 'nil by mouth' since midnight in preparation for the bronchoscopy – he last ate 16 hours ago and last drank 10 hours ago.

Evidence-based practice

Nil by mouth – for how long?

It is well known that patients who are to receive a general anaesthetic should be 'nil by mouth' before the procedure to ensure that the stomach is empty. This greatly reduces the risk of aspiration of stomach contents into the lungs if vomiting should occur. It is also wise to take similar precautions if patients are to undergo procedures which may cause vomiting (such as bronchoscopy), particularly if the patient has been sedated and may be unable to protect their airway.

Research has demonstrated that not eating or drinking for four hours is sufficient to ensure an empty stomach (Chapman 1996), and that keeping patients 'nil by mouth' for prolonged periods causes dehydration and discomfort, and can significantly affect the patients' nutritional status. Nursing research undertaken by Hamilton-Smith (1972) identified ritualistic nursing practices which resulted in patients being starved for much longer than necessary. For example, all patients on the morning theatre list were kept 'nil by mouth' from midnight, regardless of the scheduled time of their surgery. Chapman's study, undertaken 24 years later, identifies similar issues, and raises concerns that the results of nursing research are not having an impact on some areas of clinical practice.

It is important to ensure that patients are treated individually, and starved for the minimum time, to ensure safety whilst reducing discomfort. Mr Stevens arrived for his bronchoscopy having eaten nothing for 16 hours and having drunk nothing for 10 hours. This would suggest that either he had been given inappropriate, standardised instructions, or that he did not understand the instructions he had been given – this is not good care.

On the day of the bronchoscopy, his health status is as follows:

Mr Stevens has a persistent productive cough, expectorating green sputum (no haemoptysis), particularly in the morning. He is dyspnoeic on exertion, and has a very hoarse voice. His vital signs and blood test results are within normal limits for a man of his age. His chest X-ray is abnormal revealing, according to the radiologist's report, 'a left upper lobe mass, with consolidation and collapse', and his pulmonary function tests are abnormal, suggesting obstructive disease.

He is still suffering chest and back pain, of a 'sharp, stabbing ' nature. His GP has now prescribed diclofenac orally, which has been only partially effective. Mr Stevens identifies pain as his major problem.

Despite his quiet, hoarse voice, Mr Stevens is able to communicate effectively. He does not speak unless spoken to, and tends to respond as briefly as possible. He is co-operative, but appears very anxious. When questioned, he admits that he is concerned about the investigation itself, and also about his diagnosis. He is aware that his X-ray is abnormal, and thinks this could be due to, 'infection, pneumonia, cancer or anything'. He feels that he is 'in limbo – the worst bit is not knowing. It's probably not to do with the fags – actually, I'm sure it's not. Whatever it is it doesn't really matter, I just want rid of it.'

He says he feels optimistic that it will soon be all over. Mr Stevens is not aware – although the health care professionals are – that his X-ray is highly suggestive of a large central obstructing tumour, probably malignant, which clinically is inoperable, and is already causing recurrent laryngeal nerve damage.

? **Should Mr Stevens have been told that he probably has cancer? Before reading on consider the pros and cons. If so, when should he be told and by whom?**

It can be very difficult for health care professionals to decide when it is appropriate to reveal information regarding diagnosis to patients. The principles of autonomy and individuality, enshrined in the *Code of Professional Conduct* NMC 2002 would indicate that patients should be entitled to information about their condition. The amount and type of information that should be disclosed is also a matter of sensible and responsible judgement (Thompson et al 1994). In the early stages of investigation of a health problem there may be many potential diagnoses to be eliminated, and it may not be helpful to discuss all of them fully with the patient, as confusion and anxiety may result. Once a definite diagnosis has been reached, it would be crucial for Mr Stevens to be fully informed, in order that he could make rational decisions about possible treatments, if he chose to accept any.

English law does not give the patient the right to know everything about their treatment; however, judges have suggested that if a patient requests specific information, they should be given it (Carson and Montgomery 1989). Mr Stevens is clearly aware of the possibility that he could have cancer, and that this could be related to smoking, although he dismisses this. If he asks directly, 'Have I got cancer?', it would probably be most appropriate to tell him that this is quite possible, but until the results of the bronchoscopy are known, it is not certain. He should also be reassured that the results will be made known to him as quickly as possible and that he (and his daughter if he wishes) will have the chance to discuss them with the doctor.

If he does not ask, it may be because he is not yet ready to deal with this possibility, and it would be reasonable to tell him that the bronchoscopy will be able to reveal the cause of his symptoms, without mentioning cancer at this stage.

Lack of information is a major cause of dissatisfaction amongst patients with cancer (NHS Executive 1998), and it is important to be aware that the quality of communication between patients and health professionals can influence compliance with advice or treatment (Ley 1988). Thus the appropriate delivery of accurate information, at the right time, in the best available environment, is a crucial part of Mr Stevens's care.

Assessment, knowledge and skills

When Mr Stevens arrives in the day unit, the nurse's responsibility is to undertake a focused assessment of his condition. During the assessment, the patient is informed as to why the questions are being asked, and his queries are then answered in plain language. The time available for this is limited, so it is imperative that the appropriate information is acquired. The accuracy of the data obtained depends upon the patient's ability to communicate information and the nurse's skill to perceive it correctly (Stafrace 1998). In order to do this the patient must have the nurse's full attention, which means allowing time away from other distractions. This may be achieved by pulling the bed curtains around the bed area, or using an empty room or assessment area, which also provides privacy for the patient.

Practice tip

Remember that bed curtains provide only visual privacy. Conversations behind curtains can very easily be overheard. Patient confidentiality must be considered.

Well-developed communication skills are vital to good nursing practice. Some of the factors which hamper effective communication include:

- Patient anxiety about their condition
- Lack of privacy
- Patient fear because of the unfamiliar environment
- Use of professional jargon
- Pressure of time, either real or imagined
- Lack of formal training in communication skills (Buchanan 1995)

Activity 5.9

Take time to review your own communication skills, verbal and non-verbal. How effectively do you communicate? Much has been written on the subject. A visit to your library or the library website will demonstrate the large amount of information that is available.

Before beginning the assessment, the nurse should introduce herself to Mr Stevens and his daughter, and explain exactly what is going to happen. It is also important to check that neither of them have any immediate needs which should be satisfied before continuing with the assessment.

 Practice tip

Before assessing any patient, gather all the available information and make sure you have read the medical notes and referral letter so that you are aware of the clinical history and can ask the most relevant questions.

You can copy relevant data on to nursing records (to save time); for example, date of birth, address, occupation, known allergies. Remember to check with the patient that the details are still correct!

 Professional conversation:

Bob Jenkins, charge nurse

'Effective communication pathways between the primary care team and hospital-based professionals are essential to effective care, and evidence suggests that current systems are somewhat lacking!

Poor interprofessional communication can lead to inadequate symptom control, duplication of effort and wasted time, resulting in frustration and distress for patients and their families. In particular, communication between hospitals and GPs causes difficulties (NHS Executive 1998).

In some hospitals, computer-based information systems enable information to be accessed quickly, and passed from outpatient to hospital-based departments, in the future.'

Activity 5.10

Find out which information systems are in place in your areas of practice, and ensure you can use them effectively. Identify as many communication pathways as possible.

? How is information relayed to the primary care team following investigative procedures? How long does it take? Can you suggest any improvements to the current system?

The nursing assessment should include the gathering of important biographical information to ensure that all the patient's records are accurate, a review of the patient's social situation, and both psychological and physiological assessments of the patient's current health situation.

The key information required may be summarised as follows:

- Is this the patient intended to have this investigation?
- Is there any psychological or physiological reason why this bronchoscopy should not go ahead?
- Can the patient be safely discharged once he has recovered from the procedure?

If the assessing nurse can identify any cause for concern, this must be rapidly communicated to the endoscopist and the rest of the care team, as the procedure may need to be postponed or cancelled if the difficulties cannot be quickly resolved.

Psychological assessment

It is helpful to ask Mr Stevens if he understands why he has come for a bronchoscopy and if he understands what is involved. Asking Mr Stevens what he has already been told by his GP, the outpatients nurses and the consultant can be very revealing, as his knowledge and level of understanding can be assessed, and any important knowledge deficits identified.

This will also give the assessing nurse an opportunity to answer any questions that Mr Stevens or his daughter might have about the procedure, and to assess his ability to give a genuinely informed consent. Although Mr Stevens's arrival in the day unit implies his consent, written consent is required and consent can be withdrawn at any time. He might have changed his mind, or be too confused or distressed to continue.

> At the start of the interview, it is noticed that Mr Stevens is very anxious.

Most patients will be anxious when they arrive in hospital, for either treatment or investigation, and addressing this issue is an important aspect of nursing care. Whilst accepting that some anxiety is inevitable, it may be possible to reduce levels of anxiety and help the patient to feel more at ease in an alien environment.

? **What could be causing Mr Stevens's anxiety?**

Nurses must be able to recognise anxiety, and this can be manifest in several ways:

- Patients may freely admit that they are anxious, or they may be very quiet and withdrawn, or very talkative. They may appear to be aggressive.
- Physical signs may suggest anxiety, such as tachycardia, hypertension, tachypnoea, heightened startle response, or symptoms such as sweating, urinary frequency, abdominal distress, increased perception of pain.

- Disordered cognitive functioning, such as difficulty in concentrating and remembering and misunderstandings, may be due to anxiety (Spear 1996).

> **Activity 5.11**
>
> Review the effects of the autonomic nervous system.

? What are the implications of the physical and cognitive effects of anxiety for the assessment process?

Various techniques can be used to support an anxious patient:

- Cognitive interventions, such as providing accurate information in an appropriate form, has been shown to reduce anxiety (Beddows 1997). It is important to provide the amount of information that the patient is ready to accept.
- Behavioural interventions such as relaxation techniques, including controlled breathing, or guided imagery, can be helpful.
- Sensory interventions such as reducing noise and light levels, the use of massage, aromatherapy, warm baths or music.
- Pharmacological interventions such as anxiolytic drugs, which can be used on a short- or long-term basis (Fishel 1998).

Evidence-based practice

It is generally accepted by the nursing profession that giving patients information can be helpful in reducing their anxiety level, and research supports this view (Beddows 1997; Radcliffe 1993). In a small-scale study conducted in a day surgery unit, nine out of ten trained nurses identified patient empowerment and anxiety reduction as their reasons for providing information (Reid 1997). Less popular responses (50–80 per cent) included meeting the patient's needs, providing reassurance, to prepare patients for the unknown and to encourage patient choice. Other reasons were to satisfy personal accountability, encourage compliance, comply with the *Patient's Charter* (DoH 1991) and avoid litigation.

Interestingly, none of the sample group felt that information giving contributed to ease of discharge, which is clearly a key aspect of day care patient management.

? Which techniques could be helpful in reducing Mr Stevens's anxiety whilst he is attending the endoscopy suite?

Practice tip

Anxiety can be communicated interpersonally, and maintaining a calm, confident and professional approach when dealing with anxious patients can be very helpful.

Evidence-based practice

One simple and inexpensive way to reduce anxiety during outpatient bronchoscopy is the use of music. In 1995 Dubois et al, using a prospective randomised trial, demonstrated a significant reduction in anxiety levels in a sample of 21 patients who were played calming music throughout the procedure. Anxiety levels were assessed by means of physiological parameters (heart rate, blood pressure and oxygen saturation) and the patients' self-reports.

The control group who did not hear any music (29 patients) was found to be more anxious. The research also demonstrated that the staff undertaking the bronchoscopies were unable to assess accurately the level of distress being experienced by the patients during the procedure.

Physiological assessment

Pain

It is important to assess pain early in any assessment procedure, as a patient in pain is unlikely to be able to communicate in a relaxed and effective manner.

When pain is a significant problem, this should be relieved whenever possible before continuing with the assessment. Mr Stevens is troubled with pain and his current analgesic regime is not very effective. His medication should therefore be reviewed by a doctor, and Mr Stevens given appropriate advice as to how to obtain further support in his pain management (for further details see Chapter 13 on pain management).

Practice tip

Many patients who are taking analgesic medication regularly are concerned when asked to be 'nil by mouth' for a procedure, as they may miss several doses of their pain relief and suffer serious pain as a consequence. It is often possible for 'nil by mouth' patients to continue with pain relief, swallowing the medication with the smallest amount of plain water possible. If this is not possible, alternative routes can be used to administer pain relief; sublingual, rectal or injected drugs can be prescribed. It is important that pain control issues are discussed with the patient when procedures are planned, in order that the appropriate treatment can be organised and the patient can be kept fully informed.

Several measurements can be taken to assess Mr Stevens's physiological status. Temperature, pulse, respiration and blood pressure are recorded prior to the procedure, and the results provide a crucial 'baseline' against which comparisons can be made during the procedure and in the recovery phase. Any major abnormality in the initial reading may result in the postponement of the bronchoscopy. It is therefore vital that the measurements are correctly taken and accurately recorded.

Practice tip

All patients undergoing invasive procedures will require temperature, pulse, respiration and blood pressure recordings, but some patients may need additional monitoring, depending on their underlying physical condition. For example, a patient with diabetes will need capillary blood glucose measurements.

Can you measure capillary blood glucose levels? What problems could arise if a diabetic patient needs to be 'nil by mouth' in preparation for bronchoscopy?

Temperature

Disorders of body temperature may indicate that the patient has an infection, their condition is deteriorating, or that they have a problem with their thermo-regulation.

Traditionally, the temperature is recorded orally, in the sublingual pocket of the mouth, with the lips sealed. This may be difficult for patients who are dyspnoeic and mouth-breathing, or confused, when the axilla should be used as an alternative.

What is the normal range of oral temperature for an adult? Is the range different for axillary recording?

Evidence-based practice

Mercury thermometers have traditionally been used to record body temperature, however, there are problems associated with their use:

- It is time consuming to record temperature accurately using a mercury thermometer. Research suggests a minimum of five minutes to record temperature orally, and seven minutes using the axilla (Buswell 1997).
- Mercury thermometers present a safety hazard both in terms of broken glass and spilt mercury.
- Cross-infection may arise if cleaning of thermometers between patients is inadequate.

● Mercury thermometers can become inaccurate after a period of time. Research suggests 25 per cent of mercury thermometers were inaccurate after eight months of use or storage (Fulbrook 1993).

Activity 5.12

Other temperature recording devices are available such as single use disposable thermometers, electronic thermometers and infra-red tympanic thermometers. Check which types of thermometer are available in your practice area, and do you know how to use them all accurately?

Pulse

The pulse may be recorded using an electronic monitoring device or may be palpated manually. The most accessible, and therefore most commonly used site for palpation is the radial pulse.

Suggest three other sites used to palpate arterial pulses.

Before measuring the pulse, allow the patient to rest, so that the pulse rate is not artificially elevated by physical exertion. Take note of the rate, rhythm and volume of the pulse over one minute.

What is the normal range of pulse rate in an adult? Can you define 'tachycardia' and 'bradycardia'?

Blood pressure

Blood pressure is a measure of the force that blood exerts on the blood vessel walls and is usually measured in millimetres of mercury (mmHg), using a manual sphygmomanometer or electronic monitoring device.

Evidence-based practice

It is often assumed that nurses accurately record blood pressure; however, research has indicated that there is a lack of knowledge regarding its measurement, and that the procedure was performed incorrectly by a large percentage of those surveyed (Gillespie and Curzio 1998). The British Hypertension Society (Petrie et al 1997) made recommendations for good practice when recording blood pressure. In preparation the nurse should:

● Provide an explanation of the procedure to the patient.
● Allow the patient to rest for three minutes if the patient is supine or seated, and for one minute if the patient is standing.

- Position the patient correctly, supporting the arm and ensuring the upper arm is at the same level as the heart.
- Ensure that tight or restrictive clothing is removed from the arm.
- Use an appropriately sized cuff so that the bladder covers 80 per cent of the circumference of the upper arm.
- Apply the cuff evenly and smoothly on the arm with the tubing exiting from the top of the cuff, ensuring that the centre of the bladder covers the brachial artery.
- Position the manometer within three feet of the patient and at the operator's eye level

Estimating systolic blood pressure

Systolic blood pressure represents the force of the contraction that empties the ventricles of the heart, pushing blood into the aorta. Systolic blood pressure is estimated by inflating the cuff while palpating the brachial or radial artery, and noting the systolic pressure when pulsations stop.

Completing the measurement:

- Place the diaphragm of the stethoscope gently over the point of maximum pulsation of the brachial artery.
- Do not tuck the diaphragm under the edge of the cuff.
- Inflate the cuff to approximately 30mmHg above the palpated systolic blood pressure.
- Deflate the system at 2–3mmHg per second or per heartbeat.
- Systolic blood pressure is measured when a minimum of two clear repetitive tapping sounds are heard and the diastolic blood pressure is measured at the point when the sounds can no longer be heard.
- The measurement includes a recording of the blood pressure to the nearest 2mmHg, the arm used and its position.

Practice tip

Ensure the ear-pieces of the stethoscope are pointing towards your nose so they are the right way around, otherwise you will not hear anything!

Do not be alarmed if the patient is hypertensive and has tachycardia. This may be due to the anxiety of hospital admission. Have a look in the patient's notes and compare with the measurements taken in the outpatients clinic.

Activity 5.13

Review your textbook to remind yourself of the physiology relating to blood pressure regulation. Why is it important to record the blood pressure prior to an investigation such as a bronchoscopy?

Respiration

Many patients undergoing bronchoscopy will have respiratory symptoms, and may well have abnormalities of their respiratory rate, depth and rhythm. It is still very important to observe their respiration as very severe abnormalities may have recently developed, and a baseline for comparison during and after the bronchoscopy is essential. A full respiratory assessment is not appropriate at this time, but it is helpful to be aware of how such an assessment may be conducted.

Practice tip

When observing respiration, make sure the patient does not realise what you are doing. If you know somebody is watching you breathe, you will instinctively take voluntary control of your breathing. Many nurses observe respiration while holding the patient's wrist, which encourages them to think you are still counting the pulse rate.

Activity 5.14

Review the control of respiration in a physiology text. Why might Mr Stevens's breathing be abnormal?

Respiratory assessment

Respiratory assessment involves the actual observation of respiration and information related to coughing, sputum production, haemoptysis and dyspnoea. If the patient is particularly breathless, ask closed questions which can be answered with a 'yes' or 'no' response to avoid further distress. It is also very important to remember that respiratory assessment cannot be separated from cardiovascular assessment, as the two systems are closely interrelated.

A psychosocial history will reveal factors that may affect respiratory function. Note if the patient has any allergies, and if they have had any occupational exposure to asbestos, coal dust, gas fumes or other potential toxins. Does the patient smoke, or have they smoked in the past and, if so, how many packs for how many years?

The presence of cough is significant. The nature of the cough should be evaluated – listen and try to identify the character of the cough:

- Is it dry and hacking, which may indicate viral infection, early congestive cardiac failure or nervousness?
- Is the cough loose and productive, indicating possible problems in the peripheral bronchi and lung parenchyma (the essential active cells of the lung tissue)?

- Does the cough appear to stem from the upper airways, which may be indicated by a loud harsh stridor, or an audible wheeze?
- Is the cough chronic and productive, which may indicate pulmonary disease?
- Is there pain associated with the cough? If so, note the type of pain and its position.

Factors exacerbating the coughing should be explored. For how long has the cough been noticed and what factors make it worse or better? Recent onset of cough for a few days suggests infection. A cough, progressively increasing for weeks or months, may be indicative of carcinoma (O'Hanlon-Nichols 1998).

Practice tip

A persistent cough can be one of the earliest signs of a lung tumour. It is often overlooked by smokers who may have had a 'smoker's cough' for some time. When assessing patients, remember to ask if their cough has changed in any way.

Do ask if any sputum is expectorated, and note the frequency, amount and colour. Thick yellow or green sputum is usually due to bacterial infection and a rusty colour may indicate bacterial pneumonia. Frothy, liquid white or pink sputum indicates pulmonary oedema. Determine if there is any haemoptysis, and ascertain the colour, amount and how frequently this occurs.

Assess the patient for any signs of difficulty in breathing, or dyspnoea. This may be acute or chronic. Ascertain any factors which exacerbate the breathlessness, for example in relation to exertion or positioning. Has the breathlessness become suddenly or progressively worse? What could Mr Stevens do a year or a month ago that his is unable to do now? Is the dyspnoea more severe at night and is Mr Stevens able to lie down without undue distress? This will determine if he will be able to tolerate the semi-recumbent position normally used for the procedure.

When the history has been taken, the physical examination can be performed. When assessing respiratory function, it is important to observe the chest, therefore ask the patient to remove his shirt so that chest movements can be seen clearly.

Let the patient rest before the physical examination, so that observations recorded are reliable, and not affected by physical exertion.

Many respiratory abnormalities can be witnessed when assessing chest movements. Observe the rate, pattern and depth of respiration. The normal resting respiratory rate is 12 to16 breaths per minute in an adult, with expiration taking approximately twice as long as inspiration. Assess for abnormal breathing patterns or uneven rhythm or respiration. Compare the movement on both sides of the body; is there any difference in the shape or symmetry of the chest? Is the patient using accessory muscles, demonstrated by the use of the scalene, sternomastoid and pectoralis muscles when breathing?

The colour of the skin may be an indicator of respiratory status. Central cyanosis, that is, blue discoloration seen in the mucous membranes of the mouth and lips, is associated with low arterial oxygenation, which may result from inadequate ventilation.

What is peripheral cyanosis? What can cause this?

A very useful non-invasive monitoring technique, which can contribute significantly to respiratory assessment, is pulse oximetry.

Pulse Oximetry

Monitoring the haemoglobin oxygen saturation by pulse oximetry gives a reflection of the amount of oxygen available in the tissues. A probe placed on the finger or ear lobe indicates the percentage of oxy-haemoglobin present in the capillary blood, which is displayed on a monitor. Normal values of oxygen saturation for adults vary between 96 and 99 per cent. However, this may be less than 90 per cent if a patient has chronic lung disease, and this may be normal for them.

Pulse oximetry provides rapid 'real time' information about the onset of some pulmonary complications, and so can be invaluable during bronchoscopy – and many other procedures. However, to interpret the reading accurately, it is important to note if the patient is receiving oxygen therapy, and to understand the limitations of the recordings.

Evidence-based practice

Use of pulse oximetry

Pulse oximetry is now widely used in many clinical situations, as it is non-invasive and easy to establish. However, research undertaken by Stoneham et al (1994), identified a significant lack of knowledge of the basic principles of pulse oximetry amongst nurses and junior doctors, and that both groups made serious errors in interpreting readings.

There are several factors which will result in inaccurate readings (see the practice tip below). The most important point is that no direct indication of a patient's ventilation can be obtained by pulse oximetry but only of their oxygenation, thus it is possible for a previously well-oxygenated patient to have a satisfactory oximetry recording after they have actually stopped breathing!

Guidelines for oximetry use are available (Stoneham 1995) and any nurse using such equipment must ensure that they have received adequate instruction and are sufficiently knowledgeable to practice safely.

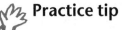 **Practice tip**

When using a finger probe, abnormal readings may be obtained if:
- The patient has poor circulation in their fingers
- The patient has cardiac dysrhythmias

- The probe is not positioned correctly
- The patient is wearing nail varnish
- The patient is shivering
- Overhead lighting is excessive

Age, gender, anaemia, jaundice and dark skin have little or no effect on the readings (Stoneham 1995).

Once the assessment is completed, any concerns that the nurse might have should be discussed with the bronchoscopist, who will then decide whether to proceed or not. In addition to physiological and psychological concerns that the assessing nurse might wish to discuss, organisational issues must be considered. The lack of a suitably experienced bronchoscopist, lack of adequate staff and facilities to deal with any emergency which may arise (pneumothorax, haemorrhage, cardiopulmonary arrest), and inability to provide safe post-procedural care remain absolute contraindications to the procedure (Belli 1999).

Results of the blood tests and pulmonary function tests performed will be available in the outpatients clinic, and these must also be considered.

Activity 5.15

1 The blood tests normally performed prior to bronchoscopy would be:
- Haemoglobin level
- Full blood count
- Urea and electrolyte levels
- Clotting screen

Find out more about these blood tests. Why are they required?

2 Arrange to visit a pulmonary function laboratory to learn about the tests and watch them being performed or, better still, have a go!

Consent – the legal and ethical implications

Before an invasive procedure such as a bronchoscopy, the person who is going to carry out the procedure is legally obliged to obtain the patient's consent. Failure to do this may result in legal action against the bronchoscopist for battery (Dimond 1995). However, obtaining the patient's consent is more than asking them to sign the appropriate form; a number of important legal and ethical principles must be observed.

Mr Stevens is prepared for bronchoscopy. He has signed the consent form, his nose and throat are sprayed with lidocaine, and he is sedated with intravenous Alfentanil, an opioid analgesic. The bronchoscopy is then performed.

Consent may be implied or expressed. Implied consent is assumed when patients take actions which imply that they agree to a procedure. Mr Stevens has arrived at the hospital ready to undergo bronchoscopy. This may be regarded as implied consent to the procedure. Implied consent is often regarded as adequate for minor procedures, such as measuring blood pressure, but it is usual practice to ensure expressed consent for more complex procedures.

Expressed consent may be verbal or written. Verbal consent is often used when administering an injection, or taking a blood sample, and is quite valid in law. Written consent is usually obtained for complex procedures, especially where there is some risk involved. It is not required in law that consent must be written, but it is generally regarded as good practice (Dimond 1995). In the event of legal action, it is much easier to prove that consent had been expressed if documentary evidence can be produced.

Regardless of whether the consent is written or verbal, certain criteria must be satisfied if the consent is to be valid:

- The patient must be able to understand what is going on and what he is consenting to.
- The consent must be voluntary, there must be no coercion, either from health care professionals, or from relatives and friends.
- The consent must not be obtained by deceit. Questions asked by the patient regarding the treatment must be answered truthfully.
- The consent must be informed. The patient must have been told in general terms about the procedure. Informed consent recognises the patient's right to autonomy and self-determination, enabling them to make valid choices regarding the acceptance or refusal of treatment (Buchanan 1995).
- It is not required in law that detailed explanations of all possible risks are given, and failure to do this will not invalidate the consent, but could lead to charges of negligence in some circumstances (Carson and Montgomery 1989).

Thus Mr Stevens must be told that the bronchoscopy will involve a small tube being passed through his nose into his airways, and that this may make him cough, but he will be able to breathe. He does not have to be told that there is a very small risk that obtaining biopsy specimens from any tumour seen may cause a major haemorrhage, or that rarely patients suffer an anaphylactic reaction to the drugs used in the procedure. However, if Mr Stevens asks directly about such complications, he must be answered honestly.

 What is the nurse's role in obtaining consent? If you are uncertain check this out.

Applied pharmacology

Lidocaine

Lignocaine is a local anaesthetic agent which is used during bronchoscopy to reduce discomfort caused by the introduction of the scope, and to suppress the cough reflex whilst the trachea and bronchi are examined. A lidocaine solution is sprayed into the nose and throat before the procedure, and additional doses are administered through the bronchoscope as the procedure progresses. Lidocaine is effectively absorbed via the mucous membranes and has a rapid onset, the effects lasting from 1½ to 2 hours.

Patients who have had their throats sprayed with lignocaine will not be able to swallow normally until the effects of the drug have worn off. To protect their airway it is important that they remain 'nil by mouth' until the drug has worn off.

Alfentanil

Alfentanil is an opioid analgesic which, when used intravenously, has a very rapid onset and short duration of action. It is therefore very useful during short, invasive procedures, to ensure that the patient is pain free and relaxed during the procedure and can recover rapidly afterwards.

As with all opioids, respiratory depression can occur, and close observation of respiratory effort is crucial. Naloxone, an opiate antagonist which acts as a respiratory stimulant, can be used to reverse the depressant effects, but serious respiratory compromise will require resuscitation and assisted ventilation.

Any drug which causes respiratory depression must be used with extreme caution in any patient who has a respiratory problem, such as Mr Stevens.

Oxygen

Oxygen is administered to patients undergoing bronchoscopy, usually nasally, to ensure that the passage of the bronchoscope does not result in hypoxia. Oxygen saturation levels are monitored by pulse oximetry throughout the procedure. Oxygen is commonly used in hospital and it is generally regarded as safe. However, it must be remembered that high concentrations of oxygen (above 24 to 28 per cent) can adversely affect the respiratory drive of some patients with chronic lung disease. Prolonged use of oxygen in concentrations above 50 per cent is thought to damage lung tissue (Fell and Boehm 1998), therefore it should be used with caution and as prescribed. Oxygen also supports combustion and consequently constitutes a major fire hazard.

? How is oxygen prescribed in your practice areas?

The nurse's role in endoscopy

The nurse has two main roles when assisting with the procedure. The first is the care and monitoring of the patient. This includes the preparation of the patient, monitoring throughout the bronchoscopy and post-procedure care, including preparation for discharge. The second important aspect of the role is to assist the endoscopist to perform the procedure correctly and safely. This includes preparing, maintaining and assisting with the equipment, handling specimens and ensuring appropriate record keeping.

Maintenance of equipment

The equipment used for all endoscopic procedures needs to be maintained in good working order to ensure that the investigations are performed safely and effectively. Specific guidelines are followed for inspection of the bronchoscope, and relevant training is required to ensure the correct care and maintenance of the equipment. The nurse needs to be familiar with the preparation of the bronchoscope, which should be inspected before use to check for faults. If there are any suspected abnormalities, the instrument should not be used. After use, correct cleaning, disinfection and storage is essential (AORN 1998), and detailed nursing knowledge of correct procedures is required.

A working party from the British Society of Gastroenterology reviewed the cleaning and disinfection of endoscopic equipment and made recommendations for practice (British Society of Gastroenterology 1988). The three essential stages that ensure the equipment is thoroughly cleaned and decontaminated are:

1 Mechanical cleaning in detergent solution
2 Disinfection
3 Rinsing

The introduction of the Control of Substances Harmful to Health (COSHH) legislation by the Health and Safety Executive, has had an impact on the cleaning of endoscopic equipment. This legislation provides maximum acceptable levels of vapour permitted in the atmosphere to protect staff working with hazardous substances. Various chemicals used for the disinfection of endoscopes are covered in the COSHH regulations. This means that the employer is legally obliged to inform all staff involved in the decontamination of equipment about the risk of exposure. They must also provide education and training regarding the safe management of these chemicals.

Activity 5.16

Familiarise yourself with the infection control policy in your area. Are there recommendations for bronchoscopic procedures? Other relevant policies include the COSHH requirement and universal precautions – these are essential for safe practice.

Assisting with the bronchoscopy procedure

The nurse assisting with the bronchoscopy should be aware of the complications which could arise during the procedure, and be familiar with the emergency procedures to follow in this instance.

Before assisting with the bronchoscopy, determine the purpose of the procedure. Is it being performed with the aim of assessment, sputum aspiration, or to obtain a biopsy specimen? This will enable the proper preparation of equipment such as specimen pots and pathology request cards. Chest X-rays are required to help locate any lesion. Often anterior–posterior and lateral chest X-rays are needed, so it is important that these are available.

? What is the difference between an anterior–posterior chest X-ray and a lateral chest X-ray? Why might both be needed?

The results of a clotting screen (to ensure that the patient has normal blood coagulation) will also be needed.

During the procedure, the flexible bronchoscope is passed into the mouth or nose and into the upper airways. Supplementary oxygen can be administered as required, and the nurse may have to assist with suctioning secretions out of the mouth, using an oropharyngeal sucker.

Care of the patient during the bronchoscopy procedure

Patients may be extremely anxious about the procedure and be in need of psychological support. Explaining what is happening to them at every stage can reduce their anxiety and increase co-operation. They need to be reassured that they will be able to breathe normally through the bronchoscope. The patient must be monitored continuously throughout the procedure.

Activity 5.17

Before reading on, make a list of the observations you would make of a patient during bronchoscopy – and why? Compare your list with a colleague!

The minimum level of observation should include:

- Level of consciousness.
- Response to the procedure, for example, pain, shortness of breath.
- Response to any drugs administered.
- Levels of patient oxygenation determined by pulse oximetry.
- Respiratory rate and depth.
- Blood pressure and pulse to assess any change in cardiac status.

Specimens and record keeping

Accurate record keeping is essential to ensure continuity of care and to provide a baseline for reference when making discharge decisions. Documentation should include the patient's condition during the procedure, with observations of blood pressure, pulse, respiration and oximetry recorded. Any biopsies that were taken, and the tests requested, should also be noted.

Practice tip

When collecting biopsies, check that the patient details are accurate on the specimen pot and the request card and that the spelling is correct. Make sure that you use a date of birth, address or hospital number as well as the name to avoid confusion. It is a good idea to label the specimen pots before the procedure, especially if several biopsies are taken.

Activity 5.18

A patient is undergoing a bronchoscopy and you are the nurse assisting the endoscopist. The procedure has progressed normally and the patient's observations have been stable throughout: pulse 78 bpm and blood pressure 140/80mmHg. The endoscopist decides to take a biopsy of a suspected tumour, which is a routine test. After this has happened, you notice that the patient suddenly appears very distressed, and is pale and clammy to the touch. You have noticed that the blood pressure has suddenly dropped to 70/40mmHg and the pulse has risen to 120 bpm.

A What does this alert you to?

At this point the endoscopist notes that there is a large amount of fresh blood pooling in the lung. The patient coughs and a large volume of bright red blood is visible, quickly covering the pillows.

B What do you think has happened?

You summon help, and prepare the resuscitation equipment while the endoscopist maintains the patient's airway with suctioning. The patient is given intravenous fluids and blood and his condition stabilises. He is taken for surgery.

The cause of this incident was major endobronchial bleeding following the biopsy of a highly vascular tumour.

Activity 5.19

Consider the following:

1 Are you aware of the physiological markers of major haemorrhage?
2 Would you know the resuscitation procedures where you work?
3 Do you know the location of the resuscitation equipment and whether it is checked and working?

It is your responsibility to ensure that you can answer, 'Yes'!

Evidence-based practice

When a cardiac arrest occurs in hospital, nurses are most likely to be first on the scene. It has been demonstrated that if the arrest is witnessed and resuscitation is started early, the patient is more likely to survive (Wynne 1993). It is therefore essential that nurses are able to diagnose cardiac arrest, know how to summon help and how to initiate basic life-support when required. Evidence suggests that a significant number of nurses are ineffective when performing cardiopulmonary resuscitation (Crunden 1991). Poor underpinning knowledge, lack of practice and hence lack of confidence, have been reported (Flisher 1992) resulting in reduced levels of competence. Lack of practice and rehearsal results in rapid deterioration of psychomotor skills (Crunden 1991; Laurent 1992). There is evidence that if staff are well trained, resuscitation occurs more rapidly, which increases the chance of patient survival (Laurent 1992). Although theoretical knowledge is important, it is crucial to practise life-support skills regularly using a manikin, preferably in a simulated arrest scenario.

Practice tip

Attend basic life-support training regularly, at least every six months. Keep updating your skills!

Patient discharge

Mr Stevens's bronchoscopy is completed uneventfully, biopsy specimens are obtained and dispatched for pathological analysis. After a period of supervised recovery and a final nursing assessment, he is allowed to leave the hospital, accompanied by his daughter.

The successful completion of a day case procedure requires the timely and appropriate discharge of the patient. Recovery may be divided into three stages:

1 Early recovery, when the patient has emerged from anaesthesia and sedating drugs, is able to open their eyes and protect their airway.
2 Intermediate recovery, when the patient is ready to go home, can stand and walk unaided, and their vital signs have been stable for at least one hour.
3 Full recovery, when the patient has resumed their normal daily activities, for example, going to work, driving (Lugay et al 1996).

Liaison with the patient's GP, practice nurse or district nurse is essential to ensure continuity of care. It is important that key information reaches the health care professionals who will be responsible for Mr Stevens, by the quickest and most reliable route. If the procedure has not gone as planned, it may be necessary to speak directly to a member of the primary care team before Mr Stevens can be allowed to leave hospital care.

To ensure that the patient has reached the intermediate recovery stage, the following points should be considered:

- Is there any evidence of physiological or psychological complications arising from the procedure?
- If the patient's throat has been anaesthetised, has his swallow reflex returned to normal?

? How should the swallow reflex be assessed?

- Does the patient know who to contact and how, if any problems arise?

? In what format would this information be most useful to the patient?

- Does the patient have access to a telephone? Can he use it?
  (Regular observation in the post-procedure phase enables rapid detection of immediate complications, but some problems can be delayed, e.g. slow bleeding, infection.)
- Does the patient have appropriate transport and escort home?
- Does the patient understand the next stage of his care? Does he need to see his GP or return to outpatients? If so, when?
  Remember that any patient who has been sedated for a procedure may well suffer some loss of memory, so information given in the immediate post-procedure phase will need to be supplemented with written information, or the repetition of information to a relative or friend.

Practice tip

Discharge planning should begin at or before admission, to ensure good continuity of care. Questions related to the patient's safe discharge need to be answered before the procedure, or before the patient is admitted. If the patient's safety is likely to be compromised after discharge, the procedure cannot go ahead.

? In your local endoscopy unit, who takes responsibility for discharging the patients?

Evidence-based practice

Research designed to identify an optimal method for determining when to safely discharge patients undergoing endoscopic procedures after conscious sedation posed the question: 'Is it possible to predict which patients will suffer pre-discharge or post-discharge complications following an endoscopic procedure?' (Lugay et al 1996).

Although it was a limited study, results suggested a close correlation between intra-procedural occurrences and post-procedure complications. Thus any patient who experiences intra-procedural events requires closer post-procedural monitoring, Also, there is evidence that age is predictive of length of time in recovery, with older patients taking longer to recover than younger patients. Thus it would seem logical to organise procedures to ensure that older patients are examined earlier in the day to ensure that enough time is available for them to recover fully prior to discharge.

It may not be possible to give the patient accurate diagnostic information following a bronchoscopy. Even if a tumour has been seen, the exact nature of the tumour is unconfirmed until results from biopsies are available. Many patients will therefore face a period of anxiety and uncertainty awaiting results. At this very stressful time, patients are often not in contact with health care professionals and rely on friends and family for support. It may be helpful to give patients and their families information regarding potential sources of support, such as patient support groups, telephone helplines and nurse specialists. Evidence suggests that such services, if the patients are aware of them, are well used. One study revealed that a nurse specialist in Glasgow received an average of eight calls per referred patient (Fennerty et al 1996).

It is also helpful to remind the patient that they can contact their GP or practice nurse for advice and support whenever they need it, ensuring that they have the relevant contact information.

Mr Stevens: 'It was all right actually – I was pretty worried about it before I came in, but to be quite honest, I don't really remember very much about it! I was glad to have my daughter with me. She asked all the questions, you know, what happens next, when will we know anything. The nurses were very good. They kept explaining things. I remember being thirsty, and having to wait for a drink, and my throat was a bit sore for a couple of days, but nothing to really bother about.

The worst thing is still not knowing – they just said I have to wait for the results. I really want to know what is going on now.'

Conclusion: developing your portfolio of practice

Reflect on what you have learned whilst studying this scenario, perhaps by reviewing the learning outcomes and concepts at the beginning of the chapter. In particular consider what you gained whilst visiting an endoscopy unit to observe a procedure, and in discussion with the endoscopy staff.

The key professional considerations related to this procedure are transferable to many investigative procedures and treatment protocols:

- Patient safety
- Reducing patient anxiety
- Effective interprofessional communication
- Effective use of resources

Activity 5.20

Write a reflective account for inclusion in your personal profile, identifying how your learning in these key areas has developed.

References

AORN (1998) Recommended practices for use and care of endoscopes *AORN Journal* 67 (1), pp. 256–61.

Bassett, C. (1997) Medical investigations 4: bronchoscopy. *British Journal of Nursing* 6 (4), pp. 592–3.

Beddows, J. (1997) Alleviating pre-operative anxiety in patients: a study. *Nursing Standard* 11 (37), pp 35–8.

Belli, M. (1999) Bronchoscopy. *American Journal of Nursing* 99 (7), pp. 24AA–24DD.

British Society of Gastroenterology (1988). Cleaning and disinfection of equipment for gastrointestinal flexible endoscopy. Interim recommendations of a working party of the British Society of Gastroenterology, Leicester meeting.

Buchanan, M. (1995) Enabling patients to make informed decisions. *Nursing Times* 91 (18), pp. 27–9.

Burgess, L. (1994) An epidemic of massive proportions. *Professional Nurse* May, pp. 566–72.

Buswell, C. (1997) Comparing mercury and disposable thermometers. *Professional Nurse* 12 (5), pp. 359–62.

Carson, D., Montgomery, J. (1989) *Nursing and the Law.* London: Macmillan Education Limited.

Chapman, A. (1996) Current theory and practice: a study of pre-operative fasting. *Nursing Standard* 10 (18), pp. 33–6.

Claxton, D. (1999) Diagnosing, Detecting and Treating Lung Cancer. *Nursing Times* 95 (20), pp. 44–6.

Crunden, E. (1991) An investigation into why qualified nurses inappropriately describe their own cardiopulmonary resuscitation skills. *Journal of Advanced Nursing* 16, pp. 597–605.

Day, J. (1998) Lung cancer: screen or prevent? *Practice Nursing* 9 (5), pp. 32–5.

Dest, V. (2000) Lung cancer. *Registered Nurse* 63 (5), pp. 32–8.

Department of Health (1991) *Patient's Charter*. London: HMSO.

Department of Health (1992) *Health of the Nation: Key Areas Handbook – Cancers*. London: DoH.

Department of Heath (1999a) *Saving Lives: Our Healthier Nation*. London: DoH.

Department of Health (1999b) *Smoking Kills*. London: DoH.

Dimond, B. (1995) *Legal Aspects of Nursing*. 2nd Edition. London: Prentice Hall.

Dubois, J., Barter, T., Pratter, M. (1995) Music improves patient comfort level during out-patient bronchoscopy. *Chest* 108 (1), pp. 129–30.

Fell, H., Boehm, M. (1998) Easing the discomfort of oxygen therapy. *Nursing Times* 94 (38), pp. 56–8.

Fennerty, A., Reid, A., O'Donnell, M. (1996) A named nurse programme for the care of patients with lung cancer. *Thorax* 51 (Supplement 3), p. A57.

Fishel, A. (1998) Nursing management of anxiety and panic. *Nursing Clinics of North America* 33 (1), pp. 135–50.

Flisher, D. (1992) Improving nurses' resuscitation skills. *Nursing Standard* 6 (50), pp. 32–5.

Fulbrook, P. (1993) Core temperature measurement in adults: a literature review. *Journal of Advanced Nursing* 18, pp. 1451–60.

Gillespie, A., Curzio, J. A. (1998) Blood pressure measurement: assessing staff knowledge. *Nursing Standard* 12 (23), pp. 35–7.

Hamilton-Smith, S. (1972) *Nil By Mouth: A Descriptive Study of Nursing Care in Relation to Pre-Operative Fasting*. London: Royal College of Nursing.

Kosco, P., Held-Warmkessel, J. (2000) Lung cancer – can early detection become a reality in the 21st century? *American Journal of Nursing* April Supplement, pp. 13–7.

Laurent, C. (1992) Arresting Facts. *Nursing Times* 88 (25), p. 23.

Ley, P. (1988) *Communicating with Patients: Improving Communication, Satisfaction and Compliance*. London: Croom-Helm.

Lugay, M., Otto, G., Kong, M., Mason, D., Wilets, I. (1996) Recovery time and safe discharge of endoscopy patients after conscious sedation. *Gastroenterology Nursing* 19 (6), pp. 194–200.

Nursing and Midwifery Council (2002): *Code of Professional Conduct*. London: NMC.

NHS Centre for Reviews and Dissemination (1998) Effectiveness matters: smoking cessation: what can the health service do. *University of York* 3 (1).

NHS Executive (1998) *Guidance on Commissioning Cancer Services: Improving Outcomes in Lung Cancer: The Research Evidence*. London: DoH.

O'Hanlon-Nichols, T. (1998) Basic assessment series: the adult pulmonary system. *American Journal of Nursing* 98 (2), pp. 39–45.

Petrie, J., O'Brien, E., Litler, W., de Swiet, M. (1997) *British Hypertension Society: Recommendations on Blood Pressure Measurements.* 2nd Edition. London: British Hypertension Society.

Quinn, S. (1999) Lung cancer: the role of the nurse in treatment and prevention. *Nursing Standard* 13 (41), pp. 49–54.

Radcliffe, S. (1993) Pre-operative information: the role of the ward nurse. *British Journal of Nursing* 2 (6), pp. 305–9.

Reid, J. (1997) Meeting the informational needs of patients in a day surgery setting – an exploratory level study. *British Journal of Theatre Nursing* 7 (4), pp. 19–24.

Spear, H. (1996) Anxiety. *Registered Nurse* July, pp. 40–5.

Stafrace, J. (1998) Assessment: the key to patient safety when undergoing an endoscopic procedure. *Gastroenterology Nursing* 21 (3), pp. 131–4.

Stoneham, M., Savile, G., Wilson, I. (1994) Knowledge about pulse oximetry among medical and nursing staff. *Lancet* 344 (12), pp. 1339–42.

Stoneham, M. (1995) Uses and limitations of pulse oximetry. *British Journal of Hospital Medicine* 54 (1), pp. 35–41.

Thompson, I., Melia, K., Boyd, K. (1994) *Nursing Ethics.* Edinburgh: Churchill Livingstone.

Wynne, C. (1993) Revival techniques. *Nursing Times* 89 (11), pp. 26–31.

Resources

📖 Further reading

Annotated bibliography

Bassett, C. (1997) Medical investigations 4: bronchoscopy. *British Journal of Nursing* 6 (4), pp. 592–3.

    This article is part of a very useful series which provides clear and concise information about a variety of medical investigations. This information will enable nurses to explain procedures to their patients more confidently, and to provide essential pre- and post-procedure care.

Belli, M. (1999) Bronchoscopy. *American Journal of Nursing* 99 (7), pp. 24AA–24DD.

    Another useful review of bronchoscopic procedure, which highlights contraindications to the procedure, discusses drugs commonly used and explains post-procedural care.

Burgess, L. (1994) An epidemic of massive proportions. *Professional Nurse* May, pp. 566–72.

    This article provides an excellent overview of the physiological, psychological and sociological effects of cigarette smoking in the United Kingdom. Thorough knowledge of this subject provides nurses with greater insight into patients' smoking habits, and may assist in the identification of effective smoking cessation strategies.

Day, J. (1998) Lung cancer: screen or prevent? *Practice Nursing* 9 (5), pp. 32–4.

    The lack of an appropriate screening procedure for lung cancer results in a poor prognosis, as many patients have widespread disease by the time they are diagnosed. In this article issues related to potential screening techniques are discussed, and the need to focus on primary prevention by reducing smoking is highlighted.

NHS Executive (1998) *Guidance on Commissioning Cancer Services: Improving Outcomes in Lung Cancer: The Research Evidence.* London: DoH.

A fascinating document which provides an overview of the research evidence underpinning recommendations currently being made by the NHS Executive, aimed at improving the outcomes in the treatment of patients with lung cancer. The available research evidence is reviewed in seven intervention categories:

1 Prevention
2 Access, diagnosis and staging
3 Multi-professional teams
4 Communication, information and support
5 Radical treatment for non-small cell lung cancer
6 Radical treatment for small cell lung cancer
7 Palliative interventions and care

Of particular interest to nursing students could be research related to smoking cessation and the role of the nurse within the multi-disciplinary team.

O'Hanlon-Nichols, T. (1998) Basic assessment series: the adult pulmonary system. *American Journal of Nursing* 98 (2), pp. 39–45.

This article is written by a North American nurse. Cultural differences in current assessment practices must be acknowledged, as many British nurses do not regularly perform chest auscultation or percussion, although there would seem to be no reason why practice should not be developed in this area. Using a case history approach, O'Hanlon provides guidelines for pulmonary assessment which would be of use to any nurse caring for patients with any form of respiratory disease.

Quinn, S. (1999) Lung cancer: the role of the nurse in treatment and prevention. *Nursing Standard* 13 (41), pp. 49–54.

Having provided a very useful overview of the aetiology, pathophysiology and treatment of lung cancer, this article focuses on the nurse's role in palliative care, reviewing the management of dyspnoea and emphasising the importance of addressing the patient's spiritual needs.

@ Web pages

'Oncolink': **www.cancer.med.upenn.edu**
'Cancer Help': **www.medweb.bham.ac.uk/cancerhelp**
'Bacup' (British Association for Cancer United Patients): **www.cancerbacup.org.uk**
'British Lung Foundation': **www.lunguk.org/index.htm**
Government Documents: **www.doh.gov.uk**

☐ Video

Practical Aspects of Fibreoptic Bronchoscopy (1991) Keymed.

6

Insights into Mental Health Nursing

John W. Rawlinson
(with acknowledgements to Tom Keen)

Introduction

This chapter, which starts with some questions and uncertainties, is intended to help you to consider 'mental health' and uses a family-based scenario to explore issues surrounding the nature of mental health problems, the impact of mental illness and service responses to mental health problems. Using the example of a family affected by mental ill health, a range of issues is raised in relation to severe mental illness, community care and intentional self-harm. What is presented within the chapter represents its author's enquiry-led processes in considering some problems and issues in the field. You may find this and the books, journals, documents and internet resources listed at the end of the chapter useful. However, the primary learning resource should be your own process of enquiry and the sense and meaning you find on that experiential journey.

Learning outcomes

After working through this chapter, considering the various issues raised and undertaking the suggested activities, you should be able to:

- Discuss the concepts of mental health and mental illness.
- Develop more empathic understanding of the experience of a person and family affected by severe and enduring mental illness.
- Discuss the development and aims of community care for people with mental health problems in order to relate them to your local circumstances.
- Adopt an approach to people with mental health problems which, while valuing their perception, recognises the importance of assessing potential risks.
- Identify some key legal aspects of mental health care.

Concepts

- Mental health
- Mental illness
- Schizophrenia
- Suicide and parasuicide
- Risk

- Therapeutic relationships
- Community care
- Mental health services
- Mental health policy
- The law and mental health

? Has the 'mental health' prefix simply become the current euphemism for 'mental illness' or does 'mental health' have some intrinsic meaning with implications for health services? If you are following, or thinking of following, the 'mental health' nursing branch, you may also like to consider its meaning for you.

? What is the knowledge base for mental health care? What could be its relationship to existing professional knowledge bases such as those in nursing, social work and psychology? Consider how 'mental health' fits in with other subject areas you have investigated or studied.

Scenario *Introducing the Page family*

Julie and Martin Page and their family live in a small house, which they own, on a council estate in an urban area. They have been married for five years. Martin is 37 and although he is a qualified engineer, he has had long periods of sickness and lost his job two years ago. Although he had some redundancy money, they now rely on Julie's earnings in their attempts to keep up with their mortgage payments. Julie is the same age and works as a sales assistant in a department store. Between them they have three children, Julie's daughter Anna who is 14, her son Matthew who is 13 and their son Jake who is 5.

Mental health

The scenario describes a relatively typical family in Britain today. No longer does the average family consist of a husband and wife, the former of whom works for 40 years and the latter who looks after their children. Many marriages break up, many families realign and many families develop around different gender roles or sexual orientations. Most people can now expect periods of unemployment. In many 'normal' families, people experience mental health problems. No longer are such problems, and those who suffer from them, confined, away from society in rural asylums. We are beginning to recognise that, instead of the 'mentally ill', the 'mad' or the 'insane' being a small separate group, quite distinct from ourselves (and from whom we must be protected), mental health problems can touch any and all of our lives.

Activity 6.1

With a friend or a partner in your learning group agree to spend at least half an hour together on this exercise. Talk about your experiences so far of mental health issues and identify personal experiences which may inform your understanding of the issues involved. Share together as much as you feel able, but if there are any difficult issues or experiences which you decide not to share, notice your responses and reactions internally.

Identify any personal needs you may have in respect of mental health issues and the resources or support you may call on in working through this chapter.

Uncomfortable or personal issues may be raised for any of us in this area. If you feel that exploring this personally, or working with this client group may touch on personal areas for which you do not have sufficient support, make sure that you discuss it with your learning co-ordinator, a friend or mental health professional.

Evidence-based practice

A survey of psychiatric morbidity among adults in private households was carried out in 2000 by the Office for National Statistics on behalf of the Department of Health, the Scottish Executive and the National Assembly for Wales.

The information obtained is available in a searchable format at:

http://www.statistics.gov.uk/downloads/theme_health/psychmorb.pdf

Navigate through this to gain an overall impression of the general scale of mental health problems, or to look in more detail at the incidence of particular problems.

The scale of mental health problems

- About a quarter to a third of the population experience distressing psychological symptoms some time in the course of a year.
- One quarter of routine GP consultations are for people with a mental health problem.
- One in four people visit their GP with a psychological problem each year, the commonest being anxiety, depression and physical symptoms with a psychological background.
- Only 10 per cent of these problems are referred by the GP to a hospital specialist 90 per cent of mental health care being provided solely by primary care.

- Mild forms of depression affect half the population at some time in their lives, although severe depression will affect only one in a hundred.
- Dementia affects approximately 5 per cent of the population over 65. This prevalence doubles every five years over the age of 65.
- In the UK over 6000 people die each year from suicide, as many as die from road accidents.
- Unemployed people are twice as likely to have depression as people in work.
- Children in the poorest households are three times more likely to have mental health problems than children in well-off households.
- Half of all women and a quarter of all men will be affected by depression at some period during their lives.
- People who have been abused or been victims of domestic violence have higher rates of mental health problems.
- Between a quarter and a half of people using night shelters or sleeping rough may have a serious mental disorder, and up to half may be alcohol dependent.
- Some black and minority ethnic groups are diagnosed as having higher rates of mental disorder than the general population; refugees are especially vulnerable.
- There is a high rate of mental disorder in the prison population.
- People with drug and alcohol problems have higher rates of other mental health problems.
- People with physical illnesses have higher rates of mental health problems.
  (Derived from Goldberg and Huxley 1992; DoH 1999b; Appleby et al 2001)

Targets for mental health

In order to deal with mental health problems and the perceived inadequacies of services over many years, a succession of key targets have been set (DoH 1992, 1999a). Currently the *National Service Framework for Mental Health* (DoH 1999b) sets the standards for mental health services in England. (Similar targets are also set elsewhere in the UK: Welsh Assembly Government 2002; Scottish Executive 1997). In the *National Service Framework for Mental Health* these standards are set in five key areas:

- Mental health promotion (Standard 1)
- Primary care and access to services (Standards 2 and 3)
- Effective services for people with severe mental illness (Standards 4 and 5)
- Caring about carers (Standard 6)
- Preventing suicide (Standard 7)

A wide range of **social, psychological** and **biological factors** has a clear link with mental health problems. This is increasingly recognised in the development of health policy

(DoH 1999a; Welsh Assembly Government 2002). 'Detailed research on the causes of mental illness has shown that the major risk factors for mental illness include:

- Poverty, poor education, unemployment
- Social isolation stemming from discrimination against people with all types of physical disabilities
- Major life events such as bereavement, redundancy, financial problems, being the victim of crime
- Genetic predisposition
- Drug and alcohol misuse
- Developmental factors such as fetal damage and injury at birth
- Poor parenting.'
  (DoH 1999a)

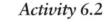

Activity 6.2

Identify relevant factors in the area in which you live or work which may affect the mental health of the local population. Where there are specific problem factors, identify any services which may provide relevant help.

Martin's mental health problems

Martin grew up living with his mother after his parents broke up when he was in his early teens. He did not have many friends at school and was not particularly academic. However, after school he went on to an engineering course at a local college. Here, he had a more active social life, drank moderately, smoked cannabis and briefly experimented with amphetamines. He had several girl-friends before meeting his first wife, whom he married when he was 23. Their marriage lasted three years, but broke down when she left after frequent rows.

In his early twenties, shortly after starting his first job, Martin began to experience difficulties relating to people at work. He was seen as difficult and argumentative, often 'blowing up' over small incidents. When he was 25, an incident occurred in which Martin, shouting unintelligibly and wielding a crowbar when approached, refused to emerge from the tunnel in which he was working.

Martin later described how he felt that the other people at work talked about him all the time and conspired to make the jobs he was doing go wrong. While he was working, he experienced voices, which be thought were those of world leaders telling him that if he was seen in public, he could be captured and tortured and that he should defend the 'cause of justice'.

Mental health and mental illness

Martin has a range of problems, some we can understand in the same terms as we understand many of the problems in our everyday lives, such as needing money, trying to make relationships work, surviving stresses and so on. Other experiences we may find more difficult to identify with, particularly experiences which seem to reflect a different perception of reality.

> ### Activity 6.3
>
> Consider the thoughts and feelings Martin described. Try to imagine how you might respond if you had such beliefs and feelings.
>
> Now reflect upon Martin's behaviour.

Hospital admissions

Martin was eventually admitted under the Mental Health Act to an acute psychiatric ward within a large district general hospital. After five weeks he was discharged, later returning to work and coping for a while without major incidents. Two years later a very similar incident occurred, followed by another admission. He was diagnosed as suffering from schizophrenia. Over the last ten years he has had four such episodes. Between episodes, he sometimes becomes rather depressed about his life.

When he married Julie five years ago, he told her about his illness, but said that he was cured. Two months after their marriage he had a relapse, and once again he was admitted to hospital for six weeks. Julie and Martin were seen for some joint sessions together and she became aware of the nature and outlook of his problem. After a further relapse he agreed to fortnightly 'depot' medication.

Professional conversation

Helen, a ward manager in an acute mental health unit

'As in general wards, the patients we have are here for shorter periods of time, often only during the acute period of their illness. About half of our patients are detained under the Mental Health Act. Making helping relationships with people, within an environment which they have not chosen, can be very demanding, but is also very rewarding.

Martin and I have had our ups and downs. Sometimes when he has been admitted here, he has been very frightened and even though he knows me quite well now, the first part of his admission when he has been "sectioned" has been particularly difficult. Usually, he has been able to come off his Section relatively quickly, and we can then sit down together and try to identify current problems and help him to deal with them. Sometimes, when he has felt low or been unable to contact Mike, the Community Psychiatric Nurse (CPN), he comes up to the ward for a chat.'

Serious mental illness and schizophrenia

Martin is described as having a diagnosis of schizophrenia. There is a range of ideas about its nature and cause and some of the opposing themes and concepts have been well and critically discussed by Keen (1999). However, the phenomenon and its sequelae are generally recognised as constituting a severe mental health problem which often has enduring consequences.

Some ideas about schizophrenia

- Genetic susceptibility

  That a predisposition to develop schizophrenia may be inherited and linked to specific chromosomes. Chromosomes 6, 8 or 22 have so far been implicated.

- Stress vulnerability and family interaction

  That the way in which families interact, particularly with higher levels of expression of emotionally charged critical responses, may be a factor, particularly in the relapse of susceptible individuals.

- Neuro-pathological

  That abnormalities in brain structure such as ventricular enlargement, temporal or frontal lobe changes may be a factor.

- Neuro-developmental

  That a lesion in the brain arising during its early development may be a factor in the development of schizophrenia later in life.

- Neuro-chemical

  That increases in levels of available neuro-transmitters such as dopamine, serotonin or glutamate may be a factor.

- Continuity v. discontinuity

  That schizophrenia may be viewed as being at the extreme of the normal distribution of experience and physiological make up (continuity theory) rather than a discreet and abnormal phenomenon (discontinuity).

- Sociological

  That the act of diagnosis can be socially constructed as labelling, and the resulting stereotyping, exclusion and stigma will, in themselves, influence both the individual's experience and others' responses.

> **Activity 6.4**
>
> **A (for all students)** Review your own reading so far about 'schizophrenia'. Identify the predominant ideas which emerge.
>
> **B (for mental health students)** Arrange a discussion about 'schizophrenia' with your peers and colleagues and note individual differences in beliefs and influences in the group.

Diagnosis of schizophrenia

Increasingly there is an international consensus on the criteria for diagnosing mental and behavioural disorders (although not about causation). There are, however, two major classification systems – *The International Classification of Diseases* (ICD-10) (WHO 1994) and the *Diagnostic and Statistical Manual of Mental Disorders* (DSM-IV-TR) (American Psychiatric Association 2000). Chapter V of ICD-10 lists 'Mental and behavioural disorders', the categories for which are shown below.

Categories in ICD Chapter V

F00–F09   Organic, including symptomatic, disorders

F10–F19   Mental and behavioural disorders due to psychoactive substance abuse

F20–F29   Schizophrenia, schizotypal and delusional disorders

F30–F39   Mood (affective) disorders

F40–F48   Neurotic, stress related and somatoform disorders

F50–F59   Behavioural syndromes associated with physiological disturbances and physical factors

F60–F69   Disorders of adult personality and behaviour

F70–F79   Mental retardation

F80–F89   Disorders of psychological development

F90–F98   Behavioural and emotional disorders with onset usually occurring in childhood and adolescence

F99   Unspecified mental disorder

           (ICD-10, WHO 1992)

> ### Activity 6.5
>
> **(For all students)** Find out attitudes to diagnostic classification systems by mental health professionals with whom you have contact.
>
> Which professionals base their approach on a diagnosis? On what do others base their ideas about mental health problems?

Diagnosis of schizophrenia

For at least a month there should be one very clear symptom from a–d below (or two or more if symptoms are less clear-cut) or two or more from e–h:

a. Experience of one's thoughts being generated from outside or taken away, echoed or broadcast to others.
b. Delusions of being controlled or influenced by outside forces.
c. Hallucinatory voices giving a running commentary on one's behaviour, or discussing one amongst themselves, or other types of hallucinatory voices.
d. Persistent delusions of other kinds that are inconsistent with one's cultural beliefs and completely impossible.
e. Persistent hallucinations of any sort (auditory, visual, tactile etc.) accompanied by vague delusions (not depressive) occurring for weeks or months on end.
f. Breaks or interpolations in the train of thought, resulting in incoherence or irrelevant speech or 'neologisms'.
g. Catatonic behaviour such as excitement, posturing, negativism, mutism and stupor.
h. 'Negative' symptoms such as marked apathy, paucity of speech and blunting of emotional responses, usually resulting in social withdrawal and lowering of social performance.
i. Significant and consistent change in the overall quality of some aspects of personal behaviour such as loss of interest, aimlessness, idleness, self-absorption and social withdrawal.
(Adapted from (ICD-10, WHO 1992)

> ### Activity 6.6
>
> **A (for non mental health students)** Identify the meaning of the terms 'delusion' and 'hallucination'. Consider the judgement which is made in applying these terms to another's experiences.
>
> **B** Read the ICD-10 diagnostic criteria, or consult the equivalent section in DSM-IV-TR, and ascertain the way in which the criteria which define 'schizophrenia' are organised.
> How might these criteria apply to Martin's experiences?

Evidence-based practice

Outcomes of schizophrenia

- 1 per cent lifetime risk in general population across all cultures.

Of these:

- 22 per cent have a single diagnosed episode with no resulting clinical or social impairment.
- 35 per cent have occasional recurrences with no or minimal impairment between episodes.
- 8 per cent experience some social impairment after the first acute episode persisting unaffected by further breakdowns.
- 35 per cent are increasingly damaged by each subsequent acute crisis so that social functioning progressively worsens.

Other negative outcomes

- Negative social reactions to symptoms and behaviour, with consequences such as stigma, discrimination, high unemployment, failed or impoverished relationships.
- Ten years shorter lifespan than the general population.
- 10 per cent of those diagnosed with schizophrenia commit suicide.
- Significantly higher risk of accidents and cardiovascular disease.
  (Frangou and Murray 1996)

Martin's coping mechanisms

Since losing his job, Martin rarely goes out. Although he has little to do with the older children, who tend to avoid him, he does appear to be very close to Jake. He spends much of his time in his shed devising and developing plans for Harmonic Interface Mechanics (HIM), a new way of preventing deterioration in the built environment which relies on the generation of a background harmonic note in tune with the soul of each building. The many rejections he has received from companies and journals to whom he has sent his ideas are convincing him of general hostility towards him. He often appears angry, shouting loudly even when on his own.

Julie wants to be able to support Martin, but feels pessimistic about the future of their marriage and uncertain of her own ability to cope. He will not discuss their marriage and becomes worked up, angry and upset when she tries to talk to him about their problems or to involve anyone else.

Assessment

Martin clearly has a long history of mental health problems. What else do we need to know in order to provide Martin with support?

Could we assess:

- His safety and the degree of risk that he might attempt suicide?
- The safety of others?
- The feelings, thoughts and perceptions of Martin and all those involved? What do they want and need?
- The severity of their distress?

> ### Activity 6.7
>
> Find out what approaches to assessment and what assessment tools, are used by professionals in your local mental health services.
>
> To what extent is the client or service user's perspective incorporated into the assessment?

Approaches to assessment in mental health have been well discussed by Barker (1997).

Struggles with treatment

During his periods of contact with mental health services, Martin has received help through talking to staff on a one-to-one basis, in groups and through some joint sessions with Julie. However, he has also received a large variety of medical treatments. These have included oral medication, in the form of tablets and syrups, and injections, which at times he refused. Sometimes he has changed his mind about treatment and stopped it because of the side-effects he experienced, particularly when it made him feel tired and lacking in energy or gave him a tremor. He has been met with a range of responses to his attempts to discuss his medication. Some staff, he felt, were too defensive, only having the goal of his taking the medication; sometimes he felt as though he were fighting a battle over medication rather than receiving help; and sometimes he felt that he was not being believed when he was talking about his own experience. Others, however, listened carefully, talked more openly and responded to his experiences. Over the years, he has found that Mike, the CPN, has been very helpful in this respect.

Treatment interventions for people with schizophrenia

A range of different treatment options are advocated for helping people with schizophrenia:

- Pharmacological intervention:
    - Anti-psychotic drugs also known as 'neuroleptics' or 'major tranquillisers' such as chlorpromazine (Largactil) or trifluoperazine (Stelazine) or newer 'atypical' antipsychotics such as clozapine (Clozaril) or olanzapine (Zyprexa). Some antipsychotic drugs are available in preparations designed for long-acting 'depot'

injections such as fluphenazine decanoate (Modecate) or flupenthixol decanoate (Depixol). Many of these drugs, however, have unpleasant side-effects which need careful monitoring, and awareness of and response to the patient's experience.

- Family management and intervention:
  - There is increasing evidence that a combination of family intervention and pharmacological intervention combined, may offer the best outlook for people with schizophrenia.

- Cognitive behavioural therapy-based (CBT) psychosocial/psychoeducational intervention.
- Behavioural approaches.
- Humanistic responses.
- Support, monitoring and supervision.
- Specific symptom coping strategies, e.g. hearing voices.
- Other psychotherapeutic approaches.

Activity 6.8

What do you know of mental health inpatient units? Find out what treatment and associated care are offered or available to people with severe mental illness in your area.

If you have the opportunity, talk to some of the service users about their experience of the treatments they have received. Identify the helpful and unhelpful aspects of the treatment and care as they have experienced it.

Evidence-based practice

The IRIS initiative

'**Early intervention**' is increasingly advocated as important in reducing the impact of psychosis. Early Intervention Services are being established in all areas as part of general mental health policy (DoH 2001a).

These services focus on:

- The early detection of the illness
- Reducing any delay in establishing intervention
- Sustaining the treatment through the critical period
- Then working with the person to recognise, cope with and prevent any relapses

Read the papers on the IRIS (Initiative to reduce the impact of schizophrenia) site on '*Management of First Episode Psychosis*' (Spencer et al 2001) and *Schizophrenia: Early Warning Signs* (Birchwood et al 2000) at: http://www.iris-initiative.org.uk/index.shtml

Policy issues – mental health services and community care

'Community care has failed'
(*Dobson 1998*)

Activity 6.9

Read the following extracts from letters in respect of the developing scenario
    Identify any underlying attitudes in the letters and discuss in your learning group how they might influence Martin's experiences.

Dear Mike,

Re Martin Page

As you know, since his last discharge from St Grevilles, this young schizophrenic man has been receiving his depot injection (Fluphenazine Decanoate 25mg fortnightly) from our practice nurse. Despite his past experiences, however, she had been finding it increasingly difficult to persuade him to continue with this and he has now missed the last two appointments. Despite her reassurances, he was complaining of putting on weight and having 'tired feelings' in his eyes, which he attributed to the medication. I gather he has still been in asking for repeat prescriptions for his Orphenadrine 50mg tds., despite previously telling me that it was 'useless'.

    I don't know if you are aware of this situation, however, I would be grateful if you would try to see him to re-establish his medication, so that we can continue to control him in the community.

Letter to the CPN from Dr Cuthbert, GP

Consider how you might respond if you were the CPN. What might be your priorities?

Dear Sir or Madam,

For the last three years, myself and my family have been living in Yew Tree Avenue, a quiet street on the Westgrove estate. Number 14 is occupied by Mr Martin Page and his wife. I gather that Mr Page is mentally ill. He is sometimes openly hostile to me and rather over-familiar to my wife and young children. I and several other residents on the estate are concerned that there needs to be more facilities for people like this where they can be properly looked after. I should point out St John's Primary School is only one hundred yards away. We would like to know why St Greville's Psychiatric Hospital is closing down when there are still people like Mr Page causing problems for himself and the community.

Letter to Blankshire Health Authority from Mr Jim Read, local resident

Consider how you might respond to Mr Read if he became aware that you were involved in Martin's care.

Historical background and context

The mental hospital has been the main focus for the treatment and residence of those with 'mental health problems' since the 1808 County Asylums Act. By the early part of the twentieth century, most asylums were thriving, but isolated communities, meeting virtually all the needs of both patients and (separately) staff. Little 'curative' treatment as such was available. From the early 1950s, although much criticised and at times overused, drugs (notably the 'phenothiazines') were developed which represented the first widely available effective treatment of the symptoms of major mental illness. Arguably, they also enabled the beginning of discharge into the community on a large scale. Since the description by Russell Barton in the 1950s of 'institutional neurosis' and sociological observation of 'institutionalisation' by Goffman (1961), further attempts have been made to reduce the isolating and damaging effects of long-term hospitalisation.

Activity 6.10

Read the following extract from the famous 'water tower' speech by the then Minister of Health, Enoch Powell, in 1961:

> There they stand, isolated, majestic, imperious, brooded over by the gigantic water tower and chimney combined, rising unmistakable and daunting out of the countryside – the asylums which our forefathers built with such immense solidarity.
>
> [Building mental hospitals . . .] is not like building pyramids, the erection of monuments to a remote posterity. We have got to get it into our heads that a hospital is like a shell, a framework to contain certain processes, and when the processes are superseded, the shell must, most probably, be scrapped and the framework dismantled.
>
> Our plans involve nothing less than the elimination of by far the greater part of this country's mental hospitals as they exist today. This is a colossal undertaking, not so much in the new physical provision which it involves, as in the sheer inertia of mind and matter which it requires to be overcome. Do not underestimate their power of resistance to our assault.
>
> . . . if we err, it is our duty to err on the side of ruthlessness. For the great majority of these establishments, there is no appropriate future use.
>
> (Powell 1961)

Talk to experienced mental health staff and/or service users and identify how NHS provision of mental health services in your locality has changed in recent years. Find out if this change is perceived positively or negatively, and why.

A range of accommodation options and settings for people with long-term mental health problems has since been developed, and the emphasis has moved to ensuring that people experiencing severe mental health difficulties can be treated in the least restrictive environment with the minimum of disruption to their lives. Mental health services have been increasingly formed around multi-disciplinary Community Mental Health Teams and current policy (DoH 2001a) includes the provision of crisis resolution services and offering home-based intervention wherever possible. This is different from community services to support people after discharge, in that it is seen as an alternative to inpatient care. Evaluative evidence (DoH 2001a) would appear to imply that similar outcomes can be achieved without the institutionalising effects of traditional services and, perhaps controversially, at a lower cost.

'Community care' has been presented as the ideal for many aspects of health care. However, this term needs further consideration as it can represent three distinct, and quite different, concepts: care *in* the community, care *by* the community and care *of* the community.

Care *in* the community Simply implies that the location of care is to be within the general community; that is, in streets, towns, villages surrounded by other aspects of community life. This concept does not, however, imply any interaction or social relationship between those in care and their neighbours or the surrounding community.

Care *by* the community Implies that those living in the community will be given care or helped and supported by others living in the local community, rather than solely by professional carers who go to their residence in order to work.

Care *of* the community Implies that the community facilities are for the benefit of that community. There is a community identity to the services and the residents of the community use them as needed. This would imply a range of mental health services for a locality from counselling to residential care.

It can be argued that present community care facilities are on the whole *in* the community, but that very little of the care is *by* the community. Resources limit care *of* the community to those who are seriously mentally ill.

Activities 6.11

1 Ascertain what current provision is made in your locality for mental health, for people with mental health problems and by mental health services.

2 Which aspects of the provision represent care *in* the community, care *by* the community or care *of* the community?

3 How might these three different concepts conflict with one another? (Consider rights, risks and resources.)

4 What sorts of care might have been options for Martin in your locality?

5 Access the *National Service Framework* and other key documents relevant to the implementation of mental health policy in your region. Identify the key elements of current policy which are influencing the services you are encountering.

The perception in government that 'community care has failed' has led to the development of new policies and directions for *Modernising Mental Health Services* (DoH 1998b). These are being established through the *National Service Framework for Mental Health* (DoH 1999b) and the *NHS National Plan* (DoH 2000) in England and through similar approaches elsewhere in the UK (Welsh Assembly Government 2002; Scottish Executive 1997). The aims of current policy are:

- To protect the public and provide effective and safe care for those with severe and enduring mental illness.
- To meet the needs of those with mental health problems who can appropriately and safely be managed within primary health and social care.
- To promote mental health in the population and help build healthier neighbourhoods. *(DoH 1998b)*

The Welsh equivalent is evident in the *Welsh National Service Framework* (Welsh Assembly Government 2002):

- Promoting social inclusion (Standard 1)
- Empowerment and support of service users and carers (Standard 2)
- Promotion of opportunities for a normal pattern of daily life (Standard 3)
- Commissioning equitable, accessible services (Standard 4)
- Delivering responsive, comprehensive services (Standards 5 and 6)
- Effective client assessment and care pathways (Standard 7)
- Ensuring a well-staffed, skilled and supported workforce (Standard 8)

The Labour Government's 'vision for mental health care' is summarised in *The Journey to Recovery* (DoH 2001b) which you can obtain, free, from the Department of Health (see list of key documents for details).

Therapeutic relationships

Think about the following questions and discuss this with your learning group before moving on to the next section:

What could you identify as essential qualities for someone working in mental health care?

To what extent do you consider *you* have these qualities?

Does the array of professional groups involved in mental health care meet the needs of those with mental health problems in today's society, or should there be a new profession of 'mental health worker'?

At the heart of mental health work, and particularly mental health nursing, is the ability to form a helpful, or 'therapeutic', relationship. A Mental Health Nursing Review identified this as the first of the core skills of mental health nursing (Butterworth 1994).

Evidence-based practice

Skills of Mental Health Nursing

It is the combination of these particular skills, together with the values and practice common to the nursing profession as a whole, which provides the unique expertise of mental health nurses enabling them to:

- Establish a therapeutic relationship which rests in a respect for others and a skilled therapeutic use of self.
- Sustain such relationships over time and respond flexibly to the changing needs of those with mental health problems.
- Construct, implement and plan a care programme.
- Provide skilled assessment, ongoing monitoring.
- Make risk assessments and judgements.
- Monitor the dosage, effects and contraindications of medication.
- Detect early signs of deteriorating mental health including potential self-harm and suicide risk, worsening physical conditions and potential threats to others.
- Prioritise work in order to respond to those most in need.
- Collaborate with all members of the multi-disciplinary team.
- Network effectively, setting appropriate boundaries to professional input.
- Manage the therapeutic environment, determined by clear awareness of such issues as safety, dignity and partnership.

(Butterworth, A., Chairman The report of the mental health nursing review team 1994)

Mental health practitioners need to be able to form such relationships with people who tend to have problems forming relationships, or who have attitudes, thoughts, feelings or behaviour which make the development of a relationship difficult. They need to be self-aware, recognising their own contribution to the development of relationships

Professional conversation

Mike, a community mental health nurse working in an inner city area

'Many of the 35 people on my case load have social problems which it is difficult for me to help them with. About 30 per cent have other problems such as drink or drugs, but it is difficult to get help for them from other services because of their mental health problems. With many of them, I have built up a therapeutic relationship over quite long periods of time and have been the only consistent professional helper they trust.

I've known Martin for about five years now, although he hasn't been on my case load all that time. My predecessor saw Martin for several years after his first admission when he was in his twenties. I first met him just after he got married and I used to see him and Julie together. I still see him when he comes up to the clinic for his injection. I have helped him to be able to recognise problems early before they get too bad. Although this doesn't always work, I think we get on well and most of the time he trusts me. If they do want help, I'm usually the first person he or Julie contacts and I can usually expedite things if he needs another specific intervention.'

The Sainsbury Centre for Mental Health (2001) has identified 67 core 'capabilities' which need to be developed by mental health practitioners if mental health services are to achieve the standards identified in the *National Service Frameworks*.

Ethical practice
- The values and attitudes necessary for modern mental health practice

Knowledge
- Policy and legislation
- Mental health and mental health services

Process of Care
- Effective communication and partnership
- Comprehensive assessment
- Care planning and review
- Supervision and CPD
- Clinical and practice leadership

Interventions
- Evidence-based
- Medical and physical care
- Psychological
- Social
- Practical
- Mental health promotion

Applications

To specific NSF/NHS Plan service settings:

- Primary care
- Community-based-care co-ordination (CMHTs)
- Crisis resolution and early intervention
- Acute inpatient care
- Assertive outreach
- Continuing care and day centres, residential and vocational programmes
- Services for people with complex and special needs, e.g., dual-diagnosis and personality disorders

Characteristics of a therapeutic relationship

Carl Rogers (1951) is usually credited with identifying and describing a set of conditions which should exist for effective therapeutic work:

1 **Accurate empathic understanding and responding:** that is, that the helper strives not only to understand how the world and his or her problems and situation is perceived by the client, but communicates this endeavour to the client

2 **Acceptance or respect also sometimes termed 'Non-possessive warmth' or 'Unconditional positive regard':** that is, that the client is not made to feel that he must please the helper or show gratitude and that the helper will not judge or be shocked by his or her situation, thoughts or behaviour.

3 **Genuineness, sincerity or congruence:** that is, that the helper is what he or she appears to be and is open in and about the relationship

(Rogers 1951)

Since the work of Rogers, these principles have been widely incorporated into approaches to counselling, therapy and 'client-centred' approaches to mental health practice.

A key skill in all these approaches is **'active listening'**. That is, having an emphasis which focuses on paying attention to what the client is saying, showing him or her that you are listening and understanding, and helping to clarify the meaning of what he or she is saying.

Elements of active listening include:

- Questioning: enabling the client to talk freely in response to open questions.
- Clarifying, checking understanding: sorting out confusion or ambiguity and encouraging the client to be specific and focus on important aspects.
- Responding: to verbal and non-verbal cues in the client.
- Noticing and being aware: not only of what is expressed, but also what is not expressed.

- Reflecting: mirroring back to the client either the sense and content in, or the feelings behind, what he/she is saying.
- Paraphrasing: listening to what the client is saying and putting the essential meaning into other words.
- Summarising: bringing together the main ideas and feelings at the end of or during a conversation.

Activity 6.12

Next time you are talking to a mental health service user about his or her experience, notice the degree to which you are 'actively listening'.

Consider how the other person would know that you are paying attention.

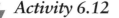

Practice tip

When you interact with clients, such as during an interview or assessment, consider the following:

- Remember that the emphasis is on listening, not talking.
- Avoid probing unnecessarily – don't 'interrogate', that is, don't ask too many questions. Is it an appropriate question – or are you are just being curious?
- Where possible ask open rather than closed questions, which allow the client to explore and develop his/her feelings/thoughts.
- Try not to ask 'why' questions: 'what', 'how', 'when', 'who', etc. questions are usually more helpful, enabling the client to be more specific about the situation, rather than trying to rationalise feelings, or explain situations which he/she does not understand.
- Avoid asking leading questions, otherwise the client explores your perspective rather than his or hers.
- Do you have permission to talk in the way you are? Be sensitive – take cues from the client.
- Don't go deeper than you can handle. You have a responsibility to ensure that you are working within the limits of your competence. Ask yourself whether you are the appropriate person to deal with a difficult issue, or whether counselling or therapy might be needed.
- If you don't have time for the answer, don't ask the question.
- Time the questions appropriately for the situation and stage of interview.
- Try to allow the person to make the decisions rather than simply giving advice.
- Notwithstanding the above, don't dogmatically refuse to give advice or avoid prescribing action, sometimes they may be the most appropriate and sensible things to do. Similarly, giving information, education, etc. may be important interventions.
- Try not to judge or blame, or use 'shoulds' and 'oughts', which reflect your frame of reference, not the client's.

- Try not to invalidate what the client feels by suggesting that what he/she feels is inappropriate, silly or that he/she feels, or should feel, something else.
- Don't say that you're 'sure that it will be all right' when you aren't! You may not be able to make it all better!

Helping interventions

John Heron (2001) suggested that in any helping roles such as nursing, teaching, social work, medicine, there are broadly six different intervention strategies. These he divided into two groups.

John Heron's six categories of intervention

Authoritative interventions

In which the practitioner tends to be dominant, assertive, interventionist:

- **Prescriptive interventions**: seek to direct the behaviour of the client, e.g., giving advice, suggesting.
- **Informative interventions**: seek to impart knowledge, meaning, or information not available to the client, e.g., giving information, interpreting.
- **Confronting interventions**: seek to raise the awareness of the client about some limiting attitude or behaviour of which he is unaware, e.g., challenging inconsistencies, giving feedback. It is important to be supportive when confronting.

Facilitative interventions

In which equality is more evident in the relationship and the role of the client is enhanced:

- **Cathartic interventions**: seek to enable the client to discharge painful emotion, primarily grief, fear, anger or embarrassment, e.g. by laughing, crying, storming, etc.
- **Catalytic interventions**: seek to facilitate self-discovery, self-directed learning and problem solving in the client, e.g., client-centred questioning and approaches.
- **Supportive interventions**: seek to affirm the worth and value of the client's person, qualities, attitudes or actions, e.g., touch, validating worth of client.

(Heron 2001)

Crisis and desperation

A week ago, after becoming increasingly frightened of his unpredictability and the effect on the children, Julie took them to stay with her mother. However, two days later, having tried to contact both his CPN and the GP, Martin made a serious attempt on his life, breaking into a neighbour's car and starting the engine after sealing the garage doors with wet sacking. He was found by the neighbour and again admitted to hospital. Julie has agreed to consider returning home to 'try again' if he will agree to accept help.

Suicide and attempted suicide

As we have seen in the incidence of mental health problems above, some 6000 people in the UK commit suicide each year. This comprises around 5000 people a year in England and Wales (10.0/100,000), nearly 900 people in Scotland (17.3/100,000), and about 170 people in Northern Ireland (9.9/100,000) (Appleby et al 2001). The prevention of suicide has therefore assumed a high priority in government targets for mental health services through the *National Service Frameworks* and the *Suicide Prevention Strategy for England* (DoH 2002a). Although each suicide is a shock for those close to the individual, suicide rarely occurs 'out of the blue'.

Evidence-based practice

Of people who commit suicide:

- 90% have been judged (retrospectively) to have some of form mental disorder
- 66% have consulted their GP in the previous month
- 60% give some advance warning
- 33% express clear suicidal intent
- 24% were in contact with mental health services in the previous year
- 11.5% were in contact with services in the previous week
  (Williams and Morgan 1996; Appleby et al 2001)

Of course it is very easy to discover these circumstances retrospectively. Clearly, we need to be able to develop some ideas which will help us identify risk prospectively. Some clear patterns are evident, and should be considered in order to guide practice.

Evidence-based practice

Groups at risk of suicide:

- Males (male:female more than 3:1) (but this varies between ethnic and cultural groups; e.g. the ratio is 14:4 in England and Wales, however, it is more common in Asian women than Asian men)
- The elderly and young men
- The divorced, widowed or single
- Social class 1 and 4
- Specific occupations, e.g., farmers, doctors, vets, pharmacists, dentists, nurses, pilots
- Those living alone

- The socially isolated, or those in rural communities
- The unemployed or retired
- Children of suicides
- Other bereavements in childhood
- People who have previously harmed themselves
- Those following recent major life event or loss
- People with mental disorders:
  - depressive illness (15% lifetime risk)
  - schizophrenia (10% lifetime risk)
  - Those who misuse alcohol or drugs (3.4% lifetime risk)
  - organic disorders, e.g., early dementia, Huntington's Disease.
  - personality disorder
- People with past psychiatric problems or family history of affective illness
- People with a terminal illness
- Those in poor physical health
  (Williams and Morgan 1996; Appleby et al 2001)

Although it is almost impossible to be certain of the intent at the time of the act of those who successfully kill themselves, this profile is a little different from those who self-harm themselves with a non-fatal outcome (parasuicide).

Evidence-based practice

Groups at risk of para-suicide

By contrast with completed suicide, these:

- Tend to be female (female:male approx. 3:1)
- Tend to be younger
- Tend to be social classes 4 and 5
- May have social problems (e.g., housing, finance, unemployment)
- Have relationship problems (e.g., marital disharmony, or break up)
- May be impulsive
- May be imitative

These profiles give indications of risk among groups. What are needed, however, are tools and questions which can be applied to individuals. As guidance to professionals in primary care, this can sometimes be reduced to a brief list of four important questions:

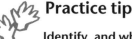

Evidence-based practice

Recognising suicide risk in primary care

1 Do you feel that life is not worth living?
2 Have you felt like acting on this?
3 Have you made any plans?
4 Have you tried before?

1 only:	(no intentions, no plans, no past history)
	See again, GP treat depression
1 and 2 only:	(intentions but no plans or past history)
	See frequently, GP treat depression and consider referral
1, 2 and 3 or 4:	(intentions and definite plans or previous attempts)
	Refer urgently, monitor closely and treat depression

(Armstrong 1997)

Practice tip

Identify, and where you are participating in clinical care under supervision, utilise, the recognised risk assessment tools in use in your area. In addition, ask yourself the following questions:

- Does the person now hope that things will turn out better or will change?
- Does he/she recognise getting some pleasure out of life?
- Does he/she feel hopeful on a day-to-day basis?
- Is he/she able to face the next day?
- Does he/she see some point in living or does he/she despair of going on?
- Does life feel a burden, and he/she wishes it would end?
- Does he/she wish he/she were dead?
- Does he/she think about ending his/her life? If so how often?
- Has he/she ever acted on such thoughts?
- Does he/she feel able to resist them?
- How likely does he/she think it is that he/she could harm/kill him/herself?
- Can he/she give a reassurance that he/she will not?
- Will he/she seek help if there is a crisis?
- Is there a risk to any one else?

The final question always seems to be subjective and intuitive: **Do I believe the reassurances or denials I am being given?**

Treatment interventions for people with depression

A range of different treatment options are advocated for helping people with depression:

- General care
- Psychosocial:
  - Cognitive behavioural therapy (CBT)
  - Support
  - Skilled helping/person-centred counselling skills
  - Problem solving
  - Coping with distress, panic
  - Offering information and other sources of help and resources
- Pharmacological intervention:
  - Tricyclic antidepressants (TCAs)
  - Mono-amine-oxidase inhibitors (MAOIs)
  - Selective Serotonin Re-uptake Inhibitors (SSRIs)
  - 'New generation' antidepressants:
    Serotonin Noradrenalin Re-uptake Inhibitors (SNRIs)
    'Dual action' Noradrenergic and Specific Serotonergic Antidepressants (NaSSAs)
  - Other antidepressants
- Physical illness management
- Self-help
  (Adapted from Armstrong 1997)

Legal issues

The legal aspects of mental health care are determined both by statute and common law. Of the former, the most relevant for mental health workers is the Mental Health Act 1983. At the time of its enactment it was seen as liberalising legislation, limiting and clarifying criteria for compulsory detention, halving the periods of detention allowed under the previous Act of 1959, enhancing patients' rights, creating more opportunities for appeal and promoting community care where possible.

Activity 6.13

Martin at different times in his life has been admitted 'for assessment', 'for treatment', detained while a voluntary patient, and discharged with 'after-care under supervision' under various sections of the Mental Health Act 1983.

Identify and examine the relevant sections of the Mental Health Act and consider how they might have affected the care Martin received.

Martin's personal reflections

'I've been in hospital several times sometimes under section, when they wouldn't let me leave hospital and insisted on me having treatment. I admit things had been getting out of hand, but I had so many problems to deal with. On top of not feeling right, them putting me in hospital against my will made me so angry. I sometimes just lashed out, I didn't mean to hurt anyone. I suppose I might have done away with myself at one point, but mostly I think I would have been OK.

I can see that I must have been quite difficult to handle and some staff, like Helen, the ward manager have been quite strict, but fair. The social workers and nurses have always tried to explain my rights and the legal situation, even though sometimes I didn't really take it in. But there were some staff who made things worse by not listening to me, or trying to play down the problems I was having.'

The Mental Health Act 1983 is now seen as being in need of reform to reflect the needs of a mental health service which is more community oriented. The demand for reform has been reinforced by a series of mental health inquiries into homicides by mentally ill people, most notably that into the care and treatment of Christopher Clunis (Ritchie 1994). A 'root and branch review' of mental health legislation, ordered by Frank Dobson, then Secretary of State for Health (Dobson 1998), was carried out chaired by Professor Genevra Richardson. The resultant proposals (Richardson 1999) suggested that the focus on compulsory admission to hospital and the point of discharge should be replaced by a wider concept of compulsory compliance with a treatment plan in community or hospital settings. This should be underpinned by reinforcement of principles of non-discrimination between compulsory and non-compulsory care, the minimum restriction of patient autonomy consistent with safety, and user participation in consensual care. Agencies and disciplines would be expected to work more closely together. A new independent tribunal should make decisions about 'admission to compulsion'. Subsequently, there was extensive further consultation through a Green (consultation) Paper on 'Reform of the Mental Health Act 1983' (DoH 1999c), followed by a White Paper outlining the new legislative framework (DoH 2000) and consultation on a Draft Mental Health Bill (DoH 2002b, 2002c, 2002d).

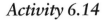

Activity 6.14

Ascertain the current stage of reform of mental health legislation as changes are announced, consulted, legislated, implemented and monitored. You can refer to the following:

http://www.doh.gov.uk/menhlth.htm
http://www.doh.gov.uk/mentalhealth/whitepaper2000.htm
http://www.doh.gov.uk/mentalhealth/draftbill2002/index.htm

Identify contentious issues, discuss how they are being tackled, and consider how they might have affected the approach to Martin's care.

Present and future – imperfect?

In summary, Martin has had over 15 years of mental health problems and is diagnosed as having schizophrenia, potentially a severe and enduring mental illness. During that time he has had periods when he has been well, has worked, married and created a family. He has also had periods in which he has been distressed, out of contact with reality and self-destructive. Julie has made her life with him and shared both good and bad times. Both of them have experienced great stress and, at the worst, he has been suicidal and she has considered leaving. They continue to make a life together, aware that there may be further difficult times ahead, but feeling that they do have support from mental health services.

Activity 6.15

Consider the effect of the experience of Martin's mental health problems and that the care offered has had on the life of each family member.

If you can do so in a facilitated group, adopt roles for each member of the family and, in role, discuss the experiences you have had.

Conclusion

Through the scenarios, we have followed Martin and Julie and their family and seen the impact of mental health problems upon their lives. By considering the questions, reading and undertaking the activities, you should have developed a good idea of the attempts by services, particularly those in your local area, to develop appropriate responses to the kind of problems they experience. You will have become aware of the changing and evolving policies and legislative framework underpinning mental health care. You should also have developed some ideas about how to respond to people with mental health problems and recognised the importance and characteristics of a therapeutic relationship.

? Now that you have had opportunities to consider some of the issues raised in mental health care, and met some of those involved as service users, carers and mental health practitioners, how do you now feel about 'mental health'. Look back over any notes you have made and reflect on the experiences you have had. How are your ideas and attitudes changing, developing, hardening, softening and so on? In what ways will any insights you are gaining in this field influence what you do in the future?

References

American Psychiatric Association (1994) *Diagnostic and Statistical Manual of Mental Disorders* (DSM-IV-TR). Washington, DC: APA.

Appleby, L., Shaw, J., Sherratt, J., Amos, T., Robinson, J. McDonnell, R. et al (2001) *Safety First: Five-Year Report of the National Confidential Inquiry into Suicide and Homicide by People with Mental Illness.* London, DoH.
www.doh.gov.uk/mentalhealth/safetyfirst/safetyfirst.pdf

Armstrong, E. (1997) *The Primary Mental Health Care Toolkit.* London: Royal College of General Practitioners.

Barker, P. (1997) *Assessment in Psychiatric and Mental Health Nursing: In Search of the Whole Person.* Cheltenham: Stanley Thornes.

Birchwood, M., Spencer, E.. McGovern, D. (2000) Schizophrenia: early warning signs. *Advances in Psychiatric Treatment* 6, pp. 93–101: via:
http://www.iris-initiative.org.uk/index.shtml

Butterworth, A. (1994) (Chairman) *Working in Partnership: A Collaborative Approach to Care: The Report of the Mental Health Nursing Review Team.* London: HMSO.

Armstrong, E. (1997) *The Primary Mental Health Care Toolkit.* London: Royal College of General Practitioners.

Department of Health (1992) *The Health of the Nation* (White Paper). London: HMSO.

Department of Health (1994) *The Health of the Nation: Key Area Handbook – Mental Illness.* London: HMSO.

Department of Health (1997) *The New NHS: Modern, Dependable.* London: HMSO.

Department of Health (1998) *The New NHS: Modern, Dependable: A National Framework for Assessing Performance.* London: DoH.

Department of Health (1998b) *Modernising Mental Health Services: Safe, Sound and Supportive.* London: DH.

Department of Health (1999a) *Saving Lives: Our Healthier Nation.* London: The Stationery Office. http://www.doh.gov.uk/ohn.htm

Department of Health (1999b) *National Service Framework for Mental Health: Modern Standards and Service Models.* London: DoH. http://www.doh.gov.uk/nsf/mentalhealth.htm

Department of Health (1999c) *Reform of the Mental Health Act 1983: Proposals for Consultation.* London: The Stationery Office, Cm 4480.
http://www.doh.gov.uk/pub/docs/doh/mentalhealth.pdf

Department of Health (2000) *The NHS National Plan.* London: The Stationery Office.
http://www.nhs.uk/nationalplan

Department of Health (2001a) *The Mental Health Policy Implementation Guide.* London: DoH. http://www.doh.gov.uk/mentalhealth/implementationguide.htm
http://www.doh.gov.uk/pdfs/mentalhealthimplowgraphics.pdf

Department of Health (2001b) *The Journey to Recovery: The Government's Vision for Mental Health Care.* London: DoH.
http://www.doh.gov.uk/mentalhealth/journeytorecovery.pdf

Department of Health (2002a) *National Suicide Prevention Strategy for England: Consultation Document.* London: DoH.
http://www.doh.gov.uk/mentalhealth/suicideprevention.pdf

Department of Health (2002b) *Draft Mental Health Bill.* London: The Stationery Office, Cm 5538–I. http://www.doh.gov.uk/mentalhealth/draftbill2002/draftbilljune02.pdf

Department of Health (2002c) *Draft Mental Health Bill: Explanatory Notes.* London: The Stationery Office, Cm 5538–II.
http://www.doh.gov.uk/mentalhealth/draftbill2002/explanatorynotes.pdf

Department of Health (2002d) *Draft Mental Health Bill: Consultation Document.* London, The Stationery Office, Cm 5538–III.
http://www.doh.gov.uk/mentalhealth/draftbill2002/index.htm
http://www.doh.gov.uk/mentalhealth/draftbill2002/draftmhbillconsultation2002.pdf

Department of Health and the Home Office (2000) *Reforming the Mental Health Act: Executive Summary.* London: The Stationery Office.
http://www.doh.gov.uk/mentalhealth/summary.htm
In PDF format: http://www.doh.gov.uk/mentalhealth/whitepapersummary.pdf

Department of Health and the Home Office (2000) *Reforming the Mental Health Act: Part 1 The New Legal Framework.* London: The Stationery Office Cm 5016–I (White Paper).
http://www.doh.gov.uk/mentalhealth/whitepaper2000.htm
Full document in PDF format: http://www.doh.gov.uk/mentalhealth/whitepaper1.pdf

Department of Health and the Home Office (2000) *Reforming the Mental Health Act: Part II High Risk Patients.* London: The Stationery Office Cm 5016–II (White Paper).
http://www.doh.gov.uk/mentalhealth/whitepaper2000.htm
Full document in PDF format: http://www.doh.gov.uk/mentalhealth/whitepaper2.pdf

Dobson F. (1998) *Frank Dobson Outlines Third Way for Mental Health.* London: DoH Press release 98/311.

Frangou, S., Murray, R. (1996) *Schizophrenia:* London: Martin Dunitz.

Goffman, E. (1961) *Asylums.* London: Penguin.

Goldberg, D., Huxley, P. (1992) *Common Mental Disorders: A Bio-Social Model.* London: Routledge.

Heron, J. (2001) *Helping The Client: A Creative Practical Guide.* 5th Edition. London: Sage Publications .

Keen, T. (1999) Schizophrenia: orthodoxies and heresies *Psychiatric and Mental Health Nursing* 6 (6), pp. 415–24.

Morgan, H. G., Buckley, C., Nowers, M. (1998) Face to face with the suicidal. *Advances in Psychiatric Treatment* 4, pp. 188–96.

Richardson, G. (Chairman) (1999) *Review of the Mental Health Act 1983: Report of the Expert Committee – November 1999*. London: DoH.

Ritchie, J. H. (1994) (Chairman) *The Report of the Inquiry into the Care and Treatment of Christopher Clunis*. London: HMSO.

Rogers, C. R. (1951) *Client Centred Therapy*. London: Constable.

Sainsbury Centre for Mental Health (Training and Practice Development Section) (2001) *The Capable Practitioner: A Framework and List of Capabilities Required to Implement the National Service Framework for Mental Health*. (A Report Commissioned by the National Service Framework Workforce Action Team.) London: The Sainsbury Centre for Mental Health.
http://www.scmh.org.uk/website/SCMH_MHT.nsf/59ae2dc0a615100a802567e4004f2d1e/dd6294343cbfb7e080256a930047a863/$FILE/The%20Capable%20Practitioner.pdf

Scottish Executive (1997) *A Framework for Mental Health Services in Scotland*. Edinburgh: Scottish Executive.
http://www.show.scot.nhs.uk/publications/mental_health_services/mhs/index.htm

Spencer, E., Birchwood, M., McGovern, D. (2001) Management of first episode psychosis. *Advances in Psychiatric Treatment* 7, pp. 133–42:
via: http://www.iris-initiative.org.uk/index.shtml

Thomas, B., Hardy, S., Cutting, P. (eds) (1997) *Stuart and Sundeen's Mental Health Nursing Principles and Practice*. London: Mosby.

Watkins, M., Hervey, N., Carson, J., Ritter, S. (1996) *Collaborative Community Mental Health Care*. London: Arnold.

Welsh Assembly Government (2002) *Adult Mental Health Services: A National Service Framework for Wales*. Cardiff: National Assembly for Wales.
http://www.wales.nhs.uk/sites/documents/334/adult-mental-nsf-e.pdf

Williams, R., Morgan, H. G. (eds) (1996) *Suicide Prevention: Mental Health Services – The Challenge Confronted. A Manual of Guidance for the Purchasers and Providers of Mental Health Care*. London: NHS Health Advisory Service.

World Health Organisation (1994) *The International Classification of Diseases* (ICD-10). Copenhagen: WHO.

Resources

📖 Further reading

Annotated bibliography of ten core texts and resources

Barker, P. (1997) *Assessment in Psychiatric and Mental Health Nursing: In Search of the Whole Person*. Cheltenham Stanley Thornes.
An updated edition of an earlier book, which outlines a range of approaches to assess-

ment in mental health care. Although the author's humanistic, person-centred perspective is well known, it deals clearly and systematically with the appropriate theoretical underpinnings of the assessment methods.

Brooker, C., Repper, J. (1998) *Serious Mental Health Problems in the Community: Policy, Practice and Research.* London: Baillière Tindall.

A comprehensive account, by experts from a range of disciplines focusing on issues and intervention strategies in the provision of effective services for people with serious mental health problems.

Gamble, C., Brennan, G. (2000) *Working with Serious Mental Illness: A Manual for Clinical Practice.* Edinburgh: Baillière Tindall/RCN.

An almost essential, practically focused book. Although, like many of the other texts, it incorporates the theory basis, this book also provides clear guidance for every-day evidence-based practice rooted in sound psychosocial intervention skills.

Newall, R., Gournay, K. (1999) *Mental Health Nursing: An Evidence-Based Approach.* Edinburgh: Churchill Livingstone.

A book focusing on the evidence base for mental health nursing. The authors argue the responsibility to provide care which is demonstrably appropriate and effective, as well as avoiding care which is demonstrably inappropriate or harmful. They argue that professional questioning and insistence on practice based on evidence, rather than custom and practice, is in itself empowering of patients.

Open University (1997) Study Pack K257. *Mental Health and Distress: Perspectives and Practice.* Milton Keynes: Open University, School of Health and Welfare.

An excellent study pack for an Open University study course which was accredited by the ENB as equivalent to the former 'Update in Mental Health Nursing' ENB 953 course.

Rawlins, R. P., Williams, S. R., Beck, C. K. (eds) (1993) *Mental Health – Psychiatric Nursing: A Holistic Life Cycle Approach.* St Louis: C. V. Mosby.

Comparable with the original 'Stuart and Sundeen' (now Stuart and Laraia 2001), a very comprehensive American textbook, with each topic area arranged around a five-domain model of self (physical, intellectual, emotional, social and spiritual).

Thomas, B., Hardy, S., Cutting, P. (eds) (1997) *Stuart and Sundeen's Mental Health Nursing Principles and Practice.* London: Mosby.

Adopting the title, although not the content of a leading American nursing textbook, this excellent book provides comprehensive coverage of the field, drawing on a range of specialist writers, and providing both underpinning principles and application to practice.

Thompson, T., Mathias, P. (2000) 3rd Edition. *Lyttle's Mental Health and Disorder.* London: Baillière Tindall.

Practically oriented, foundation level textbook aimed at pre-qualifying students. Although it bears the title of Jack Lyttle's original book, it is a completely different multi-authored text.

Watkins, M., Hervey, N., Carson, J., Ritter, S. (1996) *Collaborative Community Mental Health Care.* London: Arnold.

A collection of research-based papers discussing a range of contemporary developments and issues in community mental health care written from a variety of different professional perspectives.

Watkins, P. (2001) *Mental Health Nursing: The Art of Compassionate Care.* Oxford: Butterworth Heinemann.

A compassionate, practical book detailing how to develop relationships and work therapeutically with people in distress. Drawn extensively from the humanistic tradition

Official reports and key documents

British Psychological Society (2000) *Recent Advances in Understanding Mental Illness and Psychotic Experience: A Report by the British Psychological Society Division of Clinical Psychology.* Leicester: BPS. www.understandingpsychosis.com

Department of Health (1995) *Building Bridges: A Guide to Arrangements for Inter Agency Working for the Care and Protection of Severely Mentally Ill People (Health of the Nation).* London: DoH.

Department of Health (2000) *The NHS Plan.* London: The Stationery Office. http://www.nhs.uk/nationalplan

Department of Health (2001) *Treatment Choice in Psychological Therapies and Counselling: Evidence-Based Clinical Practice Guideline.* London: DoH. http://www.doh.gov.uk/mentalhealth/treatmentguideline/index.htm

Department of Health (2001) *National Service Framework for Older People: Modern Standards and Service Models.* London: DoH. http://www.doh.gov.uk/nsf/olderpeople.htm

Department of Health (2001) *The Mental Health Policy Implementation Guide.* London: DoH. http://www.doh.gov.uk/mentalhealth/implementationguide.htm

Department of Health (2001) *Making it Happen: A Guide to Delivering Mental Health Promotion.* London: DoH. http://www.doh.gov.uk/pdfs/makingithappen.pdf

Department of Health (2002) *Mental Health Policy Implementation Guide: Adult Acute Inpatient Care Provision.* London: DoH. http://www.doh.gov.uk/mentalhealth/inpatientcp.pdf

NHS Executive and Social Services Inspectorate (SSI) (1999) *Effective Care Co-Ordination in Mental Health Services: Modernising the Care Programme Approach.* London: Department of Health. http://www.doh.gov.uk/pub/docs/doh/polbook.pdf

Reith, M. (1998) *Community Care Tragedies: A Practice Guide to Mental Health Inquiries.* Birmingham: Venture Press/BASW.

Sainsbury Centre for Mental Health (1997) *Pulling Together: The Future Roles and Training of Mental Health Staff.* London: The Sainsbury Centre for Mental Health.

Sainsbury Centre for Mental Health (1998) *Keys to Engagement: Review of Care for People with Severe Mental Illness Who Are Hard to Engage with Services.* London: The Sainsbury Centre for Mental Health.

Standing Nursing and Midwifery Advisory Committee (1999) *Mental Health Nursing: Addressing Acute Concerns.* London: DoH. http://www.doh.gov.uk/pub/docs/doh/snmacmh.pdf

United Kingdom Council for Nursing, Midwifery and Health Visiting (2002) *The Recognition, Prevention and Therapeutic Management of Violence in Mental Health Care.* London: UKCC.

Full report: http://www.ukcc.org.uk/cms/content/Publications/ Mgt%20of%20violence%20full%20report.pdf

World Health Organisation (2001) *World Health Report 2001 – Mental Health: New Understanding, New Hope.* Geneva: WHO. http://www.who.int/whr/

NB Many Department of Health publications can be obtained free of charge from:

Department of Health, PO Box 777, London, SE1 6XH
FAX: 01623 724524; email: doh@prologistics.co.uk
Or through the NHS Responseline: 08701 555 455

Many publications from the DoH may be downloaded directly via POINT (Publications On the Internet) at: http://tap.ccta.gov.uk/doh/point.nsf/Publications

@ Web pages

NB This list of websites has been provided because of their possible value in your learning and exploration of mental health issues. However, website addresses and the material displayed on them are likely to change. No endorsement of a particular website, or its contents should be construed from its inclusion below.

Bandolier (Evidence-Based Medicine): **www.jr2.ox.ac.uk/bandolier/index.html**
British Association for Counselling and Psychotherapy: **www.bac.co.uk/**
British Journal of Psychiatry: **bjp.rcpsych.org/**
British National Formulary (BNF): **www.bnf.org.uk/**
British Psychological Society (BPS): **www.bps.org.uk/**
Centre for Evidence-Based Mental Health: **cebmh.warne.ox.ac.uk/cebmh/**
Contact – a directory for mental health: **www.doh.gov.uk/mentalhealthcontact**
Community Psychiatric Nurses Association (CPNA): **www.cpna.org.uk**
Dave Sheppard Associates (formerly IMHL):**davesheppard.co.uk/**
Department of Health (Mental Health): **www.doh.gov.uk/mentalhealth/**
Evidence-Based Mental Health: **www.ebmentalhealth.com**
Institute of Psychiatry: **www.iop.kcl.ac.uk/**
Journal of Advanced Nursing:
   www.blacksci.co.uk/~cgilib/jnlpage.bin?Journal=jan&File=jan
Journal of Clinical Nursing:
   www.blacksci.co.uk/~cgilib/jnlpage.bin?Journal=JCN&File=JCN
Medscape – psychiatry:
   psychiatry.medscape.com/Home/Topics/psychiatry/psychiatry.html
Mental Health Act Guide: **www.hyperguide.co.uk/mha**
Mental Health Foundation: **www.mentalhealth.org.uk**
Mental Health Practice (RCN): **www.mentalhealthpractice.co.uk**
Mentality: **www.mentality.org.uk/**
MIND: **www.mind.org.uk**
National Electronic Library for Mental Health (NeLMH): **www.nelmh.org/**
National Institute for Clinical Excellence (NICE): **www.nice.org.uk/**
National Schizophrenia Fellowship: **www.nsf.org.uk**

Network for Psychiatric Nursing Research: **www.man.ac.uk/rcn/ukwide/npnr.html**

NHS Centre for Reviews and Dissemination: **www.york.ac.uk/inst/crd/**

NHS University: **www.doh.gov.uk/nhsuniversity/index.htm**

NMAP (Gateway to internet resources for nursing, midwifery and allied health professions): **nmap.ac.uk**

Nursing and Midwifery Council (NMC): **www.nmc-uk.org**

OMNI (Gateway to internet resources in health and medicine): **omni.ac.uk**

Psychiatric Nursing Network/mailbase:
  www.jiscmail.ac.uk/lists/psychiatric-nursing.html

Sainsbury Centre for Mental Health:
  www.scmh.org.uk/wbm23.ns4/WebLaunch/LaunchMe

The Samaritans: **www.samaritans.org/sams.html/home2.html**

Tidal Model (Phil Barker): **www.tidal-model.co.uk/intro.htm**

WHO Guide to Mental Health in Primary Care: **www.whoguidemhpcuk.org/**

WHO *Mental Disorders in Primary Care*:
  www.who.int/msa/mnh/ems/primacare/edukit/index.htm

World Federation for Mental Health: **www.wfmh.com/index.html**

7 Insights into Learning Disability Nursing

Neil Jackson and Tony Gilbert

Introduction

This chapter will discuss general issues in relation to people with a learning disability through the medium of a developing scenario. The reader should also note that this is an important time in the relationship between people with learning disabilities and society in general. The government has just published a new White Paper *'Valuing People'* (DoH 2001) which sets out the responsibilities of government, society and public services towards this section of the community. These responsibilities are organised around four 'Key Principles: Rights, Independence, Choice and Inclusion'. A brief summary of the White Paper is included in the annotated bibliography at the end of the chapter.

The structure of the chapter can be best described as being in two parts. The first part focuses upon a range of issues that are important to the understanding of learning disability. This includes an identification of what learning disability is, its relationship with other forms of disability, key issues related to the health of people with learning disability, the importance of communication, and the role of the learning disability nurse.

The second part of the chapter develops around a scenario that involves a young woman named Cathy who is experiencing some health problems. The aim is to engage the student with the issues that might arise for a young person with learning disabilities and the type of support she may receive. At the same time, it is intended that the scenario and its related exercises will enable the student to gain an insight into the work of nurses from the learning disability branch. In particular the way in which they work with clients, carers and other professionals in the development and delivery of appropriate packages of care.

Throughout the second part of the chapter, there are sets of activities for the student to do which will help your understanding of the issues. At the same time, the scenario is illuminated through the identification of emerging questions and the use of professional conversations.

Learning outcomes

- The identification of key concepts in relation to nursing people with a learning disability.
- The understanding of the relationship between adult nursing and learning disability nursing in the context of nursing a person with a learning disability who becomes ill.
- The recognition of the importance of alliances between primary and secondary health care workers.
- The recognition of the importance of communication with all clients/patients as a prerequisite for good nursing care.
- The particular importance of finding alternative ways to communicate with people who have a learning disability or to augment spoken language.
- The recognition of the importance of anti-discriminatory practice in delivering equal health care to all.
- The understanding of the importance of access to generic and specialist health care for people with a learning disability.

Concepts

- The nursing aims for people with a learning disability
- Communication with people who have a learning disability
- Working with families
- Definition of disability
- Access to generic services
- Access to specialist services
- Advocacy and the development of autonomy
- Respect for the autonomy of people
- Health promotion and people with a learning disability
- Interdisciplinary working
- Co-working with nurses from other disciplines
- Working through families
- Sexuality and disability

Who are people with a learning disability?

The term learning disability is applied to a particular section of the population. It is the currently acceptable legal and professional term which is used to describe this section of the population. Other terms that have been used include mental handicap and learning difficulty. People within this group are often identified as

Activity 7.1

Before reading further you may like to consider your understanding of the term 'learning disability'. Who would you include in your list?

having special educational needs when they are children. Some people within this group also experience physical and sensory disabilities or they may experience neurological conditions that are often associated with learning disability, such as epilepsy and cerebral palsy (Kay et al, 1995; Wake 1997; DoH 2001). In general terms, having a learning disability is usually taken to indicate that the person is experiencing some form of developmental delay.

There are over a million people with learning disabilities in the United Kingdom and they are a group that has experienced a profound shift over the last century in the way in which services have been provided. At the end of the nineteenth century and for a substantial part of the twentieth century, people with learning disabilities were viewed as a danger to society as they were believed to lack moral controls over their behaviour, and might therefore be led into crime or immoral acts. The greatest fear was that they would endlessly reproduce, leading to an overwhelming increase of the population (Gilbert 1998). This led to a service model based upon isolated residential institutions that after 1948 became known as hospitals. For the people who remained living at home, there was the development of large 'day-time' institutions known as training centres or day centres. The second part of the twentieth century saw the development of the 'Community Care' programme. This has led to the closure of many of these large institutions, and the replacement of the residential institutions by ordinary housing and the day centres by a variety of community-based activities (Wertheimer 1996; Gilbert and Rose 1998).

> **Activity 7.2**
>
> Are you aware of people with learning disabilities who live in your home community?

This movement of people with learning disabilities from isolated and segregated services to the use of ordinary housing and every-day work and leisure facilities has been accompanied by a substantial shift in social attitudes towards people from this section of the population. This has been recently described by The King's Fund (1999) as a movement 'from care to citizenship'. This movement has also meant that people with learning disabilities are making increased use of both primary and secondary health care services in both general health care and mental health care. One continuing obstacle to people with learning disabilities meeting this potential of citizenship lies in outdated social attitudes that see individuals as dependent and incapable of making choices or decisions. The central issue for all nurses, regardless of the area of health care in which they are working, is to enable people with learning disabilities to become informed and make decisions about their own health and lifestyle. This links to the key concept in learning disability services of advocacy (McNally 1997). In many cases this will require skilled communication and knowledge of the services/resources that are available to support people with learning disabilities in the community.

What causes learning disability?

Approximately four people in every 1000 will have a severe learning disability (0.4 per cent of the population), but as many as 20 people in every 1000 will have a mild learning disability (2 per cent of the population) (Gates 1997a; King's Fund 1999). *Valuing People* (DoH 2001) provides figures for England of 210,000 people with a severe learning disability and 1.2 million with a mild learning disability. Learning disability can be caused by a number of different factors

that act upon the developing brain, which is usually taken to mean below the age of 16. These factors, genetic, infections, trauma, social and environmental influences (Watson 1997), can impact to varying degrees which, when combined with the person's social position and life experiences, can result in a complex picture. This complexity is often lost in the forms of definitions such as the idea of 'an arrested or incomplete development of the mind' which is used by the World Health Organisation (WHO 1993) and which is set within the Mental Health Act (1983).

Equally, the traditional medical/psychological approach of using the criterion of the intelligence quotient (IQ) has particular limitations and the related term 'mental age' is now considered to be derogatory. A more useful guide is a measure of the extent to which a person can perform a range of roles within society; that is, their social competence. This leads to the idea of 'support needs' (Clegg 1993), which has been incorporated into many forms of assessment that are used by professionals to determine the person's current level of functioning. The strength of this idea is that it is flexible and it does not create a hierarchy based upon the level of disability, nor at the same time does it imply that needs are stable and fixed. Instead, people can be assessed on the basis of their present circumstances. For example, a person with a learning disability who manages their own affairs, but who is presently experiencing an acute illness can be considered as having high support needs. Whereas, a person who requires daily support, but is stable with respect to the level of support needed might be considered as having less high support needs.

The idea of support needs has been incorporated into many of the assessments that are used by professionals working with people with learning disability to measure social skills and self-help skills. The ratings obtained can be used as a baseline from which to determine progress.

Disability and illness

It is important to draw a distinction between disability and illness. Disabled people are not ill, nor are people with learning disabilities. A look at the Para and Special Olympics will demonstrate this fact. As was noted earlier, the previous model of services for people with a severe learning disability was based until recently upon large hospitals.

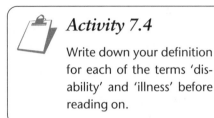

Activity 7.4

Write down your definition for each of the terms 'disability' and 'illness' before reading on.

This move brought about the medicalisation of people with a learning disability, despite the fact that learning disability itself cannot be treated medically. This led to an over-emphasis upon medical definitions of need with a denial of peoples' emotional, educational and social needs. In more recent times it has been recognised that people with a learning disability have been further damaged by the services which were established to help them (Ryan and Thomas 1987). This has occurred because these services tended to concentrate large numbers of people with learning disabilities together away from the general population, leading to social isolation, stigma and poor environmental conditions (Wolfensberger 1972). Issues central to the citizenship of people with learning disabilities; rights, independence, choice and inclusion, and the resources needed to achieve this will all depend upon the dominant social attitudes at the time (Brechin and Walmsley 1989; Redworth and Redworth 1997). Hence the importance of the government's strategy as set out in '*Valuing People*'.

This medicalisation of people with learning disabilities paralleled the medicalisation of other disabled people (Oliver 1990). Disability *per se* has been defined as either a personal tragedy or the result of social oppression, and the importance of understanding the competing definitions of disability is a key activity for any serious student of the subject (Barton 1996). Disability needs to be seen and understood within the particular historical, social and political context of a given society and the ways in which ideas of 'able-bodiedness' come to dominate. The effect of this is to include some sections of society, while other sections come to be excluded on the basis of difference. It also needs to be remembered that the experience of disability is impacted upon by other social variables such as class, gender, race and age. These in turn all have an effect upon learning disability (Brechin and Walmsley 1989).

Health and people with learning disability

People with a learning disability who have health problems should not be seen as different in any way to anyone else in the community who may become ill. They have the same rights and entitlement to comprehensive health care that meets their diverse health

> **Activity 7.5**
>
> In your practice experience to date have you yet been involved with a person with learning disability? If so, reflect on the circumstances. How was the person and family approached and cared for? It may be useful to discuss this with colleagues who have had such an experience.

needs as any other person (DoH 2001). Many children with learning disabilities will spend long periods of time in hospital, undergoing tests to identify metabolic problems or surgery to correct the physical problems which can be associated with learning disability. In adulthood there is evidence that the general medical needs of people with learning disabilities are higher than that of the rest of the population (Moss and Turner 1995), and yet there is also evidence that people with a learning disability experience difficulty accessing health care (Singh 1997). At the same time there is evidence that the experience of mental health problems may be higher in this section of the population (Gilbert et al 1998).

> **Activity 7.6**
>
> In your previous activity did issues in relation to communication come into your discussion? Identify what challenges may occur. Draw up a list of a variety of communication skills and strategies that health professionals, including nurses, need to develop to communicate effectively with a range of individuals who have learning disability.

Adult, Children's and Mental Health Nursing interventions with people who have a learning disability who become ill are the same as for any other person. However, the challenge will be in developing the skills of specialist communication in order to negotiate nursing interventions. The same issues are raised here as are apparent when nurses from any branch attempt to nurse a client or patient whose language and/or means of communication is one that they do not share. The responsibility here lies with the **nurse** to find a suitable and appropriate means of communication in order to establish a mutual frame of reference. The same is true of nursing someone with a learning disability. It is when the nurse is caring for someone who has limited or no spoken language that more communication skills are required.

There are two key processes to consider here. The first is the mode of communication, which will involve a range of observational and listening skills. It will also involve the taking of an effective communication history from either the person and/or their family or carer. This will identify the range of communication skills the person has, their preferred methods of communication, likes and dislikes, the ways they express discomfort and pain, and whether they use a sign language or an electronic aid. It is also essential to identify the range of self-help skills the person has so that it is clear what to expect.

The second key process is understanding or comprehension, and this will require the nurse to do much more than ask the person whether they understood. It is essential that the nurse is aware of the complexity of the information or instructions they are giving to the person. For example, when explaining to a person who is continent where the ward toilets are, they need to consider whether the person understands the abstract idea of 'they are at the end of the room and then turn right', even if the person states that they have understood. It would be better to take the person and show them the toilet, and to check and repeat this activity a number of times until it is apparent that the person has understood. The same can be said about a range of instructions which might be given to people with learning disability. It is easy to assume that a person who has apparently good communication skills understands all that is said to them. Equally, a common error is to assume that a person with little speech understands little (Ferris-Taylor 1997). The support of a learning disability nurse or a speech and language therapist might be useful at this time.

This requirement to offer health care equally to all has important professional and ethical consequences. These arise from the principle of justice, which is concerned with the fair distribution of resources. For the nurse to take the view that patients or clients who are not of the same ethnic background as the nurse or who have a disability result-ing in communication problems should adjust to the nurses frame of reference amounts to professional arrogance and discriminatory practice.

Learning disability nursing

The main aim of specialist nurses for people with a learning disability is to work in part-nership with the client to increase their **personal autonomy** (Kay et al 1995). Nurses trained to work with people with learning disability can be found in a range of settings such as specialist health services, social services and the independent sector. Community nurses for people with learning disabilities will often be involved in liaison work between the primary health care team or with general hospital services. Regardless of the setting, one of the primary components of personal autonomy is to increase a person's control over their own health. One of the key roles for community learning disability teams identified in the 'Valuing People' strategy is that of health facilitator. This is a role that the strategy closely identifies with learning disability nurses:

> As the first point of contact, primary care is the place where many important deci-sions are made. But for many people with learning disabilities their encounter with the primary care team may be frustrating and difficult. In order to overcome these barriers, staff from the local community learning disability team in each area will

need to take on the role of health facilitators to support people with learning disabilities to access the health care they need from primary care and other NHS services. This role may be taken up by any community learning disability team member, but learning disability nurses are well placed to fulfil this role.
(DoH 2001, Section 6.12, p. 63).

This development builds upon the learning disability nurse's role in assisting with health promotion, health education and health maintenance for people with learning disabilities (DoH 1995a). Alongside this, and complementary to this role, other activities of nurses within this speciality will include:

- Mitigating the effects of disability
- Facilitating access to and involvement in local community life
- Increasing personal competence and feelings of control
- Maximising choice
- Enhancing the contribution of others involved formally or informally in the support of the person
  (Kay et al 1995)

Activity 7.7

Considering the statement above what roles would you expect the learning disability nurse to take on to enhance the health of individuals with learning disability? Before reading on draw up your full list.

In a situation where the person with a learning disability is receiving health care from a member of the primary care team or from secondary, general or mental health services, it is not unusual for a degree of collaboration to be established between these services and the specialist learning disability services (Sines and Barr 1998; DoH 2001). This collaboration is often established through the nurses within each team. It follows that the nurse, seeking to restore optimum health to the person with a learning disability who has become her patient, may need to work closely with a specialist nurse for people with a learning disability. The rationale for this alliance is that both the nurse and the nurse for people with a learning disability share the same aim of restoring optimum health. Each nurse will bring to the alliance a common understanding of health and a complementary, but different set of skills.

In your practice experience to date have you observed any examples of this collaborative working? If so, what were the successes and challenges?

Therefore, in the scenario which is developed in the next section, one of the central issues will be to identify points of collaboration between the specialist nurse and the adult nurse. Cathy, a young woman with acute medical needs and ongoing general health needs, as well as needs related to her disability, will provide the focus for the discussion.

This alliance between Cathy and the different health care professionals will enhance the professional skills that each of them possesses. At the same time it should increase Cathy's sense of personal autonomy and her self-esteem, which has clear implications for her mental health. The adult nurse, in seeking to care for Cathy, will have to adopt communication strategies that may be new; for example, the use of sign language and 'tuning in' to Cathy's particular patterns of speech and the skilled reading of her non-verbal communication. This process, of discovering the person and what is significant to them, is a fundamental aspect of holistic nursing in any branch.

Activity 7.8

There may be other concepts, which you have already decided that you wish to explore and as you work through the text, yet more concepts may arise. Use the annotated bibliography and references at the end of the chapter to discover more sources of information. As you work through the chapter, use dictionaries to clarify words and phrases that are new to you. Dictionaries from other disciplines such as psychology and sociology may be particularly useful.

Scenario *Introducing Cathy*

Cathy is 16 years old and lives at home with her mother and father who are in their early fifties. Cathy's mother works as a journalist with a local paper and her father is a senior accountant with the local authority. She also has a younger brother Tony, who is 10 years old. The family live in a large, comfortable, detached house on the outskirts of a major city in the south of England, where Cathy attends the local comprehensive school and receives extra help from a specialist unit within the school for her learning disability.

Activity 7.9

A In order to help you picture the scenario with Cathy at school, it may be helpful to think about your own educational experiences. Were people with learning disabilities included in your schools or college; and if they were, how were they supported? Do you have any friends with a learning disability or friends who have a brother or sister with learning disability; if so, what is their experience of school?

B Try to find out about statutory educational provision for people with a learning disability within your area. Does your local education department promote the education of children with learning disability within mainstream schools or does it operate separate schools for these children? What do you feel might be the advantages/disadvantages of these two different types of educational provision?

C At the same time find out what courses are open to young adults with learning disabilities at the local further education colleges and do these lead to formal qualifications?

Cathy's experience

The problem emerges because over the last week the standard of Cathy's school-work has declined and she seems agitated at times. This has led to periods where she has become aggressive and fractious, and it has all started to happen following an incident in the playground at school, during which she fell over. Cathy's teacher has contacted her parents to express her concern. The teacher seems to be most concerned about the aggressive incidents that have taken place. She has had to intervene several times between Cathy and a boy in her class. Following a visit to her doctor, Cathy is sent to the accident and emergency department at the local district general hospital. She is also referred to a community specialist health care team for people with a learning disability because of her behaviour.

Emerging questions I

The emerging lines of enquiry can be tested and rejected or shelved, pending the arrival of new evidence. This process can be described as one of professional speculation. The first step in the process is to be clear about what we know about a situation. We then need to consider the likely reasons for any health changes or behaviour changes. On the basis of this, we can test out or explore whether our assumptions are correct. In order to do this, we need to decide what new information we need.

This is an important process as a means to begin the formal assessment of the client. It must, however, be differentiated from the expression of uninformed opinion. At this stage we are searching for guidance about the emerging problem and possible solutions to it. To help with this we may consult professional colleagues, gain evidence from the literature, records or observations.

> What is the significance of new behaviour? Before reading on consider what is meant by the concept of 'new behaviour'. What form might it take?

New behaviour can be a useful indication of a change in a person's mental or physical state. The onset of illness of any kind may be accompanied by new behaviour, as will a change in social circumstances. It is the task of the nurse, from any of the four branches of nursing, to discover the meaning of the new behaviour **for the person exhibiting it** and not to ascribe meaning to it from their own or other's framework of values. This process requires the nurse to suspend judgment and explore, with the client, the possible meanings of the new behaviour (Gates 1997b).

In the case of people with a learning disability, behaviour is often seen only as problematic and not as indicative of change or need. This approach to the analysis of the significance of behaviour will severely limit the nurse's ability to understand the significance of the behaviour and to intervene appropriately. The nurse must seek to understand the significance of the new behaviour in the context of the environment and the personal circumstances in which the person finds themselves (Donnellan et al 1988).

? How might the family view Cathy and her needs?

It is important to discover the role that Cathy plays within the family; that is, intermediary, the baby, the one who needs the care, the sensible one and so on. This can only be achieved by making an assessment not just of Cathy, but of Cathy in the context of her family. Try to discover the myths and stereotypes that the family uses to explain things that have happened to them and why they are the way they are (Dallos 1991). One means of developing this picture is to undertake a family genogram, which can help to plot and explore family relationships in a safe and non-threatening way. We will see later on in the chapter how the community nurse begins to explore the family as a unit and the effects it has on Cathy and her needs.

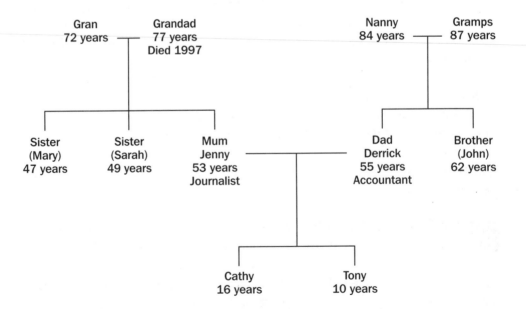

Figure 7.1 Hills family genogram (three generations)

Activity 7.10

Construct a genogram of your own family, adding details such as cultural background, religion, interests, social and health factors to build a rich picture

 How might Cathy view her needs?

Cathy's perception of her needs will provide the key to successful interventions with her. The nurse will need to discover how Cathy feels about herself and how she sees herself within the family, what role she thinks she plays, how she views other family members, how she feels about the recent incident at school and what she thinks her other needs are.

 What is the relationship like between Cathy and Tony?

The way that siblings interact in any family is of interest when trying to work with one of them. It is useful to discover and assess the significance of dyads and triads within the family; you may be helped in this process by recalling your own family. Does Cathy see herself in a protective role towards Tony or is it perhaps the other way around? Do they get on? Is there rivalry in relation to Cathy's problem over and above normal sibling rivalry? How are actual or potential conflicts resolved between them, who is the peacemaker?

 Who is closest to Cathy at school? How would this be discovered?

It is important to discover who, within the school or any other institution that is involved with Cathy, has the clearest picture of her. Discovering whom she relates with the best will enable you to access good information. Treat all information as provisional at this stage, as you may find that people have myths, stereotypes and prejudices in relation to Cathy. The task is to build up a true, comprehensive picture of Cathy and the things that are significant to her. Avoid making assumptions or absorbing the assumptions of others at this stage.

Is Cathy usually a happy person? Consider what behaviours you might expect to notice that would offer clues.

Before attempting to assess the extent of change in behaviour and its possible meanings, it is important to discover details about Cathy's personality. Is she a happy person, is she outgoing or quiet and introspective, cautious or bold?

? How has her 'new' behaviour been observed or assessed?

The first 'clue' in the scenario is the part about Cathy's behaviour changing. This is important and is the logical starting point for any enquiry. Changes in behaviour are usually assessed against a known baseline or 'norm' of behaviour. It will be useful to discover what Cathy's behaviour was like before the incident. It will be important to discover the events occurring at the point of change, and useful to find out how the change in behaviour is being monitored. Provisional hypotheses can be developed at this stage; this is a normal part of professional practice as the practitioner begins informed speculation about what might be occurring. This process is one of reflection *in* action which, along with reflection *on* action, is the key to professional practice (Schon 1983). Could the change in behaviour be caused by hormonal changes in relation to adolescence? Has a new person entered her life, either at school or at home? Has the school changed the routine in relation to Cathy? Could she be physically ill? What is the significance of the incident in the playground? A model for assessment could be used at this stage. It is important that the model used can exclude physical causes for the new behaviour.

? What is a community specialist health care team for people with a learning disability, who works in it and what services or interventions does it offer? Write down what you believe that you know before moving on.

A community specialist health care team is a collection of professional health care workers and support staff who are based administratively in secondary health care, but usually situated geographically within a local community. They receive referrals from health care workers in primary health care and, in some cases, clients will refer themselves, usually with help from their carers. The team generally works with adults, as children are usually seen within paediatric services or sometimes within a specialist children's disability team. The team can offer a range of interventions from a simple health assessment to sophisticated interventions such as cognitive-behaviour therapy (CBT). On referral to the team, it meets, discusses the needs that the potential client has, and allocates work in relation to the skill base of its members and their availability. Although Cathy is only 16 years old and still at school, it would be appropriate to make a referral to the team as Cathy is at an age when she is in transition from childhood to adulthood.

Multi-disciplinary community specialist health care teams are typically made up of:

● Nurses for people with a learning disability
● A consultant psychiatrist
● A clinical psychologist
● An occupational therapist

- A physiotherapist
- A speech and language therapist
- A social worker who works in association with the team

Some members of the team may also be care managers (Biggs 1998). Several members of the team may be part-time workers or have substantial duties elsewhere. Some members of the team may take on special advisory roles in relation to issues that arise with learning disabled people; such as incontinence, epilepsy, sexuality and mental health.

Concerns about Cathy's behaviour

Cathy's behaviour has changed at school and the standard of her work has declined. Cathy's teacher has had several 'chats' with her to try and find out what is going on. She seemed to be agitated some of the time. She keeps asking to sit down in the 'quiet' room: some of the teaching staff feel her behaviour is 'attention seeking'. Cathy is seen by the school nurse, she is reluctant to be examined and the school nurse cannot find anything wrong with her. The teacher asks the parents to come to the school and, during an informal meeting, it is discovered that the same patterns of behaviour are occurring at home. It is agreed that the parents will take Cathy to see the doctor.

The visit to the doctor does not go well as Cathy is agitated at the time and is reluctant to allow the doctor to examine her. The doctor eventually gains Cathy's consent and co-operation to allow her to make an examination. The doctor is concerned about a lack of movement in Cathy's left arm and suggests that she go to accident and emergency for X-rays and further examination. The doctor makes reference to the fact that Cathy is overweight and suggests a calorie-controlled diet. Mrs Hill agrees to this, but her husband remains quiet. The doctor suggests that a community nurse, based in the local specialist health care team for people with a learning disability, is asked to visit and make a full assessment of Cathy's needs. She agrees to make a referral to the team.

Activity 7.11

Look up the concept of informed consent (Gilbert and Dix 1995) and consider it in relation to the examination of Cathy. How does informed consent, whether implied, verbal or written, relate generally to the examination and treatment of clients or patients either in the hospital or the community?

In order for Cathy to be seen by a community nurse for people with a learning disability, her GP will normally make a referral to a community specialist health care team and the team will decide which of its members will assess Cathy's needs and work with her. The team is based administratively within a local community NHS trust, but it is geographically located near to the health centre that Cathy normally goes to. The referral takes some weeks to process.

Cathy's experience of hospital

Cathy's parents take her to the general hospital and she is diagnosed as having a fractured clavicle. The recommended treatment is that she wears a sling for her left arm and rests. Whilst in the accident and emergency department, Cathy asks the nurses several times to go to the toilet. She uses the sign language Makaton to do this. The nurses do not understand what the 'funny hand signals' mean and Cathy is incontinent of urine. This is unusual behaviour for her and she becomes quite agitated. The nurses are quite anxious in response to Cathy and the situation becomes tense. They quickly discuss the situation with the parents. The nurses assume that Cathy is regularly incontinent and ask the parents what kind of 'nappy' Cathy wears. Both parents are extremely angry that their daughter's needs have, yet again, gone unnoticed. They consider making a formal complaint.

Activity 7.12

Consult the UKCC *Code of Professional Conduct* (NMC 2002) and discuss with your colleagues the extent to which the incident in the accident and emergency department was an example of discriminatory practice. At the same time consider the following questions:

- Have you or your colleagues experienced discriminatory practice?
- What are the wider implications of excluding some people from health care?

Concerns about school

Cathy returns home but does not return to school. As the Hills reflect on what has happened to Cathy, they feel that the school should have discovered that Cathy was in pain soon after the playground incident. In their reflection they avoid the painful question of why they had not noticed Cathy's difficulties. They make an appointment to see the head teacher, and during the meeting ask to see the report of the incident in the playground. They inform the head teacher that they feel that the school failed in its duty of care to Cathy in relation to the playground incident. The meeting is a tense one and the situation is left unresolved. The GP asks the district nurse to monitor Cathy's recovery.

Emerging questions II

Again we need to engage in the process of professional speculation and to ground this with the emerging evidence related to Cathy's health needs.

> **?** Should the Hills pursue the process of making formal complaints against the NHS Trust and the school?

It needs to be recognised that all users of health and other public services have the right to complain when that service fails to meet their needs. The concept of **clinical governance** (DoH 1997) has been established in the NHS to ensure that people experience the highest standards of service possible. Instances such as that experienced by the Hills may be subject to an investigation or to a critical incident analysis. The purpose should be to learn from the experience and to take measures that will prevent a similar incident happening again rather than seeking to attribute blame. Moreover, nurses need to be aware that people who rightly complain can, nevertheless, become labelled as difficult parents and treated with more caution than they normally would be.

It is important at this stage that all concerned put energy into solving Cathy's problems rather than becoming defensive over the incident. There is a need for the nurse to acknowledge the problem but also to explore ways in which the family can place it to one side while it is being explored. This will enable the family to move on to find ways of meeting Cathy's needs.

Activity 7.13

A In order to explore the concept of clinical governance further contact your local NHS trust and identify the arrangements concerning clinical governance:
- Who has the lead role for clinical governance in the trust?
- What are the key concerns of the local clinical governance strategy?

B Try to identify the processes a complaint such as that made by the Hills family would go through and how long it would take to be resolved.

> **?** What time elapsed between the incident in the playground and the Hills being informed?

This is a key question to be answered and may form the basis of the Hill's complaint against the school. Incidents of any kind should be reported promptly to those people who have a right to know about them. Mr and Mrs Hill were informed of the incident by means of a communication book two days after the incident occurred. Incidents are normally reported quickly to parents.

What action and investigation took place following the incident in the playground?

This is another key question to be answered. The Hills will want to know that the incident was properly investigated and appropriate actions taken.

> The school saw the incident as a 'minor tussle' and nothing to worry about. Cathy refused to let the school nurse examine her and grew quite angry. The school nurse expressed the view, at the time, that Cathy did not appear to be injured. An incident report form was completed, but the information entered on it was minimal; stating time and date of the incident, and that Cathy said she was pushed over by Michael, another pupil at the school.

 What is the significance of the incident? Was it an isolated event or part of a pattern?

It will be important to discover Cathy's perception of the incident; **what meaning did it have for her,** has it happened before, is it part of a pattern of events and what is the relationship like between Cathy and the boy who 'pushed her over'. The school nurse failed to get any information out of Cathy at the time of the incident. Cathy was also quiet at home. There may be more to this incident than is at first apparent.

 ## Professional conversation

Eileen, the district nurse

'I am not sure about this, I know that we are supposed to help disabled people to be independent, but Cathy is quite vulnerable in this situation. She needs plenty of rest to ensure that the fracture heals properly and the parents need to be firm with her. I want to give clear directions to Cathy's mother, but she is not the sort of woman you direct easily. I find Cathy's father quite hostile. He still seems to be focusing on the incident in the hospital when Cathy was incontinent instead of on her needs now and in the future. The immediate issue here is helping Cathy to get over her fracture.

I am also concerned about Cathy's weight and it relates directly to family eating patterns. I think the best way forward is to get the family to modify its eating habits, but I am not sure how to achieve that. I could just "spell it out bluntly". "Mr Hill, in order to keep your daughter healthy she needs to change her diet. She seems to take her lead from you so what I am suggesting is that you change your eating habits . . ." Well, it might work, but I don't want to get a hostile response. It might work if I try to use Cathy's mum to put some pressure on Mr Hill.'

? What are the implications and possible complications of Cathy's fracture?

Cathy's fracture is one that often occurs with a young adult of this age. It is often associated with a fall and accidents are a key area identified in health policy (DoH 1995b, DoH 1998). The treatment consists of relief of pain in response to symptoms, and the use of a sling or brace to keep the shoulder as immobile as possible during the period of healing. It may be helpful to encourage Cathy to wear her coat with her left arm inside the coat. This will act as additional support and prevent the arm from swinging.

? What does Cathy understand about her weight problem?

It will be important to discover the extent to which Cathy's self-image and self-awareness have developed. If she has a sense of what someone of normal weight looks like, it can be used to set targets for her and to motivate her towards achieving them.

? What was her diet before going into hospital?

Her diet mirrored that of her father, as she seemed to enjoy her food and took portions that were rather larger than necessary. She did not drink wine with her meals, but was very fond of fizzy drinks such as cola. She liked chocolate and other sweets. She has asked if she can have a glass of wine now as she is grown up. On a recent holiday in France she saw a child who appeared to be younger than her having wine. She teases her father about this.

 What is her attitude to food?

Her attitude to food seems to be that she enjoys it and it brings her comfort when she is stressed, she enjoys snacks and has tended in the past to eat meals at irregular times. She sometimes eats according to spontaneous whims or fancies, and seems to equate food with pleasure.

 What is her family's attitude to food?

Mr and Mrs Hill use food as a reward or a treat in the household. Therefore, whenever something goes well, the family will celebrate with food and also if one of the children has achieved something, then food will be used as a reward. This will often take the form of an outing to a burger or pizza restaurant or a take-away. This is a pleasant experience for the family. However, the children have modelled the behaviour of their parents and will look for food as a reward.

Cathy's family

The family is close knit with a general stance of standing together against others. All outside views such as news on the television or radio, newspaper stories, the views of other professionals and recommendations from extended family members pass through the filter of the parent's confidently and strongly held world-view. This filter takes the form of discussion about everything in order to determine their view of whatever is at issue. The parents share a rather cynical view of life, and feel that people are generally out for themselves and what they can get. They are very concerned that their children should do well in life and believe that Cathy is as capable as Tony of achieving.

To outsiders they appear somewhat 'driven' to succeed and rather defensive, particularly in relation to Cathy. They are both fiercely protective of Cathy and yet determined to push her to her limit. As a consequence of the concern that Cathy generates, Tony gets much less attention from his parents and is sometimes just expected to get on with things. Tony resents this at times, although he does understand that in some way his big sister is different and needs extra help. Cathy loves her family dearly and is particularly attached to her father. She tends to want to please everyone in the family, but cannot achieve this. She enjoys the discussions that take place often in the house and joins in to a certain extent. Although she uses Makaton a lot, she is developing a range of speech, and the family is encouraging this very much (Hewitt and Ephraim 1994).

Cathy is overweight and her father is obese. The family eats 'well' and enjoys wine with their meals at the weekends. Cathy's father swings from 'being on a diet' to 'eating well', and his weight goes up and down. This pattern has been established over a number of years. Mr Hill has not sought professional advice regarding his obesity as he regards this as a problem that he can solve alone. Cathy's mother and father are somewhat sceptical about health care professionals who offer advice. They are well-informed and well-connected people, and note that professionals in the health service do not always seem to follow their own advice. This seems to reduce the effect of any advice that they are offered.

The community nurse's assessment

The community learning disability nurse makes an initial visit to the family home (on behalf of the multi-disciplinary team) one evening to begin the process of formal assessment. She uses a generic (multi-disciplinary) team assessment schedule to gather a range of information about Cathy and her family. At the same time, she uses a specific tool designed to assess the health needs of people with a learning disability, 'the OK Health Check' (Mathews 1996) to determine Cathy's immediate and longer term health needs. She decides that it is appropriate that the team intervenes with the family and makes an initial attempt to prioritise Cathy's needs.

Cathy's priorities

1 Healing of fracture.
2 Reduction of weight to within normal limits.
3 Change of eating behaviour through changing the family's eating habits.
4 Develop ability to manage own nutrition and monitor own weight.

Priority actions

1 Ensure that the management regime in relation to the fracture is maintained (in liaison with the district nurse).
2 Discover Cathy's understanding of what has happened to her. Check her means of communication in relation to the pain and pain control. Create a pain map for her to communicate the level of pain she is experiencing (the pain map could be devised using a continuum of faces from smiling to miserable).
3 Discover the family dynamics and networks, and use these as a base for practice.
4 Explore the family's eating patterns.
5 Commence work on the family's attitudes/behaviours to food, in particular targeting Cathy's father.

Professional conversation

Yvonne, specialist community nurse for people with a learning disability

'Well, I've been here before; the presenting problem (fracture, admission to hospital, future maintenance) is not the problem. I felt waves of hostility from Dad when I went through the door, it was as if he had a sign over his head saying, "there's nothing you, a so-called specialist nurse for people with a learning disability, can tell me about how to care for my daughter", I got nowhere near him during the first visit. His comments that "the district nurse had already told us that" and "don't you people talk to each other?" were being used to distract me away from the real question of how well the family has been and is meeting Cathy's changing needs. I managed to keep the debate, that's what it felt like, centred on the needs of Cathy and I think I scored a point when I suggested that the needs of Cathy in relation to her weight problem could not be separated from the behaviours of the rest of the family. That point was met with silence by the father, but mother quickly said, "yes, I think there are things we need to look at anyway". When mother said this, father's non-verbal behaviour told me that he was feeling distinctly uncomfortable.

I need to talk with the district nurse about the general medical issues in relation to the fracture and about diet. I think we need a joint strategy about how we tackle the wider family issues. I am concerned that the family, and in particular dad, will not listen to any advice that I have to offer in relation to Cathy's learning disability. I need to make sure that her developmental needs are being adequately met. I think I will have a talk with Cathy's teacher when I am next at the school. It would be particularly helpful to see how the school handles the parents; I might get some clues for a general approach or even work through the school as "best contact". I need to find out more about the incident in the playground. It seems logical to meet with the district nurse first to establish that I've got the priorities for Cathy's medical needs in the right order and I need to find out more about issues concerned with weight reduction . . . she'll know about it.

At the same time, I will need to begin to explore Cathy's referral with the other members of the community team. I will need to pick some of my colleagues' brains if I'm going to come up with a successful strategy here.'

Liaison with the district nurse

The specialist community nurse for people with a learning disability (Yvonne) and the district nurse (Eileen) met in the local surgery early one afternoon during the surgery's quiet period. The meeting had been initiated by Yvonne, although Eileen was very happy to meet and was about to make the same suggestion when she received the telephone call. Both nurses quickly agreed on the short-term need to help Cathy's fracture to heal and also agreed on the difficulties presented by the attitude of the parent to professional health care workers. They decided to adopt a joint strategy to support the family in supporting Cathy (Home Office 1998; DoH 2001). Eileen would focus on Cathy and on monitoring her recovery from the fracture, give or leave clear advice about diet, but would not enter into debate about the situation. Yvonne would concentrate on getting Mr Hill to realise that his eating behaviour and his scepticism about health care professionals may have a direct and negative effect on his daughter's health and general well-being.

Visit to the school and discussions with Cathy's teacher
Yvonne, the specialist community nurse for people with a learning disability met with Cathy's teacher about Cathy in general, rather than the incident that lead to the referral. She asked the parents before doing this if they minded, and was rather surprised to meet with little resistance. The story from the school was one of slow but steady progress, in line with Cathy's level of intellectual functioning.

The teacher said that she had also experienced hostility from Cathy's parents when Cathy first came to the school. She felt that it faded over time as the school showed its care and concern for Cathy to reach her potential. The teacher took the approach with the parents of honest, open discussion. If she did not know why progress was slow in a particular area, she admitted it and did not try to bluff her way through the meeting. This partnership approach seemed to work well with the Hills and they had even said that, for the first time in the long story of their daughter's disability, they felt respected.

Professional conversation Part 2: historical reflection

Yvonne, specialist community nurse for people with a learning disability

'This feels very familiar, family not trusting professionals . . . takes me back. Cathy was born in 1984. What was going on at that time? The large institutions were just beginning to close, although in the States and in Scandinavia they had gone or were going fast, so the strongest model of care around at Cathy's birth was "institution will do all". The alternative to residential care was staying at home with perhaps not much support or understanding.

At that time primary generic health care was typically not working closely with secondary specialist health care, so the family were probably given the impression that they were either to "go it more or less on their own" or submit to a long-term residential admission. The late 1970s and early 1980s was also the time of the major scandals in learning disability and mental health hospitals, and Cathy's mother in particular, as a journalist, may have been aware of all that. So the family's natural stance of "us against the rest", which was there before Cathy was born, has probably been strengthened by their experiences with professionals of one kind or another.

I need to be careful to respect their views and their experiences, and to be sure of what I can offer. I think I will adopt the strategy that the teacher has used of developing a partnership. I need to be honest and confrontative with Mr Hill about his eating habits and the effects they could have on Cathy, but it must not sound as if I am preaching to him. It may help me to have evidence about the management of fracture recovery and the need to take a family approach to long-term management.'

Joint nursing interventions by Yvonne, the specialist nurse for people with a learning disability, in conjunction with Eileen the district nurse

Yvonne's first task was to get to know Cathy through visiting her and talking with her and building up mutual trust and respect. Yvonne followed the model of nursing outlined by Peplau (1991), in which there are four phases:

1 Orientation
2 Identification
3 Exploitation
4 Resolution

In this process Yvonne focused on getting a clear picture of how Cathy saw herself, what she felt were the most important things in her life and what she would like for the future. Yvonne used a combination of spoken language, symbols and Makaton (Walker 1980) to talk with Cathy. To help in this process, Yvonne looked to other members of the multi-disciplinary team for support and advice. In particular she discussed Cathy with the speech and language therapist, who gave Yvonne advice upon the most appropriate way of working with Cathy in order to establish a level of communication and under-

standing that would enable her to put forward her feelings. This is of particular importance with abstract ideas to do with feelings or questions such as 'what would you like?'

At the same time Yvonne talked to the clinical psychologist about the best way of
designing a programme for Cathy's weight reduction. There were three key issues here:

1 What is an appropriate diet for Cathy? In this they consulted a dietician who built up
   a set of meal options from Cathy's known likes and dislikes. She also advised that
   fruit or low-calorie snacks might be used as rewards. At the same time, they looked at
   a number of exercise options that might support the weight programme.
2 The second issue related to the structure of the weight reduction programme. This
   had to be designed in a way that motivated Cathy to continue with it while at the
   same time it promoted her self-esteem and a positive body image. These issues are
   of particular importance considering her age and emerging sexuality. All of those
   concerned were very conscious not to create a programme that would make Cathy
   feel bad about herself or that would make her ill. One of the central aims of the
   programme was that Cathy should be able to keep her own record of her programme
   and her achievements. It was also felt to be important that Cathy should learn to
   manage her own rewards.
3 The third issue was how to engage Cathy's family in the programme. Here Yvonne and
   the psychologist worked on making Mr and Mrs Hill key players in the implementation and monitoring of the programme. In effect they decided that they would train
   Mr and Mrs Hill to become Cathy's personal trainers. They were going to suggest that
   Cathy went swimming at least twice a week and for a good walk as often as possible.
   This would have health benefits for the whole family (Ewles and Simnett 1995).

The resolution phase of the intervention with Cathy and her family will come about as
Cathy's ability to understand and influence her environment increases. She will in time
gain a clearer understanding of the relationship between the type and amount of food
she eats and her size and shape. She will begin to appreciate her developing sexuality
and the pleasures and responsibilities that it brings. Her family will begin to think more
about the implications of their individual behaviours and the extent to which they affect
their children. In understanding this relationship, they will hopefully use this knowledge
to help Cathy to set and achieve goals for herself. The community nurse will gradually
withdraw as the family adjusts itself. It will be important for the nurse to set some markers of change and share these with the family when change has occurred. In this way all
can see how far each has travelled.

Health promotion and health education

A referral to a specialist health care team, and subsequent work that involves a member
of the primary health care team, provides a useful opportunity for health promotion and

health education (DoH 1995a; McBean 1997). Both nurses involved will have an opportunity to make a general health assessment. Working together, a comprehensive picture of Cathy's health strengths and needs should emerge. This provides both nurses, in conjunction with the family, with a starting point for health promotion and health education activities (Ewles and Simnett 1995; DoH 1995a; McBean 1997). The focus in the case of Cathy will be around diet, exercise and sexuality. To be effective, changes in diet and exercise, aimed at the maintenance of correct weight and a balanced food intake, should be incorporated into normal daily and weekly routines and not seen as special activities for a limited period only.

The major issue in working with this family is that of influencing attitudes in order to change behaviour. Given that attitudes are strongly held this will not be easy. The tension between the mother and father in relation to diet can be used creatively. The two nurses involved will probably choose to influence the father through supporting a new dietary stance that will be taken by the mother following recent events. The proposed changes need to be seen by the family as **important rather than imposed**, which provides an example of partnerships as identified in *'Valuing People'* (DoH 2001). Information in the form of leaflets, diet sheets, alcohol unit norms, height/weight norms should be introduced sensitively. It will be much more effective if the nurses involved respond to requests for information rather than devising a pack and presenting it. It may be helpful to use a quasi-counselling approach (Heron 1990) of facilitating the development of new insights about diet and lifestyle and then offering information, support and guidance towards healthy choices. (See also Communication in Chapter 6 on mental health nursing.)

Communication skills

The issue of communication skills is a general one for nurses and midwives in all areas of professional practice. Without communication of some kind, nursing cannot take place. It is the duty of the nurse to discover what is significant to the client or patient in their care and not the other way around. It follows that the nurse must be a skilled and active listener (Heron 1990). Close attention should be paid to non-verbal communication, as this is perhaps the most reliable medium. Communication is not just directly with the client or patient, but with the context in which they live and their history. In the case of Cathy it would not have been very effective to just give written or verbal advice about diet. Once Cathy's context was understood, it became clear that the whole family's behaviour needed to change. The issues concerning the incident in the playground would not have emerged without Yvonne's ability to be creative about augmenting Cathy's communication.

Communication directly with Cathy was dominated by the need to understand a particular sign language. The communication about the basic elements of this sign language

should have taken place during Cathy's admission to the general hospital. Had Cathy been from a different ethnic background, one of the important questions that would have been asked is 'what language does she speak?'. An interpreter could then be sought. With Cathy, whose learning disability is obvious in her appearance, the question was not asked, the assumption made was that she could not communicate and the care that followed was, in respect of not helping her to use the toilet, negligent.

Conclusion

Working through this chapter and exploring the experiences of Cathy and her family will have enabled you to gain some insight into the challenges faced by someone who is growing up with a learning disability, discovering their independence and starting to make their own decisions which will shape their future.

Staff involved in Cathy's care, both in the community and in hospital, have needed to acknowledge and address the family's concerns about the way that Cathy is being understood, treated and cared for. We have seen how a lack of insight, or limitation of skill, can result in important messages being missed, and the care provided being less then adequate. There are important messages here for practitioners, which emphasise the need to liaise with, and make use of, the specialist expertise that learning disability nurses can bring to the interprofessional team. There is a particular need where a client is faced with a new or unusual challenge, for example being admitted to a general hospital.

Reflect back on the outcomes set out at the beginning of this chapter; how well have these been addressed and what will be your personal action plan be for finding out more?

References

Barton, L. (1996) Sociology and disability: some emerging issues. In: Barton, L. (ed.) *Disability and Society: Emerging Issues and Insights*. Harlow: Longman,

Biggs, S. (1998) Care management in community care – advantages, disadvantages and developments. In: Thompson, T., Mathias, P. (eds) (1998)*Standards and Learning Disability*. 2nd Edition. London: Baillière Tindall.

Brechin, A., Walmsley, J. (eds) (1989). *Making Connections: Reflecting on the Lives and Experiences of People with Learning Difficulties*. London: Hodder and Stoughton.

Clegg, J. A. (1993) Putting people first: a social constructionist approach to learning disability. *British Journal of Clinical Psychology* 32, pp. 389–406.

Dallos, R. (1991) *Family Belief Systems, Therapy and Change*. Buckingham: The Open University Press.

Department of Health (1983) *Mental Health Act*. London: HMSO.

Department of Health (1995a) *The Health of the Nation: A Strategy for People with Learning Disabilities,* London: HMSO.

Department of Health (1995b), *The Health of the Nation.* London: HMSO.

Department of Health (1998) *Saving Lives: Our Healthier Nation.* London: HMSO.

Department of Health (1997) *The New NHS: Modern and Dependable.* Cm 3807. London: The Stationery Office.

Department of Health (2001), *Valuing People: A Strategy for People with Learning Disabilities for the 21st Century.* Cm 5086. London: The Stationery Office.

Donnellan, A. M., LaVigna, G, W., Negri-Shoultz, N., Fassbender, L. L. (1988) *Progress Without Punishment: Effective Approaches for Learners with Behaviour Problems.* London: Teachers College Press.

Ewles, L., Simnett, I. (1995) *Promoting Health: A Practical Guide.* 3rd Edition. London: Scutari.

Ferris-Taylor, R. (1997) Communication. In: Gates, B. (ed.) *Learning Disabilities.* London: Churchill Livingstone.

Forchuk, C., Peplau, H. E. (1993) *Interpersonal Nursing Theory.* Newbury Park: Sage Publications.

Gates, B. (1997a) Understanding learning disability. In: Gates, B. (ed.) *Learning Disabilities.* London: Churchill Livingstone.

Gates, B. (1997b) Behavioural difficulties. In: Gates, B. (ed.) (1995) *Learning Disabilities.* London: Churchill Livingstone.

Gilbert, T., Dix, T. (1995) Informed consent. In: Todd M., Gilbert, T. (eds) *Learning Disabilities: Practice Issues in Health Settings.* London: Routledge.

Gilbert, T. (1998) Sexual health and people with learning disabilities. In: Morrissey, M. (ed.) *Sexual Health: A Human Dilemma.* Wiltshire: Mark Allen.

Gilbert, T., Todd, M., Jackson, N. (1998) People with learning disabilities who also have mental health problems: practice issues and directions for learning disability nursing. *Journal of Advanced Nursing* 27 (6), pp. 1151–7.

Gilbert, J., Rose, S. (1998) Commissioning and providing services. In: Thompson, T., Mathias, P. (eds) *Standards and Learning Disability.* 2nd Edition. London: Baillière Tindall.

Heron, J. (1990) *Helping the client.* London: Sage.

Hewitt, D., Ephraim, G. (1994) *Access to Communication: Developing the Basics of Communication with People with Severe Learning Difficulties Through Intensive Interaction.* London: David Fulton.

Home Office (1998) *Supporting Families.* Green Paper. London: The Stationary Office.

Kay, B., Rose, S., Turnbull, J. (1995), *Continuing the Commitment.* Department of Health. London: HMSO.

Mathews, D. (1996) *The 'OK' Health Check for Assessing and Planning Health Care Needs of People with Learning Disabilities.* Preston: Fairfield Publications.

McBean, S. (1997) Health and health promotion – consensus and conflict. In: Perry, A. (ed.) *Nursing: A Knowledge Base for Practice.* 2nd Edition. London: Arnold.

McNally, S. (1997) Representation. In: Gates, B. (ed.) *Learning Disabilities.* London: Churchill Livingstone.

Moss, S., Turner, S. (1995) *The Health of People with Learning Disabilities.* Report to the Department of Health. Manchester: Hester Adrian Research Centre.

Nirje, B. (1969) The normalisation principle and its human management implications. In: Kugel, R., Wolfensberger, W. (eds*) Changing Patterns in Residential Services for the Mentally Retarded.* Washington, DC: Presidents Committee on Mental Retardation.

Nursing and Midwifery Council (2002) *Code of Professional Conduct*: London: NMC.

Oliver, M. (1990) *The Politics of Disablement.* Basingstoke: Macmillan.

Peplau, H. (1991) *Interpersonal Relations in Nursing.* New York: Springer.

Redworth, M., Redworth, F. (1997) Learning disability and citizenship: paradigms for inclusion. *Journal of Learning Disabilities for Nursing, Health and Social Care.* 1 (4), pp. 181–5.

Ryan, J., Thomas, F. (1987) *Politics of Mental Handicap.* London: Free Associated Press.

Schon, D. (1983) *The Reflective Practitioner: How Professionals Think in Action.* USA: Basic Books.

Sines, D., Barr, O. (1998) Professions in teams. In: Thompson, T., Mathias, P. (eds) *Standards and Learning Disability.* 2nd Edition. London: Baillière Tindall.

Singh, P. (1997) *Prescriptions for Change: A Mencap Report on the Role of GPs and Carers in the Provision of Primary Care for People with a Learning Disability.* London: Mencap.

The King's Fund. (1999) *Learning Disabilities: From Care to Citizenship.* London: The King's Fund.

United Kingdom Central Council (1992) *Code of Professional Conduct.* London: UKCC for Nursing, Midwifery and Health Visiting.

Wake, E. (1997) Profound and multiple disability. In: Gates, B. (ed.) *Learning Disabilities.* London: Churchill Livingstone.

Walker, M. (1980) *The Makaton Vocabulary Language Programme.* 31 Firwood Drive, Camberley, Surrey: Makaton Vocabulary Development Project.

Watson, D. (1997) Causes and manifestations. In: Gates, B. (ed.) *Learning Disabilities.* London: Churchill Livingstone.

Wertheimer, A. (ed.) (1996) *Changing Days: Developing New Day Opportunities with People who have Learning Difficulties.* London: The King's Fund.

Wolfensberger, W. (1972) *The Principle of Normalisation in Human Services.* Toronto: National Institute on Mental Retardation, .

World Health Organisation (1993) *Describing Developmental Disability: Guidelines for a Multi-Axial Scheme for Mental Retardation.* 10th Revision. Geneva: WHO.

Resources

📖 Further reading

Annotated bibliography

Brechin, A., Walmsley, J. (eds) (1989) *Making Connections: Reflecting on the Lives and Experiences of People with Learning Difficulties.* London: Hodder and Stoughton.

This edited text provides a range of perspectives on the experiences of people with learning disabilities. These involve academic essays, the experiences of parents and workers, and the experiences of individuals with learning disability.

Department of Health (1995) *The Health of the Nation: A Strategy for People with Learning Disabilities*. London: The Stationery Office.

A useful summary of the ways in which the *Health of the Nation* strategy might directly relate to people with a learning disability. It suggests health can be improved through three key activities: health promotion; health surveillance; and health care.

Department of Health (2001). *Valuing People: A New Strategy for Learning Disability for the 21st Century*. Cm 5086. London: The Stationery Office.

This is the first government strategy for people with learning disabilities since 1971 and it represents a significant challenge for all those involved in public services, setting standards for achievement. The strategy seeks to end prejudice, bullying, insensitive treatment and discrimination against people with learning disabilities. It sets out to improving the life chances of people with learning disabilities by working in partnerships with them and their families and with local councils, the health service and voluntary organisations to provide new opportunities for full and active lives.

The strategy is built around four 'Key Principles': rights, independence, choice and inclusion. The development of better life chances is focused upon the following areas:

- **Disabled children and young people** Ensuring educational opportunities; health and social care while living with their families or in another appropriate setting.
- **More choice and control for people with learning disabilities** Extending direct payments and developing advocacy services; and including people with learning disabilities in the planning process.
- **Supporting carers** Increasing help and support from local agencies; increasing financial support through benefits such as the Invalid Care allowance; and a special focus upon the need of carers in ethnic minority communities.
- **Improving health for people with learning disabilities** Guaranteeing access to mainstream health care; registration with a GP; the development of health facilitators within community learning disability teams; and the development of a 'health action plan' for every person with a learning disability.
- **Housing, fulfilling lives, and employment** Greater choice with housing and the closure of the remaining long-stay hospitals; the development of leisure interests, friendships and relationships with the modernisation of local council day services; the involvement of the Learning and Skills Council; the outlawing of discrimination; the improvement of services to parents with learning disabilities; new targets for increasing the numbers of people with learning disabilities in employment.
- **Quality services** Development of local quality assurance frameworks focused upon promoting services that develop independence, choice and inclusion; the development of workforce strategies to increase the number of appropriately trained and qualified staff working in this area.
- **Delivering change** The development of effective partnerships to advise on the implementation of the programme; the promotion of research.

Gates, B., Beacock ,C. (1997). *Dimensions of Learning Disability*. London: Baillière Tindall. And also Gates, B. (ed.) (1997). *Learning Disabilities.* London: Churchill Livingstone.

Two good general readers for the field, which will provide the student who is new to learning disabilities with a useful overview and reference source.

Kay, B., Rose, S., Turnbull, J. (1995) *Continuing the Commitment*. Department of Health. London: HMSO.

A three-part report which gives a helpful overview of the role and work of specialist nurses for people with a learning disability. The resource package vignettes are particularly useful in clarifying interventions that are used.

Mencap (1997) *Prescriptions for Change: A Mencap Report on the Role of GPs and Carers in the Provision of Primary Care for People with a Learning Disability*. London: Mencap.

A useful overview of issues relating to the role and limitations of GPs and others involved in primary health care.

Mencap (1998) *The NHS – Health for all? People with Learning Disabilities and Health Care*. London: Mencap.

A good general reader on access to the NHS for people with a learning disability. It includes the results of a Mencap survey conducted in England and Wales.

Moss, S., Turner, S. (1995) *The Health of People with Learning Disability*. Manchester: Hester Adrian Research Centre.

A comprehensive overview of the general health of people with a learning disability.

National Health Service Executive (1998) *Signposts for Success in Commissioning and Providing Health Services for People with Learning Disabilities*. London: NHS Executive.

A useful guide to government thinking and strategy in relation to meeting the health needs of people with a learning disability.

Thompson, T., Mathias, P. (1998) (eds) *Standards and Learning Disability*. 2nd Edition. London: Baillière Tindall.

A useful reader which makes connections between policy and a range of contemporary developments related to services for people with learning disabilities.

Insights into Community Care

8

Cynthia Yolanda Akinsanya

Introduction

During the 1990s there were a number of significant developments in health and social care driven by key policy changes. A number of new consultative documents, White Papers and acts of parliament played a major part in bringing about changes to services. Some of these included: the *NHS and Community Care Act* (DoH 1990); *The Patient Charter: Raising the Standards* (NHSE 1992); The *New NHS: Modern, Dependable* (DoH 1997a); the *NHS (Primary Care) Act* (DoH 1997b); and *Our Healthier Nation* (DoH 1998a).

The increased emphasis on empowerment of communities to provide health care for individuals, families and carers that is specific to their needs is particularly relevant to the recommendations and to the health care professionals who are the main providers of care. Therefore, it is essential for the nurse to acquire a full understanding of these changes, their implications, and their impact on health and social care perspectives and care delivery.

Aim

The scope of this chapter is to increase awareness and understanding of aspects that may influence care delivery in the community setting. The experiences of two men living in different communities, both having diabetes, provides opportunities to explore important issues in care delivery within communities.

Learning outcomes

This chapter provides the opportunity to:

- Explore and explain the meaning of 'community' from different perspectives.
- Recognise the influences of health and social policies on the provision of community care.

237

- Distinguish those factors that contribute to the changing focus of health care with emphasis on the innovations in community care provision.
- Identify the relationship between the concepts of health, public health and social care in the historical and current context.
- Consider the impact of inter-professional and inter-agency collaboration on the delivery of health and social care.
- Outline the organisation and delivery of health care in the community and the contribution of the Primary Health Care Team to the process.
- Become acquainted with the knowledge, skills and awareness required when managing care delivery within communities.

Concepts

- Community
- Community health
- Health
- Public health
- Inter-professional/inter-agency
- Collaboration/partnership
- Networks
- Care delivery

- Consumer's choice
- Epidemiology
- Health and social care policies
- Resources
- Primary health care
- Demography
- Diabetes mellitus
- Planning and providing care

Scenario A *Introducing Mr Piper*

Mr Piper, aged 55, is a postman and lives in a rural village several miles away from the nearest town. He has recently been diagnosed as having diabetes mellitus. His care management involves himself and the multi-disciplinary primary health care team.

Scenario B *Introducing Mr Thomas*

Mr Thomas, aged 55, is a manager of a small engineering business. He was diagnosed with diabetes mellitus in his early teens. He lives in the city and attends the hospital for the greater part of his care, with only some support from the multi-disciplinary primary health care team.

Living in a community

In order for nurses to provide evidence based, competent and quality care, it is essential that they have a complete comprehension of the various terms used in the provision of health care in the community. Nurses also need to understand how members of the community multi-disciplinary team, the client and carers, interpret these terms. It has become increasingly clear that many nurses are unclear about the meaning of the different terms used in discussing concepts and theories in nursing (Akinsanya and Williams 2001).

In order to enhance team working and to ensure a seamless and improved service for individuals in need of health care, there is a fundamental need for nurses to have an extensive knowledge and understanding of the roles of other health care professionals to work alongside their colleagues.

Although collaboration within and between disciplines has long been linked with quality and clinically effective health care delivery, it is now accepted as being an essential component. The increase in health care cooperatives resulting from the implementation of successive governmental policies (DoH 1997a, 2000) also requires more integrated nursing teams demonstrating their diverse skills and working with sound ethical principles.

Activity 8.1

Communities provide an individual with life experiences:

First, how does this relate to your own travels and experiences, how different are these to Mr Piper's and Mr Thomas's experiences of village and city life?

Second, consider why communities might change over time. Talk to residents in your own neighbourhood, what has been responsible for the changes they have experienced? Why might these perceptions be important to you as a nurse? Why not discuss this with a practitioner and compare your findings with peers.

From your activity, including the review of the literature, you probably noticed that the concept of 'community' may mean different things to different people. One definition by Jones (1994) incorporates the idea of a locality (or small area) where people share common interests. These interests arise from different perspectives, such as social, cultural, political and even the idea of ownership.

From a nursing perspective the community is considered as a geographical area, or neighbourhood, in which there are different relationships in an environment that is shared by families, individuals or a social group. They all have needs that are specific and unique. Community may also be used to describe groups with interests that are common in values, beliefs or similar experiences. From a sociological perspective there appears to be general agreement on one aspect, that the word 'community' can apply either to the population of a particular geographical area or to people who share common interests other than being in close proximity.

Community relates to a set of values and norms of every-day life: mutuality, cooperation, identification and symbiosis. Jones (1994) points out that community remains central to health care professionals. In addition it is increasingly being required that services are delivered 'at a local level' to meet local community 'needs' and to 'empower' the community. The development of community care initiatives has been most important to support local health needs.

Professional conversation

Jane Stevens, district nurse

Perceptions of community

'As a nurse working within a team alongside other professionals and people from other agencies I find our varying viewpoints very interesting. They no doubt differ depending on our personal experience and background, including our education.

  With the changes brought by industrialisation, the views on community started to change, and there seemed to be a breakdown in the traditional form of association. Community types in the current sociological debate still provoke differing views. In the past the 'Gemeinschaft' and 'Gesellschaft' were the two major types. The *Gemeinschaft* was based on the traditional style of living in a pre-industrial age, characterised by small, largely self-sufficient, kinship- and friendship-based social systems, in which relationships were founded on a clear understanding of each individual's status and local standing. The *Gesellschaft* was a society characterised by individualism, in which impersonal ties were based on contact.'

  These views are supported by Jones (1994).

Activity 8.2

Building on the work you have already done, consider the demographic differences between the communities you experience every day. What are the main demographic changes that affect health?

Community care

Since the inception of the NHS in 1948 many policies have offered opportunities to do things differently, and as a result have created changes in health care delivery. Some of these policies have directly influenced the delivery of community health care. Government reports up to the late 1970s referred to community care as 'care in the community', but thereafter the emphasis has increasingly shifted to 'care by the community'.

  A succession of reports from the late 1970s signalled a new orientation towards voluntary and informal caring, and towards independent services instead of public sector provision. However, due to increase in expenditure and controversial debates about such things as funding and efficiency, the strategies were reviewed.

In 1986 the Audit Commission (the government's independent watchdog on public expenditure) attacked the high costs and widespread inefficiencies of policies for community care. The Commission also drew attention to the lack of redistribution of resources from hospital-based services to locally-based local authority and health services, and the lack of funds to ease the transition of patients to community care settings. It pointed out that people were being cared for in inappropriate, institutional settings when they could be given more appropriate and less expensive assistance in their own homes.

The year 1986 also saw publication of the *Cumberlege Report* (DHSS 1986a) which recommended monitoring of local populations, with the hope of a better focus on a 'neighbourhood' approach to nursing care delivery, providing a more ambitious local service. This led in part to an increasing focus on health care delivery in the community and a subsequent expansion in community care.

The implementation of the *NHS and Community Care Act* (DoH 1990) made it statutory to provide needs-based care for all individuals. Increasingly, the government is keen to consult on its proposed developments, but as Hawtin et al (1994) suggests, this does not always occur. Sometimes the geographical size of the area or population may be too large to enable communities to be involved in any practical sense.

Activity 8.3

Consider the possible ways in which Mr Piper and Mr Thomas might be consulted about changes in health policy in their local communities. How might such challenges be addressed?

Over time, NHS reforms have redirected the emphasis from a 'pathogenic model of care' to the 'health orientation model of care' or, to put it in other terms, from the 'acute' to 'primary' and 'community care'. Consequently, primary care has grown in importance and complexity, and this in turn has had a great impact on the delivery of community care and on the role of community health care nurses (Blackie 1998).

Community health nursing is professional nursing directed towards communities or population groups as well as individuals living in the community. It includes assessment of the environment, social and personal factors that influence the health status of the targeted population. Its practice incorporates the identification of groups and individuals within the community who require help in maintaining or achieving optimal health (RCN 1992, p. 6).

Activity 8.4

More recent policy developments have often been predicated upon a number of significant reports, government papers and acts of parliament. Although some of these now date from the middle of the last century, they are of great historical significance. Take the time to find out more about some of these by accessing the primary document or a health policy textbook. Suggestions might include:

- The Beveridge Report (DHSS 1942); National Insurance Act 1946 (DHSS); National Health Service Act 1948 (DHSS).
- NHS Re-organisation Act 1973 (DHSS 1974); Royal Commission on the NHS 1977-1978 (DHSS 1979).
- Community Care: Agenda for Action (DHSS 1986b): Working for Patients (DoH 1989b).
- The Health of the Nation (DoH, 1992); The Health Act (DoH, 1999b).

Diabetes

As the experiences of both Mr Piper and Mr Thomas unfold throughout this chapter, they will provide you with an opportunity to explore how nurses collaborate with other disciplines, to support individuals with health care needs and ensure effective transfer of care, when individuals transfer from acute settings to their own community. First, we will meet Mr Piper who has just been found to have diabetes.

Scenario A *A new experience for Mr Piper*

When Mr Piper first began to feel unwell, he had recently lost quite a lot of weight and thought that this might have had some bearing on it. He was getting out of breath, but put this down to his smoking. He seemed to be drinking a lot of water and then having to get up several times during the night to pass urine. His wife persuaded him to make an appointment at the GP's surgery in the village and following some investigations, it was confirmed that he had diabetes mellitus.

Diabetes can develop at any age and requires life-long treatment. However, effective and diligent treatment can be compatible with a full and active lifestyle. Living with diabetes does mean a lifetime of medical care. Since diabetes can affect all age groups and may present as a number of clinical symptoms which appear suddenly, or which are increasingly experienced over the longer term, health care professionals cannot address the problems in isolation.

Activity 8.5

Consider your understanding of diabetes mellitus and try setting out a definition.

Evidence-based practice

Diabetes mellitus occurs when the blood sugar level exceeds 11.1mmol/l two hours after a glucose challenge. The normal fasting blood glucose level should be 7.0mmol/l (WHO 1999).

Effective diabetes care provision calls for health care professionals who possess an in-depth knowledge of the physiological and patho-physiological basis of diabetes mellitus. Therefore it is essential for you, as a future health care professional, to become familiar with all aspects of the condition and the care management.

Diabetes mellitus is the most common endocrine disorder that affects the world's population. Situated deep in the abdomen behind the stomach is the pancreas, which contains several specialised cell types. One of the specialised cells that make up the islets of Langerhan in the pancreas is the beta cell, which produces insulin. This is a hormone responsible for the tightly controlled physio-logical regulation of blood glucose.

Activity 8.6

Based on your knowledge to date, identify the pos-sible causes of diabetes. Think about Mr Piper; he must be wondering what has caused his diabetes, what clues might there be?

In normal individuals food intake and the subsequent increase in blood glucose triggers the release of insulin. Initially, there was uncertainty over whether diabetes was due to insufficient insulin or its failure to act on the tissues, or whether it was due to the auto-immune destruction of the pancreatic islet cells that secrete insulin. It is now clear that all these possibilities exist in different forms of the disease. There is also evidence to suggest that there is a genetic component too.

When blood glucose levels increase in response to a meal, the pancreas would normally release insulin into the bloodstream to help glucose enter cells, and therefore lower the blood glucose levels. Once this takes place, homeostatic control mechanisms result in the reduction of insulin levels in the blood. In people with diabetes mellitus, insulin is either unavailable or is relatively insufficient for the body's needs. The overall aim of insulin therapy is to mimic as closely as possible the normal pancreatic response to blood glucose levels. This involves continual secretion of low levels of insulin to aid the body's metabolism of glucose (Avery 1998).

Activity 8.7

For further information read a general text such as *Principles of Anatomy and Physiology* (7th Edition) by Tortora, G. J., Grabowski, S. R. (New York: Harper & Row).

To recap, Diabetes Mellitus is characterised by high blood sugar levels that result from insufficient insulin or its inability to act. Diabetes is traditionally divided into two major types: Type 1 or insulin-dependent diabetes mellitus (IDDM); and Type 2 or non insulin-dependent diabetes mellitus (NIDDM).

Mr Thomas has had Type 1 diabetes for some years and we will return to his experi-ences in more detail in due course. Mr Piper has been newly diagnosed as having Type 2 diabetes.

Type 1 or insulin-dependent diabetes mellitus (IDDM)

People with Type 1 diabetes are no longer capable of producing the hormone insulin and rely on administered insulin therapy for survival, as in the case of Mr Thomas. This was formerly known as juvenile-onset diabetes and is thought to be caused by auto-immune destruction of the pancreatic islet cells that secrete insulin. Abnormal anti-bodies in the blood (proteins that form part of the body's immune defence system) have been found in the client with Type 1 diabetes (Howdle and Wilkin 2001).

Evidence-based practice

In auto-immune diseases such as Type 1 diabetes, it is thought that the immune system mistakenly produces antibodies directed against, and caus-ing damage to, the client's own body tissues. There is evidence to suggest that the tendency to develop these abnormal antibodies in Type 1 diabetes is due in part to an individual's genetic make up and can therefore be inher-ited. Chromosome 11 in the human genome has been reported to carry a gene associated with the development of Type 1 diabetes. Epidemiological studies propose that approximately 10 per cent of the clients with diabetes mellitus have Type 1 diabetes (Diabetes Focus 2002).

Type 2 or non insulin-dependent diabetes mellitus (NIDDM)

This is the type of diabetes that Mr Piper has recently experienced.

Until recently the mechanism responsible for NIDDM (formerly known as adult-onset diabetes mellitus), remained unclear. In this type of diabetes the client can still produce insulin, but only with an inadequate response. In addition, a major feature of NIDDM is a lack of sensitivity to insulin by the cells of the body. Under normal circum-stances, the insulin receptor signals the presence of insulin to the interior of the cells (Howdle and Wilkins 2001). Failure of insulin to act on the body's tissues (insulin

---

Activity 8.8

Many of the symptoms associated with diabetes mellitus are common to both types; however, take time to explore the differences. Considering what you know of Mr Piper so far, is there anything that might support a Type 2 diagnosis?

---

resistance) results from a defect in the insulin receptor and a lack of or impairment of this signal. NIDDM is most commonly diagnosed in adulthood and accounts for between 70 per cent and 80 per cent of all diabetes. Overall, the prevalence of diabetes in the UK as reported by most authorities is 3 per cent, which is the tip of the iceberg since at least another 2 per cent of the population is likely to remain undiagnosed.

From your enquiries, you may have already reached conclusions about the symptoms experienced during the initial stages prior to a diagnosis. Health care professionals must be aware that in confirming a diagnosis of diabetes, consideration must also be given to the Diabetes UK (2000) new diagnostic criteria that clearly identify the six main symptoms:

Table 8.1 Diabetes mellitus diagnostic criteria

- Increased thirst
- Extreme tiredness
- Genital itching
- Polyuria
- Weight loss
- Blurred vision

Scenario A *Mr Piper's symptoms*

These symptoms reflect the experieces of Mr Piper who suffers from Type 2 diabetes. He has experienced being very thirsty with a dry mouth, with increased micturition, particularly at night, symptoms commonly associated with NIDDM.

A typical presentation for a person like Mr Thomas with Type 1 insulin-dependent diabetes mellitus might also include the following signs and symptoms in addition to those set out in the table above:

Table 8.2 Typical Type 1 presentation

- Dark coloured urine
- Sweet or fruity smelling breath (like pear drops or acetone)
- Proneness to developing other infections (e.g., boils)
- Numbness or tingling in feet or hands
- Cuts or wounds that are slow to heal properly

Activity 8.9

Before reading on consider why such signs and symptoms occur.

The early symptoms of untreated diabetes mellitus are related to elevated blood sugar levels and characterised by a loss of glucose in the urine. High amounts of glucose in the urine cause increased urine output and lead to dehydration. The high glucose content in the urine leads to genital itching. The increased thirst and water consumption is due to dehydration, and the inability to utilise glucose eventually leads to weight loss despite an increase in appetite.

Diagnosis can be confirmed through a fasting plasma glucose test in which the person fasts overnight, and a sample of blood is drawn in the morning and sent to the laboratory for analysis. Tests such as the random blood glucose test and the oral glucose tolerance test (OGTT) may be used for diagnosis. As we have seen from evidence-based practice, diabetes mellitus occurs when the blood sugar level exceeds 11.1mmol/l two hours after a glucose challenge, with the normal fasting blood glucose level set at 7.0mmol/l (WHO 1999). For the purpose of ongoing monitoring, provision has been made for blood glucose monitoring with meters that are easy to operate by clients in their own home.

Activity 8.10

Find out how these tests are managed in both the GP practice and in Out Patient clinics. How are electronic blood glucose meters used in your practice areas?

Scenario A

Initially, Mr Piper was advised on modifying his lifestyle. Mrs Piper accompanied him to the surgery, but was not present when her husband was with the GP. However when the practice nurse asked her if she would like to be present while she gave Mr Piper information about diabetes, Mrs Piper said she was keen to be involved and help in any way she could. Mr Piper had no objection to his wife being present.

Expert nurses, who are confident in their clinical decision-making skills, are usually swift to notice immediate changes and responses in patient/client behaviour. These unconscious observation skills are formed from both knowledge and experience, and are valuable in identifying signs that are relevant to the decision-making process. Reassurance, respect for patients'/clients' perspectives, emotional support, alleviation of fear and anxiety are important aspects of care delivery. Patient-centred care is regarded as the optimum way of delivering health care, and may be defined as 'valuing people as individuals' (Gerteis et al 1993; Winefield et al 1996).

Patients'/clients' perspectives are also regarded as an important indicator of quality in health care (DoH 1999a). From practical knowledge of their disease, the patient/client comes to the nurse–patient interaction with his/her own understanding of normality. The patient, once a well individual, is now a 'sufferer'. The impact of a perceived lack of normality, because of illness, can lead to grief and anguish. Central to achieving the health goals is the ability of the caring professional to acknowledge this vulnerability, demonstrate consideration and instil confidence (Miller 1992).

Therefore the professionals involved with Mr and Mrs Piper should encourage and foster an environment of trust, belonging and confidence in their ability to cope. These factors will empower the patient/client to feel free to voice concerns.

Activity 8.11

Make a list of the essential factors that you will need to include in your assessment of Mr Piper and identify the methods of communication that you will use. From the scenario, you will be able to obtain some of the information you require. Try to identify Mr Piper's needs by grouping them together and then prioritising them.

Needs-based care

Consider the literature for an explanation of needs-based care and its relevance to care management. You may find the following resources helpful: Appleton, J. Cowley, S. (2000) *The Search for Health Needs.* Basingstoke: Palgrave Macmillan; Hawtin, M., Hughes, G., Percy-Smith, J. (1994) *Community Profiling – Auditing Social Needs.* Buckingham: Open University Press.

The cornerstone of the assessment process is well established to be a systematic approach in identifying the needs of the patient or client, prior to care planning and implementation. Care planning must be needs-based and patient-centred, involving the patient in decisions on care and treatment, and service planning and delivery (DoH 2000). However, this raises challenges for health professionals in today's climate where cost-effectiveness and the pressure of limited resources are highlighted.

The decisions about what care and how it is to be delivered must be based on the best evidence currently available. Hek (2000) points out that the drive for evidence-based health care and evidence-based nursing gained momentum in the latter half of the 1990s, not least as a result of the Department of Health's drive to provide

Activity 8.12

Consider ways in which you would involve Mr and Mrs Piper in care planning.

clinically effective health care (NHS Executive 1996). This is also a consequence of the recent *National Service Framework for Diabetes* (DoH 2001) publication, which gives specific guidelines for pathways, care management and delivery. To ensure the drive to effective care delivery, the professional must be responsive to and committed to implementing evidence based interventions. This is what Sue Terry, the practice nurse, must consider in her discussions with Mr and Mrs Piper.

Professional conversation

Sue Terry, practice nurse

Assessing needs

'I find that when a patient at our surgery is newly diagnosed, it often comes as quite a shock to them. This is usually followed by a sense of relief, as the reasons for the vague, non-specific symptoms become apparent. There is quite a lot of information to give to someone who is newly diagnosed with any condition and diabetes is no exception. In my role I try to put the information across in a way that helps the individual, trying to put myself in their shoes. Sometimes their response to this newly diagnosed chronic health problem is to shut off for a while and try and deny its all happening.

As I talk I show different leaflets which the person can take away. Sometimes I draw diagrams and I have quite a good collection now of teaching materials like posters. I keep on asking if they understand and ask them to repeat back, summarising what they think I have said. That way I can consider their understanding and clarify any possible misunder-standings.

It's really helpful if a family member or friend can be there, especially if that person lives with them or nearby. It's often relatives or partners, who ask the really practical questions. The key points about diabetes and lifestyle that I tend to focus on include:
healthy eating and drinking; smoking cessation; exercise; and skin care. It is essential that Mr Piper is aware of some possible complications, such as his increased susceptibility to infections. Mr Piper has been prescribed hypoglycaemic agents which will help to control his diabetes. I have therefore discussed the possible side-effects and risks of hyperglycaemia.

I took the opportunity to introduce Mr and Mrs Piper to Anne Smith, one of our district nurses who has a special interest in diabetes, she will also be involved in monitoring Mr Piper's progress. I am also in touch with the occupational health nurse for the Post Office.'

The person with diabetes is at increased risk of circulatory problems such as coronary artery disease, leading to myocardial infarct, and also to stroke. (See also Chapter 12 on rehabilitation and stroke.) Therefore appropriate diet, cessation of smoking and taking effective exercise will help to reduce the risk. The person with diabetes may develop peripheral neuro-pathy, which can lead to damage, particularly to the feet. A major effect of diabetes is the risk of blindness. Indeed, the majority of people over the age of 60 who are registered blind in the UK have diabetes.

> ### Activity 8.13
>
> Consider what lifestyle changes (if any) Mr and Mrs Piper might need to think about. Make a list, giving your rationale, before reading on.

Over the past ten years, primary care teams have been encouraged to increase the quality and quantity of the care they provide for people like Mr Piper who is diagnosed with diabetes. Experiences over the past two decades of a number of sub-specialties being involved in caring for patients has led to recognition of the increased need for coordinated diabetes specialist care.

Most of the services now involve specialist multi-professional diabetes teams, and are provided as outpatient, with some inpatient, facilities. However, there are still some problems with care management because of a lack of clear management guidelines and a lack of understanding of diabetes by the patients and by some professionals.

Some GP practices hold specialist clinics at specific times for people who have diabetes. These are often led by specialist nurses. Occasionally these are combined clinics for people with diabetes and cardiovascular problems. Group education sessions are held in some practices when guest speakers give talks on specific topics, and the clients are encouraged to share ideas and experiences.

Activity 8.14

Place yourself in the role of Sue Terry, the practice nurse who works closely with Anne Smith the district nurse. Draw up a list of speakers for your programme of monthly staff lunchtime seminars. Formulate your list before reading on.

Your list might include a podiatrist, optician, pharmacist, dietician, physiotherapist and occupational therapist. You may also have included other people who are successfully living with diabetes who have a positive attitude with helpful tips to share.

Activity 8.15

A Find out what educational information is accessible locally for the general public and people who have diabetes. What does it consist of, how is it presented and does it take account of people with specific needs?

B Find out from local GP surgeries if specialist clinics are offered, for example for diabetes or asthma. How long have these services been offered? You may like to consider your findings with a community practitioner or discuss them with your peers.

Professional conversation

Anne Smith, district nurse

Advice and monitoring

'As the district nurse, and leader of this district nursing team, I have full responsibility for the nursing care of my caseload of patients in the community. I work closely with the other members of the team and in Mr Piper's case, I liaise particularly closely with Sue Terry the practice nurse, especially regarding monitoring his progress. We are both committed to an individual approach to giving total patient care based on a needs assessment. Both of us are involved in health education and advising patients on how to develop their skills so that they can become increasingly independent.

My responsibility is to provide effective care management, thereby ensuring professional accountability for assessing and reassessing the needs of both patient and carer, fully involving both patient and carer in the process.'

Activity 8.16

Anne Smith has set out some of her responsibilities for patient care. Discuss your perceptions of her role with a community practitioner that you have contact with. How do these differ from the local arrangements that you have experienced? What protocols are used locally by district nurses in the delivery of community care?

Scenario A *Mr Piper's plan of care*

Following an assessment of Mr Piper's main needs, a programme of care needed to be developed which would focus on self-care management, symptom relief, dietary goal achievements, well-being, maintaining quality of life and preventing complications. Both Sue Terry and Anne Smith devised a plan which would provide support and guidance, and restore independence through health education and monitoring. The objectives of regular monitoring included:

- Assessing the effectiveness of treatment
- Preventing extremes of blood glucose levels
- Allowing Mr Piper to adjust his lifestyle to accommodate diabetes

Mr Piper was advised by practice nurse Sue Terry to follow specific guidelines about his diet to help control the diabetes. This was consolidated at an appointment with the dietician which both he and his wife attended. Despite his firm adherence to the dietary recommendations, his blood glucose analysis demonstrated that further therapy was needed so his GP prescribed a course of oral medication.

Activity 8.17

Take on the role of Anne Smith and look specifically at the information that you would need to build into Mr Piper's plan of care; some of what you need will have already been obtained. Think about several realistic short- and long-term goals which Mr Piper is able to sign up to. Ask a practitioner about the effects of commonly prescribed hypoglycaemic agents and include in your plan ways of dealing with any side effects. You will need to consider:

- Healthy eating and drinking
- Cessation of smoking

- Appropriate exercise
- Specific care of the feet
- Possible side-effects of the prescribed medication, for example hypo-glycaemic agents.

Discuss your plan with a peer and then check it out with a practitioner. Also look at information on diet and smoking in the chapters providing insights into cancer, nutrition and post-stroke rehabilitation (Chapters 5, 10 and 12).

Patient education is a vital part of nursing care for someone like Mr Piper, it is necessary to prevent both hypo- and hyperglycaemia. Therefore clear information on the signs and symptoms of both hyper- and hypoglycaemia, and the possible causes, must be given. Initial patient education is often carried out by the diabetes nurse specialist, with support provided when required by the community nursing team and practice nurse, who work from the PCT practice. The importance of clinic attendance and making use of the diabetic services are also essential information for Mr Piper.

Scenario A *Mr Piper – a return to health*

Regular monitoring over several months demonstrated that Mr Piper's blood glucose was now well controlled, so he continued the oral hypoglycaemic agents and continued with the dietary advice. He and his wife also decided to buy a dog with a view to increasing their activity by taking walks in the countryside.

Not everyone who has diabetes is able to continue to lead the same life as they did before. There are both economic and social sacrifices to be made in some cases, although there is considerable scope to lessen this burden. Work continues in identifying the most effective prevention and control policies (WHO 2001). Key events are set out in Table 8.3 below.

Table 8.3 Significant landmark events in the development of the WHO (2001) diabetic programme

1989 World Health Assembly Resolution 42.36: Prevention and control of diabetes mellitus

1989 Establishment of St Vincent declaration programme for diabetes in Europe

1991 WHO guidelines for the development of a national diabetic programme

1991 First World Diabetic Day, co-sponsored by WHO and the International Diabetes Federation (IDF)

1992 Special issues of *World Health Statistics Quarterly* devoted to diabetes

1993   Publication of global estimates for prevalence of diabetes and impaired glucose tolerance in adults

1994   Publication of report of WHO Study Group: 'Prevention of diabetes mellitus'

1994   First global meeting on implementation of national diabetes programmes

1995   Diabetes receives its own programme symbol at the WHO

1995   The first issue of WHO newsletter 'World diabetes' was published

1995   Establishment of official WHO/IDF working group

1996   WHO and IDF enter into regional relations in the Americas and endorse declaration on diabetes.

1997   World Health report highlights non-communicable diseases, introduces diabetes prevalence as a 'basic health indicator' for member states.
       (WHO 2001)

Planning care delivery

Over the last few decades, nursing models have been developed as a framework for care delivery in nursing practice. These models were used as a tool for clarification and enhancement of nursing knowledge. They allowed for nursing practice and care delivery to take place from a systematically constructed, more scientifically based logical approach, through assessment, planning, implementation and evaluation of care. However, working to standardised protocols is becoming more common as a means of providing effective and evidence-based care. As the Royal College of Nursing (RCN 1993) points out: 'a protocol can be described as an agreement to a particular sequence of activities that assist health care workers to respond consistently in complex areas of clinical practice'. They are also promoted as good practice developments within the government's various National Service Framework standards.

> ### Activity 8.18
>
> In order to gain a historical perspective of nursing models of care, access the following resources: Rogers 1970; Roy 1984; Orem 1985; Roper et al 1985. You will find that some of these models also provide a framework for care planning in some chapters in this book.

Protocols may be established on a uni-disciplinary or a multi-disciplinary basis and can fulfil a useful function (as in *Nurse Prescribing* DoH 1998b, c) in achieving consistency in clinical practice between health care professionals. However, protocols may also have potential to conflict with the concept of individualised patient care, appreciating that each patient/client is a unique individual with unique needs that require separate individual responses from the caring professional.

In 1991, the Department of Health launched a national research and development strategy to provide a coordinated and coherent approach to supporting evidence-based practice (DoH 1991). Initiatives were subsequently launched, including the NHS Centre for Reviews and Dissemination (NHS CRD), which provided the NHS with information on the effectiveness of treatments. The National Institute for Clinical Excellence (NICE) was also created to promote clinical excellence and cost-effectiveness. The implementation of evidence-based health care and evidence-based nursing has gained momentum in the latter half of 1990s through the Department of Health's drive to promote clinically effective health care (NHS Executive 1996). Furthermore, evidence-based health care is one aspect of the quality improvement activities of clinical governance.

Health care professionals work together to develop criteria that provide improvements in collecting community nursing patient/client assessment data in order to measure quality, appropriateness of interventions, health outcomes and information transfer across agencies. Assessment should seek to find out the individual's complete circumstances in terms of physiological, psychological, functional, social and economic status which allows for collecting in-depth information prior to forming a comprehensive picture of the patient/client for effective decision regarding the health status and perceived needs.

Clearly, a number of health care professionals are responsible for the delivery of care and to whom the referrals are made. For effective care, the person with diabetes needs to be able to access this team of professionals knowing that they will collaborate in ensuring he/she receives effective care.

> ### Activity 8.19
>
> Consider the skills of the different community team members and how they might be best utilised in the longer term monitoring of Mr Piper. For example, what role might the podiatrist have?

Diabetes care has evolved, and will continue to do so over the years. The introduction of new technical advances and changes in working practice have provided health care professionals with excellent opportunities to significantly improve the management of diabetes. Developments in research have also strengthened efforts to search for new initiatives in the treatment of people with diabetes. Due to the level of incidence, health care professionals will encounter diabetes in all clinical settings in both the acute and primary care sectors.

As a result, clinical guidelines are being systematically developed to ensure clinical effectiveness in diabetes care nationwide. The *National Service Framework for Diabetes – Standards* (DoH 2001) sets out the rationale, key interventions and an analysis of the implications for planning services based on the standards. This provides the impetus for further service developments, a summary of the standards are set out in the Table 8.4 below.

Table 8.4 The National Service Framework for Diabetes – Standards

In summary these standards relate to:

Prevention of Type 2 diabetes
- In the population as a whole
- To reduce the inequalities in the risk of developing Type 2 diabetes

Identification of people with diabetes
- to identify people who do not know they have diabetes

Empowering people with diabetes
- People of all ages will receive a service that encourages partnership in decision making, supports them in managing their diabetes, and helps them to adopt and maintain a healthy lifestyle, involving parents and carers as appropriate

Clinical care of adults with diabetes
- High quality care throughout their lifetime
- Support to optimise the control of their blood glucose, blood pressure
- Minimise risk of complications of diabetes

Clinical care of children and young people with diabetes
- Consistently high-quality
- Support to optimise the control of their blood glucose and their physical, psychological, intellectual, educational and social development
- Smooth transition of care from paediatric diabetes services to adult diabetes at an appropriate age, agreed with them

Management of diabetic emergencies
- Agreed protocols for rapid and effective treatment of diabetes emergencies by appropriately trained health care professionals
- Management of acute complications and procedures to minimise the risk of recurrence

Care of people with diabetes during admission to hospital
- People admitted to hospital, for whatever reason, will receive effective care of their diabetes, being involved in decisions concerning the management of their diabetes wherever possible

Diabetes and pregnancy
- Empower and support women with pre-existing diabetes and those who develop diabetes during pregnancy to optimise the outcomes of their pregnancy

Detection and management of long term complication
- Surveillance for the long-term complications of diabetes
- Effective investigation and treatment of people who develop long-term complications of diabetes to reduce their risk of disability and premature death
- Integrated health and social care

(DoH 2001)

Scenario A *Mr Piper – adapting to life with diabetes*

Mr Piper has made good progress over the first six months since his diagnosis, his weight is stable, he has made an effort to control his diet and appears to tolerate well the hypoglycaemic agents that he has been prescribed. He has tried to cut down on his smoking but so far without success. Anne Smith is now considering discharging Mr Piper as he is well and has no problem monitoring his own blood glucose levels. He works as a postman and the occupational health nurse has agreed to provide any support he might need. He feels fit but knows all about looking out for potential complications. He has also bought an identification bracelet and carries glucose tablets with him just in case of a hypoglycaemic episode.

? Who are the most likely members of the multidisciplinary team to whom referrals will be made to ensure Mr Piper will enjoy continuity of his diabetes care?

Scenario B *Diabetes – every-day life for Mr Thomas*

Unlike Mr Piper, Mr Thomas has had diabetes for many years and the approach to his care and treatment has changed significantly over the years. He has had to make a number of adjustments to his lifestyle, but generally has remained healthy. At 55 he has recently gained promotion at work, becoming manager of a small manufacturing business.

Mr Thomas still remembers clearly how ill he was when he was 13. His GP had referred him straight to the local hospital where the diagnosis of diabetes mellitus was confirmed. He started on insulin therapy straight away, and remained in hospital until his condition was stabilised and he and his mother had learnt how to manage the insulin therapy. At first his mother used to help with the injections, but he quickly learnt to manage it all himself. Now that his mother has died, he lives alone. He still visits the Diabetic Clinic in Out Patients for annual checks.

Last week Mr Thomas was admitted to hospital after making contact with his GP. His non-fasting venous plasma glucose was extremely high, far above the normal, and he needed regulating with immediate crisis care intervention. He had not experienced illness like this since the age of 20 and was extremely worried.

The individuals seen most often in hospital are generally those with poor management of their diabetes or those with secondary complications. Therefore the overall aim of the multi-professional team is to help in facilitating self-management and control once again, allowing for self-adjustment and return to the normal lifestyle, so as to reduce morbidity, mortality and hospitalisation.

The key requirement in case management is to take a holistic approach to care. To see the whole picture, nurses ask challenging questions to identify priorities. The process of decision making must include client-centred goal planning, as this encourages the multi-professional team members to work in partnership with the patient/client to achieve the desired outcome. Goal setting encourages and enables the patient/client to move forward from dependency to a self-management routine. In the acute environment the speed of decision making is crucial, especially for patients in need of insulin therapy.

> **?** Many patients with insulin-dependant diabetes mellitus, like Mr Thomas, present with acute symptoms. What assessments would nursing and medical staff need to carry out, and what immediate treatment would Mr Thomas require to return his blood glucose level to normal? You may wish to refer to a general text on diabetes. The following resources may also be useful: Chambers et al (2001); Jerreat (1999).

Scenario B

Mr Thomas's admission, with an episode of hyperglycaemia with ketoacidosis, included a full assessment of his general condition and range of specific laboratory tests.

Although the clinical signs may have been evident, it is important to confirm the degree and nature of hyperglycaemia with laboratory tests. Blood glucose must be raised in the range of 25–40mmol/1 for a diagnosis of ketoacidosis to be made (Higgins 1994). Since, in this condition, plasma glucose exceeds the renal threshold, glucose is always present in the urine of patients with ketoacidosis.

Scenario B *Mr Thomas's immediate needs*

The aims of Mr Thomas's immediate care management after assessment included measures to:

- Correct the fluid and electrolyte disturbances
- Correct low intracellular and raised extracellular levels of glucose
- Reduce the blood pH
- Reduce accompanying fear and anxiety

Although fluid replacement can lower blood glucose levels significantly, insulin replacement is necessary to allow glucose to enter the body cells and inhibit ketogenesis (ketone formation). This is achieved using a sliding-scale insulin regime during which capillary blood glucose is tested at appropriate intervals and an intravenous infusion of insulin is adjusted according to the blood glucose levels. It is essential that the team are familiar with protocols in hospital for the treatment of ketoacidosis (Hand 2000).

This regime continues until the urine is free of ketones. It is only then that blood glucose can be maintained within the normal limits with subcutaneous insulin and the patient is re-educated to self-manage once again. Insulin is most commonly given between two and four times a day, the regime being agreed after consultation with the patient.

Practice tip

Whenever you are caring for a patient in practice consider what form of insulin the patient receives to familiarise yourself with the full range. Insulin is measured in units, the unit being a measure of weight: 24 units = 1mg. 'U100' insulin is so called because there are 100 units of insulin in 1cc of solution. There are a range of preparations of insulin including synthetic and animal origin, some short, some medium and others long acting. Try to discover the rationale for the insulin regime for each person.

An increase in availability of injection devices that fit into cartridges has enabled most patients to use these rather than conventional syringes. This administration method saves time and assures accuracy of the dose. The patient also receives information during the self-management education process to identify symptoms of an insulin reaction that can come on suddenly (Diabetes Focus 2002; Diabetes UK 2000 web pages).

Self-management is an essential process that helps to prepare the patient for discharge. Adequate arrangements for the discharge of patients from hospital are regarded as a priority, and should be considered and planned towards from the day of admission. The importance of discharge planning is emphasised in 'Caring for People' (DoH 1989c). *The NHS and Community Care Act* (DoH 1990) established the 'care management approach'. The recommended policies give guidance on service delivery across the statutory and independent sectors.

Activity 8.20

Consider your understanding of the concept of 'care management'.

One of the main people to whom referral may be made is the nurse, perhaps in the role of clinic nurse, district nurse or practice nurse. The concept of nursing diagnosis is a successful clinical initiative as identified by Thorddsen and Thorsteinsson (2002). Nursing diagnosis is internationally accepted as a crucial step in a systematic and individualised care plan. It is a clinical judgement about individual, family or community responses to actual or potential health problems/life processes. Nursing diagnosis provides the basis for selection of nursing interventions to achieve outcomes for which the nurse is accountable (NANDA 1994)

All the issues need careful consideration in the development of a plan of care for people with diabetes requiring treatment in hospital. Professional carers therefore need to have a conceptual understanding of what quality nursing assessment entails (Skidmore 1997;

Watson and Wilkinson 2001). The care planning system must ensure that the standard of nursing documentation is consistent with professional and legal requirements.

The BDA (1993) have developed comprehensive guidelines to facilitate this process. These were used to ensure that the essential requirements for Mr Thomas's care were met during his stay in hospital. These are set out in Table 8.5 below.

Table 8.5 Recommendations for caring for people with diabetes in hospital

Health professionals should:

1 Explain to patients and carers what is going to happen throughout the hospital stay and how their diabetes will be managed until discharge.

2 Discuss any necessary change of treatment with the patient.

3 On admission, establish the patient's routine regarding insulin, tablets, blood-glucose monitoring and food.

4 Inform the diabetes team about the admission.

5 Discuss whether the patient would like to manage aspects of his or her monitoring and treatment.

6 Allow patients to keep snacks and emergency anti-hypoglycaemic food supplies in their locker and ensure that snacks are available when necessary.

7 On admission, inform the patient of meal times and offer advice on how to order food.

8 Ensure that patients are updated on all aspects of diabetes management and that they have written guidelines on blood-glucose monitoring, injection technique and the treatment of hypoglycaemia.

9 Ensure that only staff who have attended an appropriate training programme carry out blood-glucose testing.

10 Follow the blood-glucose monitoring quality assurance programme that should exist in every hospital. Poorly performed tests are dangerous and expensive.

11 Ensure that the correct timing is entered on the drug chart for oral hypoglycaemic agents and insulin, as they must be given to patients before food.

12 Aim to re-establish the patient's usual treatment as soon as possible, especially if insulin is given intravenously.

13 Be aware that particular attention needs to be given to pressure-area care for people with diabetes.

14 Check that arrangements have been made for the patient to have regular follow-ups for diabetes.

(BDA 1993)

The management of diabetes during a patient's stay in hospital requires a set of vital skills from all health care professionals. Elimination of apprehension is important as Mr Thomas is fearful of experiencing a further hypoglycaemic attack. From the beginning every aspect of care management must be discussed with him. Effective communication and information giving facilitate the establishment of a good relationship, and in turn this allows for meaningful decision making.

Empowerment is an extremely important consideration in any patient care discussion. The word empowerment appears in many philosophies of care and many see it as the ultimate in a patient-centred approach. The shift from the 'medical model' of planning and delivering care has enabled nurses to embrace care that is individualised and respects the uniqueness of being human. However, as Wright (1995) claims, this still can be misunderstood, the degree to which empowerment affects nursing action is unclear.

> ### Activity 8.21
>
> Take the opportunity to observe nurses interacting with patients and relatives, in what ways do the clients give their consent to the interventions carried out? Reflect on behaviours such as use of language. How do nurses empower and disempower their clients. In what way has Mr Thomas been empowered?

The requirement to obtain informed consent prior to care delivery is stated in nursing policy documents (UKCC 1996, 2001). The Nursing and Midwifery Council (2002) requires that the practitioner '. . . must obtain consent before . . .' giving treatment or care (p. 4).

Scenario B *Mr Thomas's preparation for discharge*

Mr Thomas spent time with the nurse prior to his discharge home as she needed to ensure that he understood the specific information on his treatment plan. She also checked that the date of the follow-up appointment to attend the diabetic clinic had been made and took time out to discuss any concerns that Mr Thomas might have. This included ways in which he was committed to achieving his individualised self-care targets. They discussed and agreed ways in which he could participate in meeting goals relating to:

- Adequate diet – deciding upon food type, amount and timing of meals.
- Physical activity.
- Insulin therapy – the dose and timing of insulin injections. Also how to change doses based on self-monitoring.
- Strategies for maintaining his target values for blood glucose, blood pressure and weight.

Mr Thomas's acute problems may have been due to the additional stress of his new job. He had possibly underestimated the need to make adjustments to his insulin intake, which had resulted in his admission to hospital with acute complications.

Evidence-based practice

Currie et al (1996) identified two main admission groups for people with diabetes: Diabetes-related causes and non-diabetes-related causes. Diabetes-related causes can then be further divided in two subgroups: acute complications and chronic complications. These are set out in Table 8.6 below.

Activity 8.22

Mr Thomas had been admitted to hospital with 'acute complications'. Consider the different complications listed below, which ones apply to Mr Thomas? Reflect upon their aetiology.

Table 8.6 Diabetes-related causes for hospital admission

Long term/chronic complications	Acute complications
• Coronary heart disease	• Diabetic ketoacidosis
• Cerebrovascular disease	• Hyperosmolar non-ketotic coma
• Neuropathy and peripheral vascular disease	• Hypoglycaemia
• Eye complications	
• Renal disease	

(Currie 1996)

Scenario B *Mr Thomas's follow up arrangements*

Further assurances were given about arrangements for follow-up visits and continuing assessment reviews, Mr Thomas was still worried that something similar might happen again. The frequency of follow-up visits will be based on his general well-being and goal achievement. To ensure continuity and give Mr Thomas peace of mind, it had been agreed from the outset that he should be given the option of being referred to the community care team. Therefore Anne Smith, district nurse, was approached well before discharge because of her specialist interest in diabetes.

Evidence-based practice

Appropriate referrals

The Audit Commission, in a report entitled *First Assessment – A Review of District Nursing in England and Wales* (Audit Commission 1999), highlighted the number of inappropriate referrals that the service receives. Research evidenced that between 6 and 11 per cent of all referrals are unnecessary and that the most likely reason is that health professionals may have a poor understanding of the service due to unclear referral criteria.

Ineffective referral criteria can create great difficulties in communication of information when the care of a patient/client is transferred from hospital to the community or vice versa. The introduction of the primary care groups (PCGs) that arose from the White Paper; *The New NHS – Modern, Dependable* (DoH, 1997a) created initiatives, allowing nurses to become more involved and to work in partnership with GPs to improve services for the

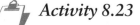

Activity 8.23

Find out whether criteria exist locally for referral to the community nursing team. Think about the needs of Mr Thomas, what issues must be considered in relation to his referral?

community. One of the main objectives of the PCG was to ensure clarity and equity to the population, by introducing referral criteria and encouraging collaborative working, resulting in similar services being offered to all patients, depending on their needs (Vafeas 2000)

The Audit Commission's review of district nursing also noted the variability in assessment information. It suggested that the quality of assessment information could be improved through the use of standardised, condition-specific forms which prompt the assessors to seek and record general assessment information as well as information specific to the patient's condition (Audit Commission 1999).

Referrals may occur directly from the hospital ward or through a district nurse liaison system, requesting assessment or follow-up care. Referral criteria were drawn up in response to the Audit Commission's Report (1999) with the aim of reducing the number of inappropriate referrals and providing patients with a more efficient service.

Table 8.7 Criteria for referral to the district nurse

- The patient must be thought to have a specific nursing need that requires the expertise of a qualified nurse. Referrals will only be accepted where there is clearly a need for skilled nursing interventions.

- All referrals must include patient's name, address, date of birth, GP, telephone number, contact details and anticipated nursing need. A printout of the patient's details should accompany a referral from GP surgeries.

- Referrals to the district nursing service will only be accepted if the patient is housebound, that is, only able to leave home by ambulance, or if there is a nursing reason that makes a home visit more appropriate. As the patient's condition improves, he or she might be required to visit the practice nurse at the surgery or a specialist clinic run by the district nursing team.
- Patient and carers must be made aware of referral to the district nursing service and have given their permission.

Referrals will be categorised as

- Urgent contact deemed necessary within four hours (must not be misused).
- Non-urgent contact made within 24 hours and visiting date agreed.
- Routine contact within 48 hours and visiting date agreed.
- The referral must not give the patient any false indication of when and how often the district nurse will visit. This will be decided on contact with the patient at the initial assessment.
- Any referral for home help, meals on wheels, day care and help with personal hygiene, bathing, getting up and putting to bed must be referred directly to social services.
- Any referrals for equipment that might be required for longer than 16 weeks must go to the disability living team. This equipment includes commodes, raised toilet seats and hoist. Community nurses must not be expected to move any immobile patients during nursing intervention without the use of a hoist (following a moving and handling assessment). In addition, the district nurse will assess a request for advice on pressure-area care. Special equipment might be required for a short time.
- Referral for continence promotion will result in full assessment before any decision is made regarding the treatment available, with continence being the goal and pads a final or short-term option.
- Any referral for wheelchair or chiropody service must be made directly to the GP. Toenail-cutting arrangements must be made privately by the patient or carer.
- All interventions will aim to provide the highest quality of care within the available resources.
- Due to the complexity of a full nursing assessment, which can take up to two hours including full documentation, consideration must be given to the patient's real needs before referral to the service. The referral process will be audited by giving feedback regarding appropriateness of the referral, either in writing or verbally.
- Referrals for prescribing of medication/dressings will only be considered if the patient is currently being seen by the district nursing service (in accordance with the local trust protocol).

(Suggested by Vafeas 2000)

? Considering concepts such as consumer's choice, collaboration, care delivery, resources, what is your view of the criteria stated above? How appropriate is Mr Thomas's recent referral to the community services? Were there alternatives?

Increasingly, since the changes brought about by PCGs and PCTs, specialist diabetes clinics have been set up collaboratively to improve early detection and provide effective surveillance. About half of the diabetic population regularly attends such specialist facilities. The main group attending the hospital are diabetics in younger age groups and those with established complications requiring particular surveillance and treatment.

Nurses often see patients referred by other professionals or who are self-referred. The increasing autonomy of nurses is being accomplished by a greater willingness of health professionals to share expertise and work across previously rigid boundaries.

The recommendations of the *Cumberlege Report* (DHSS, 1986a) provided opportunities for reviewing the community nursing services. Further changes for community care were then influenced by *Caring for People* (DoH, 1989c) and the *NHS and Community Act 1990* (DoH 1990), which required the caring services to co-operate more effectively in planning and delivering individualised packages of care.

Providing care for people with diabetes is a team effort not only involving members of the multidisciplinary team, but also the client, their relatives and/or carers. One reason given for the reform of the NHS in the early 1990s was that service provision was fragmented and lacked cohesion. Reforms (DoH 1997a, 1997b) have continued to strive for improvements in service delivery. As Cook (2002) indicates, collaboration within and between disciplines has long been linked with quality and clinically effective health services. Collaborative working is central to effective care delivery.

In the current climate of care delivery, caring professionals are under increasing pressure not only to provide comprehensive services, but also to be conscious of cost, assure quality and provide value for money. Assessment of quality in nursing care has been inhibited by the lack of apparent criteria for evaluation including parameters for measurement. The Department of Health (1989a) specified in 'A Strategy for Nursing' the importance of evaluation and emphasised the need for nurses to become familiar with quality assessment techniques to measure good practice.

At the core of the community care policies that were implemented in the 1990s lies the concept 'consumer's choice', which is a powerful and persuasive notion for professionals involved in care delivery. This is as important today as it was in 1990. The *NHS and Community Care Act* (DoH 1990), required that health care within the community must be delivered by skilled, knowledgeable and competent teams of professionals, working in collaboration with each other to give effective, efficient, comprehensive and appropriate needs-based quality care to clients and individuals. *The NHS Plan* (DoH 2000) again emphasised the need for staff to collaborate in the patient's best interest and not be constrained by restrictive practices. Nurses, midwives and health visitors do work flexibly and imaginatively with others and roles continue to expand. They are guided by the *Code of Professional Conduct* (NMC 2002) and are required to work within their scope of professional practice (UKCC 1996).

Conclusion

With increasing numbers of people who are predicted to become diabetic, it is essential that strategies for collaborative working are further enhanced. Estimated epidemiological statistics predict that if current trends continue, the number of people with diabetes will more than double from 140 million to 300 million in the next 25 years (WHO 2001). In the United Kingdom alone there are 1.4 million affected, with an estimate that the prevalence will double by 2010. Statistical information for the United States indicates that there are around eight million people with Type 2 diabetes who do not know it.

In order to continue to promote a positive approach to diabetes care management, there is increasing interest in guidelines to improve the quality of care for the diabetic individual. Clinical effectiveness needs constructive guidelines that are formulated from sound research findings. The fundamental importance of a rigorous high-quality research programme within the NHS has been recently renewed. *The National Service Framework for Diabetes* (DoH 2001) sets out the governments commitment to the development of services for people with diabetes.

Many of the new approaches to care management and delivery strongly influenced by *The New NHS: Modern, Dependable* (DoH 1997a) have since been taken forward by the requirements of the *The Health Act* (DoH 1999b) and *The NHS Plan* (DoH 2000). Interdisciplinary teamwork, coordination and integration remain a major theme. The need for collaborative working with commitment to effective care delivery has to be the objective of every health professional wherever care is delivered.

Community care is now fully involved in the assessment and treatment of an increasing range of health issues and conditions. The roles and scope of district nursing continue to expand in the management and delivery of patient care. The specialist care needed for patients such as Mr Piper or Mr Thomas requires that all practitioners have a good understanding based on sound knowledge and are accountable for the care delivered.

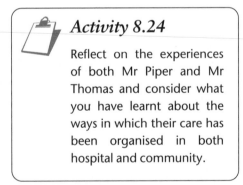

Activity 8.24

Reflect on the experiences of both Mr Piper and Mr Thomas and consider what you have learnt about the ways in which their care has been organised in both hospital and community.

Both Mr Piper and Mr Thomas were provided with care that allowed them to develop their own self-management, skills which helped them towards full independence. Although they were cared for in different parts of the service, many of the interventions and care management processes were similar. Empowering Mr Piper and Mr Thomas to achieve their overall goals required accurate assessment, developing trust and ensuring participation, skills essential for nursing practice.

References

Akinsanya, C., Williams, M. (2000) *Perspectives in Teaching & Learning.* Unpublished manuscript in press.

Audit Commission (1986) *Making a Reality of Community Care.* London: HMSO.

Audit Commission (1999) *First Assessment: A Review of District Nursing Services in England & Wales.* London: HMSO.

Avery, L. (1998) Diabetes mellitus Type 1 and 2: an overview. *Nursing Standard* 13 (8), pp. 35–8.

Blackie, C. (1998) *Community Health Care Nursing.* Edinburgh: Churchill Livingstone.

British Diabetic Association Diabetes Service Advisory Committee (1993) *Recommendations for the Management of Diabetes in Primary Care: A Vision of Recommendations for Diabetes Health Promotion Clinics.* London: BDA.

Cook, L. (2002) Triple integration nursing. *Nursing Standard* 14 (52), pp. 33–4.

Currie, C. (1996) Patterns of in- and outpatient activity for diabetes district survey. *Diabetic Medicine* 13 (3), pp. 273–80. Cited in Cradock, S. (1999) The hospital care of patients with diabetes. *Nursing Times* 4. 28 April, 95 (17), pp. 52–3.

Department of Health and Social Security (1986a) *Neighbourhood Nursing: A Focus for Care.* Report of the Community Nursing Review (The Cumberlege Report). London: HMSO.

Department of Health (1989a) *A Strategy for Nursing.* London: DoH Nursing Division.

Department of Health (1989c) *Caring for People: Community Care in the Next Decade and Beyond.* London: DoH.

Department of Health (1990) *The NHS and Community Care Act 1990.* London: HMSO.

Department of Health (1991) *Research for Health: A Research and Development Strategy for the NHS.* London: HMSO.

Department of Health (1997a) *The New NHS: Modern, Dependable.* London: HMSO.

Department of Health (1997b) *NHS (Primary Care) Act 1997.* London: The Stationary Office.

Department of Health (1998a) *Our Healthier Nation.* London: DoH.

Department of Health (1998b) *Nurse Prescribing: A Guide for Implementation.* London: DoH/NHSE.

Department of Health (1998c) *Implementating the Scheme across England.* Department of Health 1998/32. London: DoH.

Department of Health (1999a) *The National Survey of NHS Patients: General Practice 1998.* London: The Stationary Office. www.doh.gov.uk/public/gpnhspres.htm

Department of Health (2000) *The NHS Plan: A Plan For Investment, A Plan For Reform.* London: The Stationary Office.

Department of Health (2001) *National Service Framework for Diabetes – Standards.* London: HMSO.

Diabetes UK (2000) *New Diagnostic criteria for Diabetes Summary of Changes Factsheet.* London: Diabetes UK. www.diabetes.org.uk

Gerteis, M., Edgeman-Levitan, S., Daley, A., Delbanco, J. (1993) *Through the Patient's Eyes.* San Francisco, CA: Jossey Bass.

Hand, H. (2000) The development of diabetic ketoacidosis. *Nursing Standard* 8 November, 15 (8), pp. 47–52.

Hawtin, M., Hughes, G., Percy-Smith, J. (1994) *Community Profiling - Auditing Social Needs.* Buckingham: Open University Press.

Hek, G. (2000) *Evidence-Based Practice: Finding the Evidence.* London: RCN.

Higgins, C. (1994) Laboratory backup. *Nursing Times* 90 (32), pp. 45–8.

Howdle, S., Wilkin, T. (2001) Type 2 diabetes in children. *Nursing Standard,* 17 January, 15 (18), pp. 38–42.

Jones, L. J. (1994) *The Social Context of Health and Health Work.* Basingstoke: Macmillan Press – now Palgrave Macmillan. Cited in *Journal of Community Nursing* 14 (11), pp. 19–22.

Miller, J. F. (1992) *Coping with Chronic Illness.* 2nd Edition. Philadelphia, PA: F. A. Davis.

NANDA (1994) *Nursing Diagnosis: Definitions and Classifications.* Philadelphia, PA: North American Nursing Diagnosis Association.

NHS Executive (1992) *The Patient Charter: Raising the Standards.* London: HMSO.

NHS Executive (1996) *Promoting Clinical Effectiveness: A Framework for Action in and through the NHS.* London: NHSE.

Nursing and Midwifery Council (2002) *Code of Professional Conduct.* London: NMC.

Royal College of Nursing (1992) *Nurses and Skill Mix: What are the Issues.* London: RCN.

Royal College of Nursing (1993) *Code of Practice for Handling Patients.* London: RCN.

Skidmore, D. (1997) *Community Care: Initial Training and Beyond.* London: Arnold.

Stewart, M., Belle Brown, J., Weston, W. W., McWhinney, J. R., McWilliams, C. L., Summers, J. (2001) Caring in nursing: a different interpretation. *Journal of Advanced Nursing* 35 (6), pp. 926–32.

Thorddsen, A., Thorsteinsson, H. (2002) Nursing diagnosis taxonomy across the Atlantic Ocean: congruence between nurses' charting and the NANDA taxonomy. *Journal of Advanced Nursing* 37 (4), pp. 372–81.

United Kingdom Central (1996) *Guidelines for Professional Practice.* London: UKCC. Council for Nursing, Midwifery and Health Visiting.

United Kingdom Central Council for Nursing, Midwifery and Health Visiting (2001) *Requirements for Pre-Registration Nursing Programmes.* London: UKCC, p. 9, Nursing competencies.

Vafeas, C. (2000) Referral criteria. *Nursing Standard* 14 (45), pp. 39–41.

Watson, N., Wilkinson, C. (2001) *Nursing in Primary Care: A Handbook for Students.* Basingstoke: Palgrave Macmillan.

Winefield, H. R., Murrell, T., Clifford, J., Farmer, E. (1996) The search for reliable and valid measures of patient-centredness. *Psychology and Health* 11, pp. 811–24.

World Health Organisation (1999) *Definition Diagnosis and Classification of Diabetes Mellitus and its Complications.* Geneva: WHO.

World Health Organisation (2001) *Report of the Expert Committee on the Diagnosis and Classification of Diabetes Mellitus Diabetes Care.* Geneva: WHO pp. 1183–1197.

Wright, J. (1995) Can patients become empowered? *Professional Nurse* June, 10 (9), p. 599.

Resources

📖 Further reading

Appleton, J., Cowley, S. (2000) *The Search for Health Needs.* Basingstoke: Palgrave Macmillan.

Chambers, R., Stead, J., Wakley, G. (2001) *Diabetes Matters in Primary Care.* Oxford: Radcliffe Medical Press.

Jerreat, L. (1999) *Diabetes for Nurses.* London: Whurr Publishers.

Orem, D. (1985) *Nursing: Concepts of Practice.* 5th Edition. St. Louis, MO: Mosby.

Rogers, M. E.(1970) *An Introduction to the Theoretical Basis of Nursing.* Philadelphia, PA: Davis.

Roper, N., Logan, W., Tierney, A. (1985) *The Elements of Nursing.* 2nd Edition. Edinburgh: Churchill Livingstone.

Roy, C. (1984) *Introduction to Nursing: An Adaptation Model.* 2nd Edition. Englewood Cliffs, NJ: Prentice-Hall.

Tortora, G. J., Grabowski, S. R. (2002) *Principles of Anatomy and Physiology.* 7th Edition. New York: Harper & Row.

Official reports and key documents

Department of Health and Social Services (1942) *The Beveridge Report 1942: Full Employment in a Free Society.* London: HMSO.

Department of Health and Social Services.(1946) *National Insurance Act.* London: HMSO.

Department of Health and Social Services (1948) *National Health Service Act 1946.* London: HMSO.

Department of Health and Social Security (1974) *NHS Reorganisation Act 1973.* London: HMSO.

Department of Health and Social Security (1979) *Royal Commission on the NHS: A Service for Patients: Conclusions and Recommendations.* London: HMSO.

Department of Health and Social Security (1986b) *Community Care: Agenda for Action.* Griffiths, R. London: HMSO.

Department of Health (1989b) *Working for Patients: The Health Service Caring for the 90s.* London: DoH.

Department of Health (1992) *The Health of the Nation: A Strategy for Health in England.* London: HMSO.

Department of Health (1999b) *The Health Act.* London: HMSO.

@ Web pages

Department of Health – diabetes resource: **www.doh.gov.uk/nsf/diabetes.htm**
Department of Health: **www.doh.gov.uk**
Diabetes Focus (2002) **www.focusondiabetes.com/script/main/art/asp**
Diabetes Mellitus (2000) **Medline medicine.net.com**

Diabetes UK: **www.diabetes.org.uk**
Joslin Diabetes Centre – educational website: **www.joslin.harvard.edu/education**
NHS Direct Online: **www.nhsdirect.nhs.uk**

Insights into Nursing Older People in the Community

9

Carolyn Gibbon and Alison Cochrane (with acknowledgements to Rosemary Sargeant)

Introduction

Frail elderly people within the population are now recognised as a client group with their own special needs and barring life threatening disease or disability, people are generally living longer than in previous generations. However, the impact of this may mean that certain individuals, whilst living to a greater age than perhaps their parents did, may also experience longer periods of frailty with a consequent need for greater and more varied amounts of care. This, then, has implications as to where that care is given and by whom. There are a number of factors to be considered when making these decisions, and ideally the care needs of the individual should be the main determinant. However, in our current Western society the decisions are increasingly being influenced by economic considerations.

This chapter sets out to explore these factors as they impinge upon the experience of Vera, her family and those caring for her. Vera is frail and elderly and eventually leaves her own home to live in a nursing home. The care she receives along the way will be influenced by standards discussed by Bowers (1999), *The Health Advisory Service* 2000 (1998) and laid out in the *National Service Framework for Older People* (Department of Health 2001a).

Learning outcomes

This chapter will enable the student to:

- Develop an understanding of the main issues related to being frail and elderly.
- Explore the impact of grief on individuals.
- Discuss the psychological and physiological effects of ageing.
- Explore the use and effects of pharmacology with the frail elderly.

- Identify the roles of the members of the multi-disciplinary team and explore the ways in which continuity of care is maintained.
- Identify various tools used to assess the needs of frail, elderly people and how the findings are used to plan and evaluate care.
- Understand the issues related to care management within a person's own home and within a nursing and/or residential home.

Concepts

- The ageing process
- Degenerative disorders in old age
- Increasing dependency
- Loss and grief associated with moving home
- Bereavement – loss of spouse
- Adaptive mechanisms
- Continuing care for older people

- Needs and risk assessment
- Pharmacological interventions
- Care management
- Legal and ethical issues
- Multi-disciplinary team
- Financial issues
- Social constructs in relation to older age

Scenario *Vera's experience*

Vera Jenkins is 87 years old, widowed and currently lives in her own 3-bedroomed semi-detached house which she and George purchased when they were newly married. They had one son, Matt, who Vera seldom sees. He is divorced with no children and lives abroad.

George was a Chartered Accountant, he managed their personal finances and ensured that Vera would have some additional savings set aside to supplement her State Pension. Since George died, Vera has found it increasingly difficult to cope with every-day life. She has become physically frail and is experiencing mild confusion and disorientation which she finds distressing.

Defining what is meant by 'elderly' and 'frail' is not easy as each can be approached from a variety of perspectives. Wade (1996) points out that 70-year-olds have different needs from 90-year-olds, yet each group would be classed as 'elderly'. The word 'frail' also invokes images of varying degrees of dependence. Therefore it is essential to consider the impact that the use of these terms can have.

Activity 9.1

Construct your personal definition of the words *elderly* and *frail*. Are there any gender differences in your definitions? Determine if your ideas are supported by research.

Incidence

It was in 1821 that records began to be compiled in relation to how long individuals live. Currently there are ten and a half million elderly people in the United Kingdom, with two-thirds of those being women. This difference increases with age as older women live even longer than men. Over the age of 60, 58 per cent are women; over the age of 75, 67 per cent are women; and over the age of 90, 80 per cent are women (Bernard and Meade 1993). This trend continues with projections for the year 2011 estimating 9 per cent of the total population will be men aged 75 years, whilst 11 per cent will be women (Social Trends 2001). This is largely due to a reduction in mortality and increases in life expectancy since the start of the twentieth century.

> ## Activity 9.2
>
> Information about population trends in localities can be found at
> http://www.statistics.gov.uk
> Try looking at the projections for your local area. What are the implications for caring for older people?

Receiving primary care

Over the last 3 months social services have become involved in Vera's care following a telephone call from her neighbour Mrs Barker. Mrs Barker has tried to help Vera by taking her a hot meal on a regular basis. This has received a mixed reception, depending on Vera's mental state and the fact that she sometimes perceives it as an affront to her pride and ability to cope. Mrs Barker believes that professional intervention is now needed, as she is only able to offer limited support because of her own family commitments.

Activity 9.3

A Consider how you might respond in similar circumstances, try putting yourself in Vera's shoes.

B Vera has been demonstrating that she is going through the *grieving process*. Make notes on what you understand by this (see Chapter 14 on paliative care; and Ffoulkes 1996) in relation to grieving.

Social services have alerted Vera's GP who, on visiting, is concerned about Vera's deteriorating condition. Vera clearly stated, 'you are not going to put me in the workhouse, I can manage'. Whilst respecting her wishes, he decided to maintain close contact with social services and reassess the situation on a regular basis.

What does Vera mean by the *workhouse*? What association do some elderly people believe exists between workhouses and health care?

Activity 9.4

Read Webster (2001) *Caring for Health: History and Diversity*, chapters 2 and 3.

Matt, Vera's son, was contacted by Mrs Barker, who thought he ought to know what was going on. Matt recently contacted social services and explained that although at present he was unable to fly home, he would if the situation required it. He was keen to know whether residential care would be the answer, but social services explained that this could only be considered in discussion with Vera and that this had not yet been put to her. Social services instigated a care package whereby a care worker provides support to Vera in her own home for a couple of hours each day.

Activity 9.5

Social service provision is vast and may vary from area to area. Collect examples of care packages from your own locality and consider the ways in which they are able to address individual needs.

Visits from the district nurse

Vera is becoming even more frail and far less mobile. She is now unwilling to leave the house, so her care worker does her shopping and collects her pension. Her immobility, combined with her deteriorating mental state and reduced motivation, means that Vera spends long periods of time just sitting in her chair. As a result her troubles are compounded by the development of a small sacral pressure ulcer. The discovery of the pressure ulcer was quite by chance when the care worker noticed a stain on Vera's dress which she first associated with incontinence. The GP was informed and a district nurse now visits daily to dress the ulcer.

Activity 9.6

There continues to be a great deal of debate surrounding *nurse prescribing*. Make notes on what you understand by this term and what you believe may be the advantages and disadvantages of nurses prescribing medications and dressings.

Read Humphries and Green (2002) *Nurse Prescribing*.

The nurse has also provided pressure relieving aids as well as trying to encourage Vera to move around a little more. Vera has also been referred to the community physiotherapist, who has agreed to visit to assess her mobility and see if she requires a walking aid.

Pressure ulcers

The term pressure ulcer, pressure sore or decubitus ulcer is defined in Mallet (2000) as any area of damage to the skin or underlying tissues caused by direct pressure or shearing force. They cause pain and discomfort, delay rehabilitation and can cause disability and death.

There are four main causes of pressure sores:

- Pressure
- Shearing forces
- Trauma or friction
- Moisture

Assessment of the risk of developing a pressure ulcer is vital and the nurse must take into account factors such as age, nutritional status, circulatory status, mobility, dependence level and mental awareness (Royle 1992). To assist in this process there are a number of assessment tools that can be used. However, the Norton Score is an assessment tool devised specifically for use with older people. Criteria focus on the general physical condition, the mental state, activity, mobility and incontinence, and a score is awarded for each section. A total score is then given, with the lower the score the greater risk the patient has of developing pressure ulcers.

It is vital that attention is paid to the **prevention** of pressure ulcers and Royle (1992) recommends the following strategies:

- Assess the patient for risk factors.
- Ensure regular changes of position to relieve pressure on vulnerable areas such as the heels, sacrum, elbows, or shoulders.
- Maintain good standards of hygiene.
- Prevent mechanical, physical or chemical injury.
- Ensure adequate nutrition and hydration.
- Promote continence.
- Careful positioning.
- Use devices to equalise pressure over pressure points.

Activity 9.7

A number of care plans have the Norton Score already printed on them as an *aide memoire*. Observe the tool and become familiar with the criteria for assessment.

- Inspect the skin several times a day.
- Promote mental alertness and orientation.
- Educate the patient, family and care givers in skin-care measures.

Pressure ulcers take many different forms and a grading system has been devised to grade the level of severity (Royle 1992).

Table 9.1 Levels of pressure ulcer severity

Grade 1	There is redness, warmth and slight erosion of the epidermis. It will go white when touched
Grade 2	There is shallow ulceration with redness and heat and does not blanch when touched
Grade 3	The ulceration is deep, foul-smelling with a necrotic base
Grade 4	The ulcer involves all layers of the skin, the underlying muscles, and may involve the bone or joints. It is deep

All ulcers should be examined closely to determine the extent and depth of tissue involvement. It is then measured in centimetres and recorded. Regular inspection then determines the stages of healing.

The healing process has several recognised phases and these are noted in Table 9.2 below.

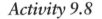

Activity 9.8

Read Russell (2000) 'Understanding the physiology of wound healing and how dressings help'.

Table 9.2 Pressure ulcer healing process

Stage 1	**Inflammatory process** Cells are released to help in clot formation
Stage 2	**Granulation** Occurs in deep dermal wounds as new tissue is laid down
Stage 3	**Epithelization** Occurs quickly in small wounds, occurs when squamous cells migrate across the wound surface
Stage 4	**Remodelling/maturation** This stage may take from 2 days to 2 years to take place. Vascularisation decreases, collagen matures and the appearance of the granulation tissue changes from red to white.

Vera has a sacral pressure ulcer that the district nurse has assessed as being Grade 2. This will need treatment and there are a number of products available, including topical agents to clean and/or protect ulcers and dressings to assist in the healing process. The sore is treated with a hydrogel as there are some exudates. A dry dressing is placed over this, and the ulcer is checked on alternate days and the findings noted on the care plan. There is a great deal of literature on this topic, but consult your local tissue viability nurse as a resource person.

Activity 9.9

Read Dealey (1999) *Care of Wounds*, Chapter 2.

Referral to the consultant

The care worker and district nurse are very concerned as Vera is becoming increasingly frail and confused. The GP again visits Vera and, after spending some time talking to her, makes a referral to a consultant with a specialist interest in older people at the local district general hospital. It is hoped that the consultant will be able to establish the reason for Vera's physical and mental decline, this assessment needs to take place before considering whether Vera may be safer living somewhere other then her own home.

The GP writes a letter of referral to the consultant

Dear Dr Smart,

Re: Mrs Vera Jenkins, 2 Holly Cottages, Castleberry, TU15 1SH. Age 87

I visited Mrs Jenkins today who is frail. She has been deteriorating both mentally and physically since the death of her husband George, six months ago from an MI. Both social services and the district nurse are now expressing concerns about her ability to manage at home. I would value your opinion regarding the cause of her deterioration. I am not convinced that this is necessarily the onset of a dementing illness and feel the need to exclude depression in the light of her recent bereavement before any decision is taken regarding possible consideration for residential care. Mrs Jenkins is reluctant to take any form of medication, and therefore no antidepressants have as yet been prescribed. I have spoken with the son who lives abroad. He is intending to return in two months time and it would be helpful if a case conference could be arranged around this time.

Presenting Symptoms

Mrs Jenkins has enjoyed relatively good health over the years. Following a difficult birth, she only had the one child. It is a source of disappointment that she was unable to have more children. There have been no significant episodes of ill health.

More recently there have been considerable physical changes which have led to her current state of frailty. She is 160cm tall but only currently weighs 52kg, having lost approximately 13kg since the death of her husband.

I have found Mrs Jenkins to be mildly confused and disorientated, and when spoken to she is either tearful or over-cheerful. Mrs Jenkins was distraught following George's death, but at first appeared to be coping. She has always kept herself 'tidy' but has recently started to look unkempt, and on a number of occasions has been seen wearing inappropriate clothes for the weather. One of her great interests is her garden and this has started to look neglected. She continues to go to the local shops, but frequently returns having forgotten what she had gone for in the first place.

I look forward to hearing from you.

Dr H. Monroe, General Practitioner

? **How and why do our bodies alter with age?**

According to Jones (1996) the 'body develops to maturity and then declines slowly'.

For Vera this decline has been taking place over many, many years. Vera has enjoyed good health, except for her pressure ulcer, and now Vera is experiencing the normal physical changes associated with the ageing process.

When considering the ageing process, a number of variables, such as good health, being a non-smoker, and exercise, must be taken into account. Whilst these variables may delay ageing, there are no guarantees. Physiological changes may begin in adulthood, whereas for some individuals they may not occur until after 70 years of age (Black 1992).

Black (1992) notes that when reviewing physiological changes, the nursing assessment is important and takes place in three parts:

 Activity 9.10

Review the extensive chart in Black (1992, p. 39) on physical and functional changes related to ageing and note the nursing implications.

Also review Barker (1998, pp. 19–32) for biological theories of ageing.

- **Interview** This takes time due to slower functioning, reduced energy and/or memory deficits. Information may need to be collected on several different occasions.
- **Observations** Looking at the individual can reveal a great deal of information. Smell may detect unusual breath, excretory or skin odours. Touch to determine strength, flexibility, texture and temperature. Hearing to detect quality of speech or respirations.
- **Examination** Inspection and palpation and findings carefully recorded.

Physiological changes

- **Skin** This 'thins' and becomes less elastic with reduced vascularity. The superficial blood vessels are less efficient in dilating and contracting to regulate body temperature. Older people are at greater risk than younger people of developing hypothermia. Wound healing is retarded, especially as feelings of heat, pressure and pain are not as acute.

> Vera is found wandering at night and there is great concern that she could become hypothermic.

> This can be seen with Vera and the development of her pressure ulcer.

- **Skeleton** Bones become weaker and the vertebrae compress leading to a loss of height. They also change shape and, because of altered mineralisation, also change texture (Barker 1998). Osteoporosis (bone loss) begins to take place from about 40 years of age and is thought to be related to exercise, diet and hormonal changes. This combination leads to increased risk of bone fractures.

  Jones (1996) notes that reduced muscle activity can lead to respiratory movements being reduced, with an increased risk of chest infections.

> Joints and muscles are also affected and Vera would be finding it more difficult to move about and may even find it painful. Vera has not been eating properly, yet attention to diet, especially the need for proteins, potassium, calcium and Vitamin D, may slow this process down (Black 1992).

- **Cardiovascular** Barker (1998) notes that degenerative diseases of the heart and blood vessels are the most common effects of ageing. Calcification of the blood vessels cause pulse and systolic pressure to increase (Jones 1996).

> Currently Vera tends to sit for long periods and has periods of heightened activity when distressed. These need to be moderated so that she enjoys a balance of activity and rest.

- **Gastrointestinal** The gastrointestinal tract alters with age, and saliva and digestive secretions decrease in volume (Jones 1996). Tooth enamel becomes thinner and teeth may become brittle (Black 1992) or dentures may not fit properly. This combined with less sensitivity to smell and taste may result in inadequate intake of food. Reduced intestinal peristalsis and duller nerve sensations can cause missed signals for defaecation (Black 1992).

> Vera is currently taking an inadequate diet due to a lack of interest in food caused by her distress. Thus she is at risk of developing digestive problems and constipation.

- **Genitourinary** In some older people the filtration functions of the renal system slow down. Bladder capacity reduces from 500ml to 250ml, leading to frequency and nocturia (Black 1992). The generalised weakening of muscles affects the bladder, making it more difficult to empty, and can cause urine retention. For Vera a reduction in oestrogen following the menopause causes the pelvic floor muscles to relax, leading to problems of stress incontinence or dribbling.

- **Special senses** Barker (1998) notes a number of issues in relation to the senses. The lenses in the eye harden with age and become increasingly opaque, leading to cataracts. The ear is affected because of loss of hairs on the cochlea and vestibule.

  > Vera will find diminished perception of sound, pitch and amplitude and her balance will also be affected.

  Taste buds degenerate with age leading to the loss of taste perception, which in turn affects salivation, mouth cleanliness and appetite.

  > This is an added problem for Vera.

- **Nervous system** This changes with age as the brain reduces in weight and response times slow down. Short-term memory may be affected, but changes are very individual and only a minority may develop dementia (Barker 1998).

  > Vera will be at risk of a greater susceptibility to hazards and be less aware of pain.

- **Reproductive system** Testosterone reduces in men leading to hypertrophy of the prostate, slow erection and thinner pubic hair (Black 1992). Ovulation stops with the menopause as oestrogen production ceases. The female reproductive organs atrophy, and the vagina is less vascular and moist but more alkaline.

Activity 9.11

The ageing process is not confined to physical and biological changes. Read the overview of psychological and sociological theories in Black (1992) *Ageing and Health*, pp. 43–4.

Ongoing deterioration

Vera continues to deteriorate, she needs lots of encouragement to wash and change her clothes and she remains tearful. The consultant, having assessed Vera, has diagnosed a moderate dementia with an overlying depression. There is no doubt that

George's recent death has caused Vera much distress, but Vera has also said how worried she is about her ability to remember things and cope with what seems normal every-day activities. In fact she thinks she is going mad. The consultant has commented in his report to the GP that it is this level of insight, which is often apparent in the early stages of dementia, that is likely to be contributing to Vera's depression. He believes that Vera's willingness to talk about her loss will over time help relieve some of the effects of her depression, but he has suggested that the GP prescribe a mild anti-depressant.

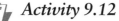

Activity 9.12

Consider the differences between sadness and depression and then compare and contrast the symptoms of dementia with those of depression. You will find that some are similar whilst others are quite different. Why might it be important for the District Nurse who has been visiting Vera to be aware of these differences?

Read Holden and Woods (1988) *Reality Orientation*, chs 1 and 4; and also the *National Service Framework for Older People* (DoH 2001a) Standard Seven in relation to mental health in older people.

A number of different health and social services practitioners have now become involved in Vera's well-being. It is important that the activities are coordinated so that Vera receives the best possible care and that there is no disparity or duplication in the services provided. This is *multi-disciplinary* working, health and social services practitioners usually work in a team – the *multi-disciplinary team*. Ovretveit (1993) defines a multi-disciplinary team as, 'a group of practitioners with different (multi-disciplinary) professional training, employed by more than one agency (multi-agency), who meet regularly to coordinate their work, providing services to one or more clients in a defined area'.

Vera has so far had contact with the following health care workers:

- Social worker
- District nurse
- Occupational therapist
- General practitioner
- Consultant with a special interest in older people
- Community physiotherapist
- Home care workers

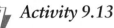

Activity 9.13

Recalling your own experience of practice in both institutional and community settings, consider the measures taken to ensure that communication remains effective between different members of the multi-disciplinary team. Which professional takes the lead role and why?

Read Ovretveit (1993) *Coordinating Community Care.* You will also need to access Department of Health (2000) *Partnership in Action* the action plan to implement the recommendations of the NHS taskforce on staff involvement

---

A care manager is appointed to co-ordinate decisions that are taken to ensure that Vera receives the most appropriate care. The care manager will have had training in case management, which provides the skills to draw together the assessments made by each practitioner and formulate a care plan.

The person appointed as a care manager needs to be very competent with a high level of experience and training. Ovretveit (1993) states that the care manager has '. . . responsibilities for assessing, coordinating and liaising with all the services a client needs for his or her assessment, treatment and care'. The use of care (or case) managers was put forward by Griffiths in 1988, with a view to providing better support for individuals in their own homes and therefore preventing unnecessary admission to hospital or a nursing home.

Social services have appointed the social worker as the care manager for Vera who now, due to increasing concerns for Vera's safety, reconsiders the possibility of residential care, an option previously put forward by Matt, Vera's son. The social worker spends time with Vera, putting forward options and providing her with information which might help her to make an informed choice. Vera is still convinced that she wants to remain in her own home, but agrees to participate in an assessment of her daily living and safety needs. Social services are therefore able to carry out a needs assessment and decide to use a tool based on the *Clifton Assessment Procedures for the Elderly (CAPE)* (Pattie and Gilleard 1981).

Below is an extract from Vera's CAPE assessment. The criteria for scoring is zero for no assistance, 1 for some assistance, and 2 for maximum assistance (see pages 290–1).

CAPE scale	Findings	Score
1 **Bathing and dressing**	Needs prompting to wash. Needs assistance with getting in and out of the bath	1
2 **Walking**	Walks slowly, but steadily	1
5 **Disorientated**	Unable to always know where she is or to find her way around	2
6 **Dress and appearance**	Appears dishevelled and unkempt	2

The CAPE results suggest there are high levels of dependency with an indication of deteriorating mental health. The care manager decides to contact Matt to discuss the situation with him. Although the idea is again put to Vera, she is still reluctant to consider leaving her home.

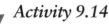

Activity 9.14

How appropriate do you think the CAPE assessment is for identifying Vera's needs? Find out what assessment tools are used by your local social services department, consider whether they would be as suitable for assessing Vera's needs.

Table 9.3 Essential criteria for the assessment of need

The care manager selected the CAPE needs assessment as being the most suitable for assessing Vera's needs, however others may have proved as suitable. Whichever tool is selected there are essential assessment criteria which the Department of Health and Social Services Inspectorate (1993) say should be included in all assessments of need. These include:

Biographical details Date of birth, address, marital status, and so on.

- **Self-perceived needs** What are Vera's perceptions of her needs?
- **Self-care** These cover basic activities such as washing and dressing, shopping, cooking, using the telephone and dealing with money.
- **Physical health** This will help to identify whether the direct involvement of health practitioners is required.
- **Mental health** This will look at indicators that will help to determine an individual's mental state. A more detailed assessment may need to be carried out by a mental health practitioner.

Table 9.3 (continued)

- **Use of medicines** This will seek to identify what, if any, medication is being prescribed. For example, the individual could need regular medication for a chronic condition such as diabetes, or medication that might be used more intermittently, i.e. for arthritic pain or headaches. Help may be required from a doctor or a pharmacist.

- **Abilities, attitudes and lifestyle** This area focuses on the individual as a whole and determines what social networks are important to the individual.

- **Race and culture** It is important that care workers have an understanding of each individual's culture and background. This is an aspect of assessment that in the past has not always been effectively addressed, the findings of the Black Perspectives Sub-Group (1998) which considered the needs of black clients in residential care identify important lessons to be learned.

- **Personal history** In Vera's case her recent bereavement has direct relevance for her immediate care needs, it is important to acknowledge the quality of her relationship with Matt, her son. Other issues might best be explored later. A full personal history can be important, but the assessor should be guided by what is volunteered rather than attempting to construct an in-depth study.

- **Needs of carers** This is an area which has often been neglected in assessment. Whilst Vera has no carers as such, the amount of support currently provided by her neighbour Mrs Barker should be ascertained. Aspects to be considered should include the carer's relationship with the patient, the nature of care provided, their commitment and willingness to continue providing this in the long or short term.

- **Social network and support** This goes beyond the work of immediate carers and includes the input from a wider field. For example, Vera collected her pension at the same time on the same day every week, and the post office staff would know this and may express concern if she failed to arrive or appeared at a different time/day with no explanation.

- **Care services** What services are already being provided?

- **Housing** Individual preferences should be respected, but location, access and facilities will need to be considered when supporting someone in their own home.

- **Finance** It is important that each individual is in full receipt of their full social services benefits and entitlements. Tact is required when inquiring about the financial situation, but it can have a bearing on what assistance is provided. The Court of Protection may need to be approached where an individual is unable to cope with their own financial affairs.

- **Transport** This is vital in enabling services to get to people, or people to services.

- **Risk** A risk assessment is vital and includes risks associated with environmental hazards, and risks associated with physical or mental illness or disability; for example, gas fires, falls, epilepsy, challenging behaviour or psychotic episodes.

Increased support

The needs assessment helps to determine the care plan that is required and clearly is tailored to the individual. The immediate care plan for Vera includes increasing the amount of time the home care worker spends with her and maintaining the daily visits from the district nurse, who will keep the GP informed of developments pending the setting up of a case conference. This will consider the best ways of meeting Vera's longer term needs. The social worker who is the care manager will monitor the care package and has agreed to contact Matt. He explains that although Vera can be supported at home in the short term, her interests need to be considered with a view to longer term care. He is asked when it might be convenient for him to return to the UK. It is agreed to hold the case conference in two months time. Vera is invited to attend and time is taken to explain to her what will be discussed, the nature of the questions that she may need to consider, and the options that might arise. She is delighted to hear that Matt is coming home.

? In your notes about the multidisciplinary team you should have the phrase *Case Conference*. What do you understand by this?

The care manager will chair the case conference to which Vera and Matt are to be invited. The decision to call a case conference has resulted from concerns over Vera's ability to live safely at home: it would appear impossible for her to continue living in her own home for much longer. Prior to the case conference, the care manager meets with Matt and Vera to discuss some of the options. Vera is understandably distressed about any thought of possibly losing her independence and security. She is tearful about the thoughts of leaving the house and its associations with George. Matt is able to reassure Vera that any move into residential care could be temporary and may be the best short-term option. Vera admitted that she had recently become distressed and frightened at night, she keeps thinking that she can hear people breaking into the house. She agrees that she may feel safer with others around, at least for a while. With advice from the care manager Matt and Vera are able to visit a number of residential homes. At the one Vera liked best, there happened to be a resident who she had previously known through George's work. The home also had a nursing home facility for those residents requiring such care; however, currently there were no vacancies.

All the health and social care practitioners involved in Vera's care are able to be present at the case conference. Occasionally it is impossible for all the practitioners to meet and so a telephone conference may take place instead. Mrs Barker has also been invited to attend part of the meeting with Vera's permission. All those present now have the opportunity to meet with Vera and Matt to discuss their assessments, review the current plan of care, and consider the longer term implications.

The outcome of the conference is that Vera is banded as Band 5, which means that whilst she is very dependent, she does not yet require 24-hour nursing care, which is Band 6. This decision is important at this stage not least because of the financial implications. Classed as Band 5 means that social services pay, whereas Band 6 means the local health authority pays. At this stage Vera will receive intensive support at home with a review every six weeks. However, a nursing home is located as it seems inevitable that Vera will need this type of care sooner rather than later.

Activity 9.15

Currently there is a great deal of discussion about free nursing care and who will be eligible. The Government's policy on this continues to evolve, but already there are marked differences between Scotland and England and Wales. See: http://www.doh.gov.uk/coinh.htm

Find out what criteria exist locally which might determine different levels of banding for clients in need of residential care.

A more intensive care package is now instigated to fill the gap between the current situation and Vera being able to move into the nursing home. The home care worker now visits daily, for two hours in the morning and two hours in the late afternoon. She also does Vera's shopping and helps Vera wash and bathe. The Women's Royal Voluntary Service (WRVS) are also involved in delivering a hot lunch through 'meals-on-wheels', provided under contract with social services three days a week. Mrs Barker has agreed to provide a meal on each of the remaining days. Vera generally pays for this service herself, but sometimes she forgets and Mrs Barker has stepped in and paid the volunteer who delivers the meal.

Activity 9.16

Make notes about your local WRVS. Who are they, what services do they provide and how are they co-ordinated?

The district nurse continues to visit on a daily basis to dress the pressure ulcer, ensure Vera has taken her medication, and continually assess Vera's situation. The GP has decided to prescribe Vera with the anti-depressant paroxetine 20mg to be taken once a day in the morning to try to lift her mood.

? The GP has prescribed Vera with the anti-depressant paroxetine (Seroxat). What do you understand by this? What would the district nurse caring for Vera need to know about this medication and why?

The effects of medication in older people

A study by the Royal College of Physicians (1992) demonstrated that 87 per cent of individuals over 75 years of age were receiving regular drug treatment, and of these 44 per cent were taking three or more different drugs daily. It is also worth noting at this point that the same study highlights a number of potential problems associated with the prescribing of medication for older people. These include:

● A disease process may present itself differently, its symptoms being masked by the medication being prescribed for something else. This could lead to an incorrect diagnosis being made. For example, the use of analgesics to control pain elsewhere might mean that the chest pain associated with myocardial infarction is not recognised, or medication used to reduce inflammation might result in the absence of pyrexia in a chest infection.
● The ways in which medicines are metabolised within the body can be affected by the ageing process in a number of ways:
  ● Oral medication may be absorbed more slowly.
  ● Lower cardiac output may reduce the speed at which medication is transported throughout the body.
  ● Effects of medication may be potentiated where plasma albumin levels are low. Many drugs bind themselves to a plasma protein like albumin. When levels are reduced the proportion of unbound medication in the plasma increases, so enhancing the effect of the drug and leading to potential overdose.
  ● Many drugs are deactivated in the liver and then excreted via the kidneys. Therefore, where liver and kidney function is reduced, excretion may be slowed so that drugs might remain in the body longer and their effects be lasting.
● Where there is multiple pathology, drugs may be prescribed to alleviate a problem but their action might have an unwanted effect elsewhere which has to be counteracted by another drug. The older person with a number of different illnesses can then end up receiving a cocktail of medication where each drug counteracts or potentiates the effects of another.

Activity 9.17

Investigate the effects of ageing on the ways in which drugs are metabolised by the body. Consider these effects in relation to *absorption, distribution, metabolism* and *elimination*.

Read Trounce and Gould (2000) *Clinical Pharmacology for Nurses*, ch 21.

Professional conversation

Jane Swift, district nurse

Medication concerns

As Vera's district nurse, I am constantly on the look out for the unwanted side-effects of prescribed medication amongst the older people I visit. I need to find out what patients are currently taking as sometimes they may have been prescribed something by one doctor who is unaware that something else has been prescribed by another. Believe me, it can happen! I also check out the "over the counter" medications people are taking on top of their prescribed medication. You just wouldn't imagine what people do without realising the dangers. Local pharmacists are getting much better at spotting potential problems and give jolly good advice. It is not surprising that the incidence of adverse drug reactions rises with age, especially after 65 years. There are a number of reasons for this. First, there are increasing numbers of drugs that older people need to take because they often have several different illnesses, but it's often not appreciated that the different drugs used to treat these multiple illnesses may be toxic when taken together. Second, there is often poor compliance with dosing regimes, I often find different tablets all mixed up in the same container, you really have to keep your eyes open. Third, physiological changes associated with ageing mean that dosages used for younger people may require adjusting when prescribed for an older person. Although I can only prescribe a limited range of medicines myself, I am well aware of the actions of those drugs regularly prescribed by doctors to older people. I do let the doctor know straightaway if I think a patient is receiving too high a dose or it is affecting them adversely. That's what professional teamwork is all about. There is a check-list that the doctors and nurses I work with often refer to, you too may find it helpful.' (See Humphries and Green (2002), *Nurse Prescribing*.)

Activity 9.18

Read the following information in conjunction with DoH (2001) *Medicines and Older People*, p. 11.

Promoting safe drug use

- Why is the drug prescribed? Are there any alternative methods that can be used, for example, a gentle back rub?
- Is the drug still required? It may have been prescribed many years ago.
- Is the smallest dose prescribed? Older people tend to take longer to excrete the drug. An accumulation of the drug within the body may lead to adverse reactions.
- Is the patient allergic to the drug? A known allergy may have been overlooked or may not have been reported. Be alert for new symptoms when a patient has been taking a particular medication for some time. Check if they are using 'over the counter' drugs as well.

- Does a particular drug interact with others that are prescribed? Regularly review the literature accompanying drugs.
- Are there any special instructions for taking the drug? For example, with milk, after a meal.
- Is the method of administration appropriate? The patient who finds it difficult to swallow tablets may find it easier to take the medication in liquid form. Also, consideration needs to be given to how the drug is packaged.

(Adapted from Eliopoulos 1997)

Activity 9.19

Read Chapter 35 in Eliopoulos (1997) and make brief notes on particular points to be aware of, for example when giving medicines to Vera.

Crisis at home

It is unclear as to what happened, but the neighbour Mrs Barker reported unusual isolated noises in the night. When the home care worker arrived the next morning, Vera was wandering around the house very disorientated. She was also very cold, as though she had been up all night, which may have been the case. She was also clutching one of George's jumpers. Vera looked as though she had been crying for some time. The home care worker suggested to Vera that she may like to go back to bed, but she refused to go, so the Care Worker wrapped Vera in her dressing-gown and put slippers on her feet whilst she telephoned the social worker and the district nurse.

Activity 9.20

Place yourself in the role of the district nurse and with the information available to you, make a brief assessment of the current situation. What measures would you now take to ensure Vera's safety and best meet her needs?

The district nurse discussed the situation with the GP and agreed to meet the care manager at Vera's home to carry out an assessment. She found that Vera is experiencing interrupted sleep patterns, which could make her more at risk of falling. Wandering at night could also lead to hypothermia.

Activity 9.21

Read Standard 6 in the *National Service Framework for Older People* (DoH 2001a) with regard to falls and older people, and determine what actions can be taken to prevent falls occurring.

Vera is becoming more and more distressed and agitated, and this is seen by her crying and clutching George's possessions. She also appears to be unsure of where she is and the correct time of day, although Mrs Barker thought that this is worse at night.

Vera is currently totally dependent on the help provided by her home carer and from Mrs Barker, the neighbour. Vera appears to find it difficult to initiate or sustain a conversation and appears to have lost interest in day-to-day events. This in turn is causing distress to Mrs Barker, who feels powerless to help Vera.

The care manager discusses the situation with the district nurse and carries out another assessment called the 'Mini-Mental State' (Folstein et al 1975). The maximum score on this assessment is 30 points, Vera scores very low, which appears to confirm concerns about her level of orientation and her vulnerability.

The 'Mini-Mental State' assessment focuses on:

1 **Orientation** – time, place, person, event. (Score max. 10 points)
2 **Registration** – the individual is given three objects to remember, they are then asked to repeat the list three times and after a short period has elapsed, asked to again recall the three objects. (Score max. 3 points)
3 **Attention and calculation** – subtracting numbers. (Score max. 5 points)
4 **Recall** – asked to state three objects learned earlier. (Score max. 3 points)
5 **Language** – asked to name a pencil and watch, give a three-stage command, and so on. (Score max. 3 points)
6 **Reading** – reading a sentence and doing what it states. (Score max. 2 points)
7 **Three-stage command** – person takes paper in left (or right) hand, folds it in half and puts it on the floor. (Score max. 3 points)
8 **Copying** – asked to copy a diagram of a pair of intersecting pentagons. (Score max. 1 point)

Accessing residential care

A telephone case conference urgently took place to review the care package, including discussion with the GP and with Matt, Vera's son. Because all were in agreement that Vera would be at risk if she remained at home, the decision was made to transfer her to a nursing home within the next 24 hours. When this was put to Vera, rather than increasing her agitation, the news appeared to have a calming effect. Even though Vera was unwell, it was essential that she was given the facts and that she should feel involved in her own care. The district nurse wanted to ensure that Vera had an advocate, and did not feel lost or vulnerable at a time when it must have felt like all the decisions were being made without her involvement. The district nurse made sure that as far as she was aware, Vera's interests were taken fully into account and that Vera was able to give informed consent for the move.

Activity 9.22

Think of an example where you have observed a nurse acting as an advocate in order to ensure that a vulnerable person's interests are protected.

Advocacy and informed consent

Nurses provide care in a wide variety of settings, and at all times they are expected to abide by the *Code of Professional Conduct* (NMC 2002). The *Code* requires that:

You are personally accountable for ensuring that you promote and protect the interests and dignity of patients and clients.

Kendrick (1996) states that there is a clear directive between this statement as cited previously (UKCC 1991), and the main elements of advocacy. In other words the nurse becomes an 'active voice' for patients when, for whatever reason, they are unable to state their own interests.

A number of authors have discussed how health care delivery is largely about power (see Kitson 1991; Mackay 1993; Kendrick 1994), they have identified situations where invariably the doctor has the last word. There is also a great deal of evidence to suggest that patients often feel the need to comply with a doctors suggestion, but become distressed when they feel their own wishes are ignored. In such situations patients will often seek the help of nurses even though, paradoxically, they are often regarded as the doctor's assistant.

Informed consent is when a patient is given full information by a competent person so that he/she can accept or reject a course of treatment. The nurse should be able to act as the patients advocate in these circumstances, thereby ensuring that the individual is provided with the information and time needed to explore the options available to them (Kendrick 1996). Nurses therefore need to explore for themselves the issues around advocacy and informed consent. This is a challenging area and case studies can be very useful for exploring your own views and for realising that there may not be any definite right or wrong answers (see also Chapter 5).

In Vera's move to a nursing home, who acted as the advocates, how were her interests protected?

> Vera was accompanied by the care manager and Mrs Barker. They were greeted by Mrs Shaw the Matron of Holyrood Nursing Home, and shown to a comfortable room where they could talk. Mrs Shaw and the social worker decided to carry out a further needs assessment using CAPE (see p. 281). This enabled a comparison to be made against the previous CAPE assessment findings.
>
> - Vera knew who she was and her age, but was uncertain of which day it was.
> - She was uncertain of her actual birthday and gave a date which later turned out to be Matt's birthday.
> - She knew where she was, but thought that she was visiting someone.
> - Vera knew the name of the nearest city and the prime minister, but not the US president.
> - Vera also knew that the national flag contained the colours red, white and blue.

The CAPE relates to four sub-scales which observe physical disability, apathy, communication difficulties and social disturbance. The criteria for scoring is based on zero for no assistance, 1 for some assistance and 2 for maximum assistance. However, there is some criticism of the assessment tool in relation to its validity and reliability (see Bowling, 1997, pp. 36–7).

> The outcome of the assessment would indicate that Vera's problems largely relate to her fragile mental state and recent physical frailty. It is not entirely certain what is causing the deterioration, but there are signs associated with both an early dementing illness and the depression probably resulting from her recent bereavement. The outcome of the assessment has indicated a degree of physical and mental deterioration, some disorientation, sadness, agitation and loss of memory. The information gathered was used to develop a plan of nursing care for Vera.

 Activity 9.23

> The nurses in your practice area will use a philosophy or framework to guide the way in which they systematically assess, plan, implement and evaluate care. Their approach may be based around one or more models of care, try and find out why one model may have been selected in preference to another, what would they describe as their philosophy of care?

 You will notice the term 'confusion' has not been used to describe Vera's problems, why do you think this term is best avoided?

Table 9.4 The CAPE behaviour rating scale findings

CAPE scale	Findings	Score
1 Bathing and dressing	Needs prompting to wash, some assistance needed to get into and out of bath	1
2 Walking	Walks slowly but steadily without aid	1
3 Incontinent of urine/faeces (day or night)	Never	0
4 In bed during the day	Never	0
5 Disorientated	Sometimes forgets where she is	1
6 Dress and appearance	Often needs prompting to select clean and/or appropriate clothes	2
7 Outside activities	Sometimes needs help crossing the road	1
8 Carries out activities in the home	Was independent until recently, now requires prompting to cook, clean and prepare food	1
9 Engages in purposeful activity	Often appears preoccupied, sits alone for long periods and tends to forget to carry out everyday tasks.	2
10 Socialises with others	Has some difficulty establishing relationships	1
11 Accepting of ideas	Appears to go along easily with what is suggested	0
12 Correctly interprets what is being communicated	Usually quickly and correctly interprets what is being communicated to her	0
13 Communicates effectively	Has some difficulty being understood as speaks very quietly	1
14 Acts appropriately in relation to others during the day	Always	0
15 Acts appropriately in relation to others during the night	Has been found wandering at home during the night	2
16 Accuses others of doing her bodily harm	Never	0
17 Hoards apparently meaningless items	Has large collection of paid bills in her handbag	1
18 Disrupted sleep pattern	Sometimes appears to have difficulty getting off, then wakes in the early hours	2

(Adapted from Pattie and Gilleard 1981)

Professional conversation

Rosalynd Shaw, matron, Holyrood Nursing Home

Models of care

'You may be familiar with models of nursing care, but I had to try and sit down and think about how these might lend themselves to the nursing home situation. We looked at Roy's (1976) 'Adaptation Model of Nursing' where the focus is on how a patient adapts to the changed environment, change in circumstances and mental and/or physical, changes. We also considered using Orem's (1991) 'Self-Care Deficit' Model, where the emphasis is on determining what a patient can or cannot do. The aim then is to correct the deficit, through varying degrees of nursing intervention, to enable the patient to regain a higher level of independence. It is about enabling and empowering patients. Several staff were familiar with this model, but after a lot of discussion we all eventually agreed to use the Roper, Logan and Tierney 'Activities of Living' Model (1990). The assessment within this model has a number of similarities to the needs assessment and it provided us with a useful framework for operating the nursing process. We then based our documentation around the model and this seems to have served us well. The local hospitals use this, so many of the bank staff we get are already familiar with it which ensures continuity. Having used this approach for several years, I guess we need to see whether it's still applicable or whether something else may be more beneficial. Staff nurse Davies is currently doing a literature search.'

Activity 9.24

Taking note of the information already provided in the scenario and using care plan documentation from your practice area, take the role of Staff Nurse Davies who is Vera's named nurse. Document a nursing assessment and then construct a plan of care for Vera's first three days at Holyrood Nursing Home. Consult Walsh's (1998) book on care plans in both the community and mental health for guidance. Before you commence your plan, remember to give the district nurse a ring – she may have some helpful tips about that pressure ulcer and information about the medication that Vera has been prescribed.

Staff Nurse Davies identified the following issues as problematic for Vera:

● Disorientated and anxious at times, forgets to take medication, eating very little
● Has some reluctance to socialise with others
● Assistance is needed with hygiene and dressing
● Pressure ulcer of 1cm diameter on buttocks with scab, needing treatment.
● Disrupted sleep pattern

The care plan must aim to improve the situation through a holistic approach to nursing care. This must address needs such as hygiene, dressing, nutrition, mobility and sleeping. It must also consider social needs, with time set aside for communicating socially 'one-to-one' until Vera feels more comfortable with other people. The whole plan will need to be reviewed on a regular basis – at least weekly and updated as necessary.

? Who else would you involve in your plan of care? You have already contacted the district nurse. The bereavement counsellor and the tissue viability nurse could provide help, but how would you make use of their expertise? You may wish to involve others in your plan of care, for example the local hairdresser or a volunteer from Vera's local church.

Extract from Vera's care plan

Date: 6 June
Problem: Disorientated in time and place
Goal: To become reorientated to time and place by 10 June
Intervention: Place Vera's personal items in her room
Encourage Vera to join the other residents at mealtimes and in group discussions
Give Vera time alone – about 1 hour a day
Evaluation: 11 June
Vera recognises family photographs
Vera enjoys lunchtime, but prefers to be on her own at breakfast
Vera still has some difficulty with group discussions

? Some nursing homes may use *Care Pathways or Care Management* rather than nursing models. What do you understand by these terms?

The care plan provided for Vera has been devised using a nursing model of care which has provided the framework for a needs assessment. The framework focuses on *nursing* which fails to take account of the contribution of other care workers (Walsh 1998). Also, there are problems associated with a multitude of written, sometimes overlapping reports, as each professional seeks to maintain their own records. To overcome this issue, care management has been introduced in the United Kingdom with a view to 'streamlining' care, improving communications, preventing

Activity 9.25

Enquire about the use of care pathways in your practice area. Does your area have a care pathways coordinator who may be able to help you with this activity? Can care pathways be adapted for use elsewhere? Do all practitioners contribute to the documentation?

overlaps between practitioners and setting standards. Care pathways are increasingly being used in nursing homes for the same reasons.

When Vera moved into the Nursing Home she was upset and slightly disorientated. Staff worked hard at helping her to settle by introducing her to other residents and placing some of her personal items from home around the room. She was encouraged to eat her meals with the other residents and join them in the lounge as far as possible, but time was also set aside for Vera to be alone. Inclusion in the social activities was encouraged, although Vera was not pressurised, perhaps surprisingly Vera was soon found to enjoy a short game of Bingo. Accompanied by Staff Nurse Sue Davies, she also started to go for short walks around the garden. Vera started to talk about George, she often used to tease him about how little he knew about plants and he would tease her about her knowledge. Definite improvements were being noted. Although Vera has made good progress, she has not regained her appetite and has lost a further 5kg, she now weighs 46kg.

Activity 9.26

As Staff Nurse Sue Davies, use the information you have available to assess Vera's nutritional status and decide on the measures you would take to improve it.

You are advised to make reference to Chapter 10 on nutrition.

Evidence-based practice

Nutrition

In 1998 the British Nutrition Foundation recommended estimated average requirements (EAR) for all age groups. This is an estimate of the average requirement for energy or a nutrient. In Vera's case she will require 1810 kcal per day to meet the EAR for energy, also her nutritional requirements will have altered from when she was younger. For greater detail see:
http://www.nutrition.org.uk/Facts/energynut/requirements.html

Calorie intake also tends to focus on the average healthy adult, but as nutritional intake declines it becomes virtually impossible to take in adequate amounts of essential vitamins, iron, protein and calcium. Dudek (1997) states that caution should be used when adopting dietary guidelines for older people. It is vital that these guidelines are individualised because for elderly frail people, the focus is on improving the quality of life and some of the guidelines may be inappropriate. For example, lowering fat intake may not be appropriate if the person is at risk of malnutrition. Similarly, reducing sodium intake may not necessarily be important as it would limit food choices and may make food less palatable. If older people are only moderately overweight, trying to lose weight may be a lost cause, again because of reasons already mentioned.

The following information may further inform the plan of care:

- Vera has difficulty in chewing and as her dentures do not fit properly, she finds meat difficult to eat. The dentist is making new dentures.
- Vera tends not to eat much fibre and may be at risk of constipation.
- Whilst Vera is not too keen on fruit, she sometimes enjoys bananas and oranges.
- Because of Vera's state of mind when she first arrived at the nursing home, she was fed by a member of staff at each meal time. Gradually, she was encouraged to feed herself and as she started to feel more sociable and independent, she joined other residents in the dinning room.
- In a reminiscence group she revealed how she and George used to enjoy a glass of sherry on a Sunday. A small glass of sherry was introduced each evening and her appetite slightly improved.
- From your nutritional assessment, what goals have you identified and how will these now be incorporated into the care plan?

Staff Nurse Davies reported that:

- It had been important to ask Vera, Mrs Barker and Matt what foods Vera liked.
- It was essential to try and plan a balanced diet to facilitate weight gain.
- Help from the community dietician was very important in determining a plan.
- Nursing intervention was aimed at providing small, attractive meals high in nutrients.
- Fibre was increased as well as fluid intake to prevent constipation.

Over time there was a marked improvement in nutritional intake and mental state. Vera regained the 5kg she had previously lost within a month.

Activity 9.27

Improving Vera's nutritional status will also help to improve her general health. Make short notes on the terms 'health', 'health education' and 'health promotion'.

Read Bernard (2000) *Promoting Health in Old Age.*

Statistics would indicate that individuals are living longer, as are people with varying degrees of physical and/or mental dysfunction (Social Trends 2001). The scope for health promotion is enormous and never more so than for older people in general. Health promotion aims to improve the health status of individuals and the societies within which they live. In Vera's situation promoting health will ensure that she maintains a reasonable level of physical and mental health that is sustained by the environment where she is now living. Many older people will feel that it is a waste of time having health care workers discussing how to maintain and improve health, as they frequently believe alterations in health are due to 'getting old'. Yet the benefits can be huge in terms of enjoying life and being positive about the future.

Health care workers need to take into account that many older people have sensory difficulties such as poor eyesight and/or impaired hearing. The memory may not be as sharp as it once was. They may be experiencing symptoms associated with a physical or mental illness. The environment will also have an impact, choice of diet may be restricted and opportunities for exercise limited.

It is important to establish goals, as with any other health promotion activity. Dodge and Knutesen (1994) identify the need to:

- Maintain functional capacity
- Prevent premature institutionalisation
- Maintain informal networks of care (for example family, care givers)
- Maintain quality of life.

They also warn of the need to be aware of potential barriers such as health professionals holding negative attitudes about ageing, or elderly people themselves being fatalistic about their health. Increasingly it is being recognised that certain strategies can encourage healthy lifestyles, such as sound nutrition, moderate alcohol intake, regular exercise, not smoking and adequate amounts of sleep (Dodge and Knutesen 1994).

Scenario

Vera does not smoke but does need to pay attention to her diet, exercise and getting enough sleep.

- **Diet** – the dietician was asked for advice.
- **Exercise** – a programme of gentle stretching exercises was drawn up increasing from gentle mobility to walks round the garden.
- **Sleep** – it was decided not to prescribe a mild sedative. Vera soon appeared to benefit from a combination of diet, exercise and company.

 ### Professional conversation

Sue Davis, staff nurse

Reminiscences

'Health promotion in elderly people can be problematic as it does not always come high on the agenda in a nursing home. We have often tended to concentrate on keeping people comfortable and getting the residents involved in activities in the afternoon. Then I read an article by Granville (1996) and there were some similarities to Vera because she is a bit forgetful at times. Anyway, I talked about the article to my colleagues and we felt we could help Vera. So what we aimed to do was to promote her self-esteem, we could facilitate her friendships and social contacts, and hopefully optimise her mental health. How we set about this was to set up a reminiscence group once a week in the lounge. We also invited residents from the next-door residential home and three of their residents now regularly attend.

A rotating programme has been developed and it is in three parts. The first part we talk about school days, childhood, the Depression and the Second World War; the second part is about working, marriage, having children and events like the Queen's Coronation. The final part is when we talk about the years since then. This is sometimes more difficult as many of the residents have better memories of the earlier years than the latter ones! We try to use old photographs, clothes, music or anything the residents may bring with them, and every couple of months we use the minibus and take them to the museum. The residents really enjoy these sessions and it is interesting to see how they become more lucid and sometimes quite animated.

In Vera's case she found it painful to talk about children as she only had Matt. It would appear that she was unable to have any more, which must have been hard for her and George when the expectation after the war was to have children. What was fascinating though was when she talked about the garden. It seemed to take her mind off George for a little while. Her thinking is really clear, she says she once met Vita Sackville-West. Vera has now become friendly with another resident Joan, and they go for sojourns in the garden when the weather is fine. I'm so glad I found that article because we have been able to make a real difference.'

Activity 9.28

Reflecting on your previous knowledge about the community multi-disciplinary team, how may the team now caring for Vera have changed since moving to in the Nursing Home?

The roles of other professionals

Although Vera has now moved into a nursing home, there are a number of professional care workers who have a regular input into Vera's care. You will already have a list of which personnel were involved earlier and you will have determined what their roles were then. In the nursing home the personnel may or may not be the same however; there may be more but different involvement. When considering the multi-disciplinary team, it is automatic to name the doctor, the social worker, and the physiotherapist. These individuals are regarded as 'direct' carers. In a nursing home setting there is an army of 'indirect' carers. These are the kitchen staff, cleaners, caretakers, hairdressers and many others.

 Who are the care workers now involved in Vera's care and how have they been prepared for their role?

In 1994 the United Kingdom Central Council for Nursing, Midwifery and Health Visiting established a project group to look at continuing care for older people. The main objective was to consider the ways in which 'care in institutional and non-institutional settings, is accessed by older people and aims to promote and maintain maximum potential for self-care.' (UKCC 1997). The document also aimed to encourage all nurses and health visitors to reflect on how they provide continuing care for older people. The main areas for consideration included:

- Appropriate education, induction and clinical supervision
- An organisational culture that is committed to continuing care
- Positive attitudes expressed by nurses and health visitors towards older people
- Supportive and committed management processes
- Respect for the contribution of other members of the care team
- Appropriate delegation and supervision.

They also identified the areas where, it was felt, nurses and health visitors could make a positive contribution to continuing care. First, the need for specialist practice skills has been recognised for some time and there is a great deal of potential for nursing homes to become clinical development units, with an emphasis on teaching and research, similar in manner to teaching hospitals. Second, the report recognised the need to develop tools for needs assessment and review. Third, the need to promote and maintain health in order to reduce illness and dependency. Finally, it is crucial that carers work in partnership with older people and every effort is made to reduce petty jealousies that surround professional boundaries.

Since then other task forces have been set up by the government to also look at the continuing care of older people. These documents have already been mentioned, but it is worth returning to them and reading them in conjunction with the UKCC (1997) document.

Activity 9.29

Obtain your own copy of this important document as it will act to guide you in reflecting on your own practice: UKCC (1997) *The Nursing and Health Visiting Contribution to the Continuing Care of Older People.* London: UKCC.

Vera appears to have settled well into Holyrood Nursing Home, but there is every indication that she may soon be able to be reaccommodated within a residential care home. Thankfully she has made good progress and appears not to require the level of nursing care originally envisaged. Vera has mixed feelings about another move, but she likes the thought of living nearer friends. Vera talks with Matt on the phone and a case conference is set for Monday week.

Activity 9.30

With the information you have, what is Matt's role in Vera's care? What support is available for Matt? Think about a family you know which has an older member living in residential care. Make brief notes on the family's role in relation to this older person.

Conclusion

Having worked through this chapter, you will have experienced many of the challenges which Vera Jenkins, her son and neighbour have each had to meet. Central to the support available has been the ability of the multi-disciplinary team to communicate with each other and involve Vera and others when assessing, planning and delivering the care that Vera needed, both in the community and in a residential setting.

The scenario has raised many issues which nurses working with older people need to consider. You will no doubt have been able to make comparisons with the care of older people that you have witnessed or been involved in delivering. Many decisions that older people have to make happen at a time when they are at their most vulnerable. The nurse has a duty to protect and safeguard their interests, giving an older person the time and the information that they need in order to come to a decision which could affect the rest of their lives. These can be tough decisions and they are not always appropriately managed.

Now reflect back on the outcomes which are set out at the beginning of this chapter, and consider how much you have learnt. Think about the questions that remain unanswered and the ways in which you intend to address them.

References

Allott, M., Robb, M. (1998) *Understanding Health and Social Care: An Introductory Reader.* Milton Keynes: Open University Press.

Bernard, M., Meade, K., (1993) *Women Come Of Age.* London: Edward Arnold.

Black Perspectives Sub-Group (1998) Black perspectives on residential care. In: Allott and Robb. *Understanding Health and Social Care.*

Bowers, H. (1999) *Standards for Health and Social Care Services for Older People.* Brighton: Pavilion Publishing.

Bowling, A. (1997) *Measuring Health.* Milton Keynes: Open University Press.

Dealey, C. (1999) *Care of Wounds.* Oxford: Blackwell Science.

Department of Health and Social Services Inspectorate (1993) *Care Management and Assessment: Practitioners Guide.* London: HMSO.

Dodge, J., Knutesen, P. (1994) Enhancing health and function in late life. In: Webb, P. (ed.). *Health Promotion and Patient Education.* London: Chapman&Hall.

Dudek, S. G. (1997) *Nutrition Handbook for Nursing Practice.* 3rd Edition. Philadelphia, PA: Lippincott.

Ffoulkes, M. (1996) Loss and bereavement in later life. In: Wade, L., Waters, K. (eds). *A Textbook of Gerontological Nursing.* London: Baillière Tindall, ch. 6.

Folstein, M. F., Folstein, S. E., McHugh, P. R. (1975) Mini-mental state: a practical method for grading the cognitive state of patients for the clinician. *Journal of Psychiatry and Research* 12, pp. 189–98.

Granvill, G. (1996) Promoting health in older people. In: Wade, L. and Waters, K. A textbook of *Gerontological Nursing*: London: Baillière Tindall.

Griffiths, R. (1988) *Community Care: Agenda for Action* (Griffiths Report) London: HMSO.

Health Advisory Service 2000 Project Team (1998) *'Not because they are old': An Independent Enquiry into the Care of Older People on Acute Wards in General Hospitals.* London: HAS.

Jones, H. (1996) The impact of ageing. In: Wade and Waters. *Gerontological Nursing.*

Kendrick, K. (1994) An Advocate for whom – doctor or patient? How far can a nurse be a patient's advocate? *Professional Nurse* 9 (12), pp. 826–9.

Kendrick, K. (1996) The challenge of advocacy: a moral response. In: Wade and Waters. *Gerontological Nursing.* London: Baillière Tindall.

Killick, J. (1998) Listening and life-history work. In: Allott and Robb. *Understanding Health and Social Care.*

Kitson, A. (1991) *Therapeutic Nursing and the Hospitalised Elderly.* Harrow: Scutari Press.

Mackay, L. (1993) *Conflicts in Care: Medicine and Nursing.* London: Chapman and Hall.

Mallet, J. (2000) *The Royal Marsden Hospital Manual of Clinical Nursing Procedures.* 5th Edition. Oxford: Blackwell Science.

Marr, J., Kershaw, B. (1998) *Caring for Older People.* London: Arnold.

Nursing and Midwifery Council (2002) *Code of Professional Conduct.* London: NMC.

Orem, D. (1991) *Nursing: Concepts of Practice.* 4th Edition. St Louis, MO: Mosby Year Books.

Pattie, A. H., Gilleard, C. J. (1981) *Clifton Assessment Procedures for the Elderly (CAPE).* London: Hodder and Stoughton.

Roper, N., Logan, W., Tierney, A. (1990) *Elements of Nursing.* Edinburgh: Churchill Livingstone.

Roy, C. (1976) *Introduction to Nursing: An Adaptation Model.* Englewood Cliffs, NJ: Prentice-Hall.

Royal College of Physicians (1992) *Drugs and the Elderly*. London: HMSO.

Royle, J. (1992) Caring for the Patient with a Disorder of the Skin. In: Royle, J., Walsh, M. (1992) *Watson's Medical – Surgical Nursing and Related Physiology*. London: Baillière Tindall.

Social Trends (2001) *Number 31*. London: HMSO.

United Kingdom Central Council for Nursing, Midwifery and Health Visiting (1992) *Code of Professional Conduct*. London: UKCC.

Wade, L., Waters, K. (1996) *A Textbook of Gerontological Nursing*. London: Baillière Tindall.

Wade, L. (1996) New Perspectives on gerontological nursing. In: Wade, L., Waters, K. (eds) *Gerontological Nursing*. London: Baillière Tindall.

Walsh, M. (1998) *Models and Critical Pathways in Clinical Nursing*. London: Baillière Tindall.

Webb, P. (ed.) (1997) *Health Promotion and Patient Education: A Professionals Guide*. Cheltenham: Thounes.

Resources

📖 Further reading

Barker, K., (1998) The ageing process. In Marr, J., Kershaw, B.(eds). *Caring for Older People*. London: Arnold.

Bernard, M. (2000) *Promoting Health in Old Age*. Milton Keynes: Open University Press.

Black, M. (1992) Ageing and Health. In Royle, J., Walsh, M. (eds). *Watson's Medical–Surgical Nursing and Related Physiology*. London: Ballière Tindall.

Department of Health (2000) *Partnership in Action*. London: HMSO.

Department of Health (2001b) *Medicines and Older People*. London: HMSO.

Eliopoulos, C. (1997) *Gerontological Nursing*. Philadelphia, PA: Lippincott.

Holden, U. P., Woods, R. T. (1988) *Reality Orientation*. Edinburgh: Churchill Livingstone.

Humphries, J., Green, J (2002) *Nurse Prescribing*. Basingstoke: Palgrave Macmillan.

Ovretveit, J. (1993) *Coordinating Community Care*. Milton Keynes: Open University Press.

Russell, L. (2000) Understanding the physiology of wound healing and how dressings help. *British Journal of Nursing* 9 (1), pp. 10–21.

Trounce, J., Gould, D. (2000) *Clinical Pharmacology for Nurses*. Edinburgh: Churchill Livingstone.

Webster, C. (ed.) (2001) *Caring for Health: History and Diversity*. 3rd Edition. Milton Keynes: Open University Press.

Annotated bibliography

Bernard, M., Meade, K. (1993) *Women Come of Age*. London: Edward Arnold.
    A book that embraces the wider world beyond nursing and encourages all health care workers to do just that. As women live longer, the inequalities in their lives become greater.

Department of Health (2001) National Service Framework for Older People. London: HMSO

A great deal of work has already been carried out by the NHS and social services to improve care for older people. This National Service Framework (one of a series) continues the work and is important reading for students caring for older people in the community, in hospitals and the independent sector.

Health Advisory Service 2000 (1998) 'Not because they are old': An Independent Enquiry into the Care of Older People on Acute Wards in General Hospitals. London: HAS.

This is a report that presents the findings of an inquiry into the care of older people on acute wards in general hospitals. The aim of the inquiry was to seek and bring together the views of older patients, their significant others, ward staff and managers about the care given. Fifteen recommendations are made to enhance care including a National Service Framework for Older People.

Ovretveit, J. (1993) Coordinating Community Care. Milton Keynes: Open University Press.

The author of this text has written extensively in this area. Highly recommended to develop an understanding about how health care workers can work together and provide quality care.

Wade, L., Waters, K. (eds) (1996) A Textbook of Gerontological Nursing. London: Ballière Tindall.

This text is written by a number of 'experts in the field' and has been used extensively in the development of this chapter. It is ideal for student nurses in providing them with a wide range of insights into caring for older people. The text also includes clinical discussion points and extensive references.

Official reports and documents

Department of Health (2000) Partnership in Action. London: HMSO.

Department of Health (2001a) National Service Framework for Older People. London: HMSO.

United Kingdom Central Council for Nursing, Midwifery and Health Visiting (1997) The Nursing and Health Visiting Contribution to the Continuing Care of Older People. London: UKCC.

@ Web pages

Department of Health: **www.doh.gov.uk/nursing.htm**
Essence of Care: **www.doh.gov.uk/essenceofcare/**
National Care Standards Commission: **www.doh.gov.uk/ncsc/index.htm**
National Service Framework for Older People:
　www.doh.gov.uk/nsf/olderpeople.htm
Reuters Health (daily news service on health issues): **www.reutershealth.com**

For related articles the following websites may be helpful:

British Nutrition Foundation: **www.nutrition.org.uk**
Free Nursing Care? **www.dih.gov.uk/coinh.htm**

Nursing Standard: **www.nursing-standard.co.uk/index.html**
Nursing Times: **www.nursingtimes.net**
Population Trends: **www.statistics.gov.uk**
Residential care: **www.nursingresidentialcare.com**

There are a vast number of organisations that can provide help and advice for older people and their carers. Many of these organisations have local addresses and the reader is directed in the first instance to the telephone directory or the local library.

The following are only some examples where assistance may be available for your studies.

Age Concern: **www.ace.org.uk**
Benefits Agency: **www.dss.gov.uk/ba**
British Association for Counselling: **www.bac.co.uk**
British Geriatric Society: **www.bgs.org.uk**
British Red Cross Society: **reccross.org.uk**
Citizens Advice Bureau: **www.nacab.org.uk**
Council for Voluntary Services: **www.nacvs.ord.uk**
National Association of Bereavement Services: **www.directions-plus.org.uk**
National Association of Widows: **www.directions-plus.org.uk**

10 Insights into Meeting Nutritional Needs

Pam Jackson

Introduction

Nutrition is of fundamental importance to life. This chapter will explore a number of aspects of nutrition. It will consider what the current guidelines for healthy eating are, and how to implement them. It will look at the factors that influence food choice and food consumption, and provide guidelines on how to undertake a nutritional assessment, and policies to prevent malnutrition in hospitals. Finally, it will look at the importance of good nutrition in the prevention and management of other health problems, such as constipation and wound healing.

Learning outcomes

This chapter will enable the student to:

- Discuss the basic nutritional principles of nutrients and energy.
- Explore and name the components of a healthy, balanced diet.
- Outline the factors which may influence food choices in the elderly, in both hospital and community settings.
- Recognise the need for assessment of nutritional status, and know how to carry out a simple nutritional screening test.
- Outline six strategies for promoting appetite and suggest ways of optimising nutritional intake.
- Discuss the consequences of malnutrition.
- List ten factors that can contribute to constipation, and discuss its management.
- Identify eight intrinsic factors and four extrinsic factors that may contribute to the development of pressure ulcers and discuss their management.
- Suggest five strategies that could be used to improve nutrition in hospitals.

Concepts

- Nutrition
- Balanced diet
- Malnutrition
- Dehydration
- Constipation
- Ageing
- Bereavement
- Loneliness
- Pressure ulcers

- Screening
- Assessment
- Health education
- Healthy eating
- Food choices
- Nutrition in different ethnic groups
- Adjustment
- Community support
- Motivation

Scenario *Introducing Jack*

Jack is an 82-year-old man, living alone since the death of his wife, in a house in the old part of town. He does not eat well and has recently lost weight.

 Activity 10.1

Consider the factors that affect your food choice and food consumption. Then think about those factors that might affect what Jack eats.

 Activity 10.2

In your practice placement, find out what factors interfere with normal eating and drinking.

Jack's wife, Hetty, died six months ago, less than a year after the couple had celebrated their diamond-wedding anniversary.

? Consider how Jack might be feeling now. How might this affect his health?

Table 10.1 Factors that affect food choices

- **Physiological changes** Jack is 82 years old. There is physiological deterioration in most body systems with increasing age, and slower structural repair. In the gastrointestinal system there are reductions in secretion, absorption and motility, and impaired ability to metabolise and synthesise. Other systems have similar deterioration, such as reduced senses, muscle weakness, reflexes and so on. Jack's loss of appetite may partly be due to these effects of ageing. (For a more detailed discussion of the effects of ageing, see Chapter 9 on older people.)

Table 10.1 (continued)

- **Psychological factors** Jack is feeling very low following the death of his wife. This can affect appetite and lead to anorexia. (For a more detailed discussion of the effects of bereavement and depression, see Chapter 9 on the older person.)

- **Socioeconomic factors** Jack feels lonely and isolated. He has no one to eat meals with. He only has his pension to live on.

- **Cultural factors** His wife has always done the shopping and cooking.

- **Cognitive factors** Jack does not know what constitutes a healthy, balanced diet.

- **Psychomotor ability** Jack is physically able to care for himself, but lacks experience of such things as shopping and cooking, and his motivation is low.

- **Resources available** Jack has a kitchen with a stove for cooking, but has difficulty getting to the shops.

- **Health and disease** Jack has enjoyed quite good health, but is currently suffering from constipation and a sore mouth.

- **Convenience** Jack is likely to choose foods that require little preparation or cooking.

- **Drug-nutrient interactions including alcohol** Some drugs interfere with normal digestion.

In hospital there may be other factors:

- **Environmental factors** such as unfamiliar food, strange surroundings and smells, and reduced access to food and drinks.

- **Loss of independence** Reduced choice over types of meal and timing.

- **Effects of treatment** May reduce appetite.

- **Institutional factors** Change in routine, and mealtimes.

- **Increased nutritional requirements** Due to illness, surgery or trauma.

Hetty had always looked after Jack, doing all the shopping and cooking, as he was always so busy running a 'pub'. Jack became a publican after the War, and only retired ten years ago. He still enjoys a drink and smokes 20 cigarettes a day. Jack has one son who lives abroad. Although Jack has enjoyed quite good health, he always seemed to get a couple of colds each winter. Since his wife died, he has tended to neglect his health, and has been suffering with constipation for the past few months.

 Why might Jack be suffering with constipation? Think about this before moving on to the next section.

Table 10.2 Causes of constipation

Normal defaecation can be defined as the regular and easy passage of a soft, well-formed and complete stool. There is a wide range of normal frequency, from three times a day to three times a week (Brocklehurst 1990). If a person has difficulty with evacuation of faeces, they are said to be suffering from constipation.

Constipation can be caused by a wide range of factors:

- **Self-induced** Such as a diet that is poor in fibre, eating too little, not drinking enough, lack of exercise/immobility, ignoring the call to defaecate, or unnecessary use of laxatives
- **Environmentally-induced** Such as poor toilet facilities, travel or admission to hospital
- **Drug-induced** Such as many analgesics, anticholinergics, aluminium-based antacids, antidepressants.
- **Disease-related** Such as neurological disorders, muscular deficiencies, obstruction, endocrine or metabolic disorders or psychiatric problems.
- **Psychological** Such as depression.
- **Local tissue factors** Such as haemorrhoids, or weak pelvic floor muscles.

See Winney (1998) for further information.

Activity 10.3

Think about people who were constipated that you have met in your practice placements. What specific factors may have contributed to their constipation?

Jack went to the chemist to buy a laxative, to try and alleviate the constipation. The pharmacist at the Chemist shop overheard Jack asking for a laxative. He advised senna, 1–2 tablets, but also suggested that Jack might find it helpful to see the practice nurse at his local surgery.

 How do laxatives work?

 What is the role of the pharmacist at a chemist shop?

 How might the practice nurse help Jack manage his constipation? You may like to review your answer to this question having read Table 10.3.

Table 10.3 Management of constipation

- **Increase fibre intake** Cereals, especially porridge and bran types, grains and wholemeal bread, fruit and vegetables, pulses and beans. Stools that are high in fibre are bulkier and have a higher water content, and are therefore softer in consistency, and easier to expel. The fibre also provides a more acidic environment which is conducive to normal gut flora activity.

  It is often difficult to effect a change of diet, as many people are resistant to changing lifetime habits. However, this can be done by suggesting the gradual introduction of high-fibre cereals, encouraging brown/granary/wholemeal bread instead of white, and trying to increase the number of servings of fruit and vegetables.

- **Increase fluid intake** Minimum intake of 1–1.5 litres a day. Inadequate fluid intake reduces the stimulus for intestinal activity and triggers a greater absorptive response in the colon, leaving the stool hard and dry. Some fluids stimulate bowel activity, for instance fruit juices, real ale and tea. (As Jack enjoys a drink, the mention of real ale may encourage him.)

- **Increase activity level** Exercise and general mobility help prevent constipation, by stimulating smooth muscle activity in the gut, and aiding the process of defaecation.

- **Re-establish regular bowel emptying** Ignoring the call to stool leads to increased water absorption from the stool due to prolonged transit time, and reduced response to gut activity.

- **Avoid unnecessary use of laxatives** Stimulant laxatives such as bisocodyl should only be used short-term, as the large bowel becomes insensitive to their action, and then stronger laxatives will be needed to effect the same result. Ideally, suppositories or micro-enemas should be used in preference to laxatives, as they will only have a local action of irritating the mucosa and lubricating the passage.

For further reading on the effectiveness of laxatives in the elderly, see the NHS Centre for Research and Dissemination systematic review (2001), commissioned by NICE.

Jack still misses his wife and finds it hard to cope without her.

Activity 10.4

Consider what effect this may have on Jack's appetite and nutritional status, before reviewing the following.

Jack never did visit the practice nurse but because he is feeling lonely, he decides to write to his son:

'. . . I still miss your mother very much and sometimes I find the silence almost unbearable. I can picture her in the kitchen with her apron on, busy baking an apple pie for dinner. I can smell it even now! I don't seem to have much of an appetite these days and there doesn't seem much point in getting a meal when there's just me. Anyway, your mother never let me in the kitchen, so I wouldn't know how to cook even if I was feeling hungry. I still go down the 'King's Head' most evenings for a couple of pints and my pack of cigarettes, but other than that I can go for days without seeing anyone.'

 Do you know what constitutes a healthy, balanced diet? You may like to think about what you know before reading on.

Table 10.4 What constitutes a healthy, balanced diet?

The following recommendations for healthy eating have been made by the National Task Force for nutrition in the document *8 Guidelines for a Healthy Diet,* published in association with the Department of Health (DoH), Ministry of Agriculture, Fisheries and Food (MAFF), by the Health Education Authority (HEA), in 1997.

- **Plenty of vegetables and fruit** About a third of your food intake. Aim to eat at least 5 servings of vegetables and fruit a day, as they are rich in fibre and vitamins – especially dark green and orange fruit and vegetables.
- **Plenty of starchy foods** About a third of your food intake, as they are rich in fibre, vitamins and minerals, and a good energy source, e.g. pasta, rice, potatoes, bread, especially wholemeal varieties.
- **Regular meat, fish and alternatives** Eat moderate amounts of these foods, as they are a good source of protein, vitamins and minerals. Choose lean meats. This group includes eggs, pulses, soya and nuts. Eat fish at least twice a week, especially oily fish, such as salmon, tuna, mackerel and sardines, as these are rich in Omega-3 fatty acids, which help reduce the risk of heart disease.
- **Regular milk and dairy foods** Eat moderate amounts of these foods, as they are all good sources of protein and calcium. Choose low-fat alternatives if possible, except for children under 5 years of age.
- **Not too much fat** Eat in small amounts and not too often. Fat is a good source of energy and fat-soluble vitamins. Try to avoid saturated (animal) fat.
- **Not too much salt** Avoid adding salt at the table and reduce salt in cooking (microwave cooking avoids the need for salt), as salt increases the risk of hypertension.
- **Infrequent sugary foods** Eat sparingly, as they increase the risk of dental caries.
- **Maintain physical activity** This can take a variety of forms such as regular exercise through sport or work, and through everyday activities.

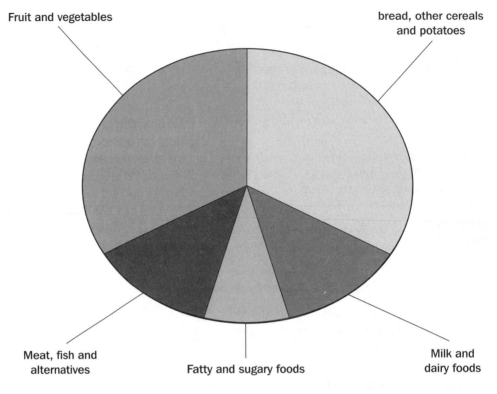

Fruit and vegetables

bread, other cereals
and potatoes

Meat, fish and
alternatives

Fatty and sugary foods

Milk and
dairy foods

Figure 10.1 Healthy-eating plate

(Reproduced with permission from the Health Education Authority)

Activity 10.5

A Find out what the Health of the Nation targets are and see how many of them link with the nutrition guidelines above. (Also, see Chapter 12 on rehabilitation, for more on the Health of the Nation targets.)

B Work out a balanced healthy menu for Jack over two or three days, taking into account his age and lifestyle.

C Find out what facilities related to nutrition are available for the elderly in your community. For example: Meals on Wheels, luncheon clubs, help with shopping (see Chapter 9 on older people).

Jack lacks any appetite and finds it hard to motivate himself to eat.

Why is food important? Consider your response before moving on.

Why is food important?: nutrition science

Food is absolutely essential for life. Human metabolism is a complex process which is constantly active, and which relies on a supply of specific chemicals, or nutrients. These provide energy, and maintain structure and function. Many of these chemicals can be synthesised by the body, but some cannot; these are called essential nutrients, that is, we have to ingest them as we cannot synthesise them. Broadly, there are three categories of essential nutrients:

- **Minerals** Usually only required in small amounts, e.g. iron and calcium or, in very small amounts, (trace elements), e.g. iodine.
- **Organic compounds** Synthesised in the food chain, but not by humans. These include essential fatty acids, vitamins and essential amino acids.
- **Organic precursors** Necessary as the substrates for synthesis of organic compounds needed by humans. If the diet does not provide sufficient precursors, the body is unable to synthesise the compounds needed for maintaining structure and function.

The chemical compounds present in food fit into one or more of the following categories:

- **Nutrients** Carbohydrates, fats, proteins, vitamins, minerals and water
- **Energy sources** Carbohydrates, fats, proteins and alcohol
- **Other compounds** Additives and toxins for example.

As can be seen, several food groups appear in more than one category. They can be used for a variety of purposes, depending on the individual requirements. Maintenance of a stable metabolic state requires sufficient energy and nutrients to satisfy metabolic demand. If food intake is restricted, the body's energy requirements to maintain metabolism will take priority over other activities such as maintaining structure and function.

For more detailed explanations and further reading about major food groups and metabolism see Chapter 9 for discussion of estimated average requirements (p. 294) and either Barasi (1997) or Garrow and James (1999).

> Jack's lack of motivation and poor appetite are hindered by feeling constipated, and by a sore mouth, caused partly by his dentures no longer fitting properly, and possible vitamin B deficiency.
> Jack has lost 12kg in weight: a year ago he weighed 68kg He is 1.75m tall.

 What effect can a sore mouth have? (See Holmes (1996) for information on oral care in older patients.)

How would you describe Jack's current weight?

 What is Body Mass Index (BMI)? Calculate Jack's BMI. Is it normal? (See Table 10.5 for an explanation.)

> **Activity 10.6**
>
> Work out the percentage weight loss: is this significant? If so, in what way? (See Bond, 1997, ch. 3.4.)

Table 10.5 Body mass index

Body Mass Index measures height and weight and is used as an estimate of fatness. It is calculated in the following way:

$$BMI = \frac{Weight\ (kg)}{Height^2\ (m)}$$

Body mass index is a better indicator of fatness than weight alone and is commonly used in nutritional assessment tools. It is considered to be a stable, easily performed and sensitive measure of malnutrition, including for hospitalised and frail elderly. However, the figures should be interpreted with caution in this age group, as the published norms are based on young adults. In the elderly, there is often reduced muscle mass as well as fat.

The suggested classification of BMI in the UK is as follows:

Less than 19	underweight
20-25	normal weight
26-30	overweight
31-40	obese
40 +	severely obese

There is a relationship between BMI and health outcome, with the greatest risks of ill health associated with the higher and lowest BMI.

 In cases where height is difficult to measure, are there other parameters which could be used instead? What is a demispan? (See Bond, 1997, p. 68 for details.)

> Jack walks down to his local 'pub', most evenings, for a couple of pints and a pack of cigarettes. This is his only regular social contact.

 Where does the responsibility lie to survey health needs of the elderly? Which health professionals might be involved?

The publican became concerned for Jack's welfare after he had not been in for a couple of days. Jack was found at home, having fallen on the floor. He appeared dehydrated, rather confused, and complained of soreness over his hip. There was very little food in the house, and a half-empty carton of stale milk on the kitchen table. Jack was admitted to the Elderly Care Unit of the local community hospital for investigations. The ambulance paramedic's assessment notes state that Jack is 82, malnourished and mildly confused. He was found on the floor, where he had remained, immobile for several hours.

? As Jack's named nurse, you would undertake a nutritional assessment on his admission to hospital. What would you need to find out and why? (See below for more information.)

Nutritional screening and assessment

Nutritional Screening should be carried out with all patients coming into hospital, to identify those with, or at risk of, malnutrition. Factors included in a screening tool may include weight and height (BMI), appetite (especially recent changes), diet, ability to eat and drink and swallow, gastrointestinal function (such as constipation or diarrhoea), mental condition and medical problems.

Activity 10.7

Find out if a nutritional assessment tool is used in your practice area and carry out an assessment.

? What strategies are in place in your practice area to deal with malnutrition? (For example, dietitian referral, access to 'sip feeds'.)

The Department of Health published patient-focused benchmarking for health care professionals in February 2001, and food and nutrition were one of the eight identified areas (DoH 2001). This document, known as the *Essence of Care*, encourages trusts to be active in improving and raising the profile of nutritional screening and assessment, as a means to reducing malnutrition. It is a valuable resource, which can be used to help improve quality of care as it focuses on fundamental elements of care that matter most to patients.

Activity 10.8

Visit the DoH web pages at:
http://www.doh.gov.uk/essenceofcare/intro.htm and see if any of the other 7 identified areas are pertinent to this scenario.

Nutritional assessment tools have been developed to try and identify patients at risk of malnutrition but, at the current time, very few have been validated.

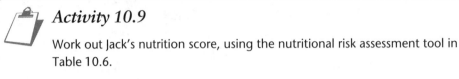

Activity 10.9

Work out Jack's nutrition score, using the nutritional risk assessment tool in Table 10.6.

 What are the implications of using unvalidated tools? (See Pattison et al. 1995, pp. 54–5.)

Table 10.6 Nutritional risk assessment tool

Elderly Care Unit:

Multidisciplinary Nutrition Assessment Tool

Complete on admission and as the patient's condition changes

Height (or estimation): 1.75m

Date of scoring	/ /	/ /	/ /	/ /

Weight (kg)	56			

Section 1: Mental State   Score

- alert and orientated 0
- confused 1
- cognitive impairment 2
- unconcious 3

1			

Section 2: Appetite/intake

- good intake (3 meals/day)/tube fed 0
- reduced intake (½ meals eaten) 1
- poor intake (¼–½ meals eaten) 2
- appetite nil/NBM/inadequate tube feed 3

2			

Section 3: Ability to eat and drink

- independent – self fed with no aids 0
- independent using feeding aid 1
- needs assistance to eat/drink e.g. food cut up/ prompt to swallow 2
- unable to feed without full assistance 3

0			

Section 4: Diet

- normal 0
- special e.g. low potassium or modified diet
  e.g. soft/puree 1
- nausea/vomiting/diarrhoea for >2days 2
- severe vomiting/diarrhoea (4+episodes/day) 3

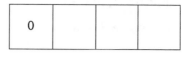

Section 5: Clinical/medical factors

- none 0
- current/recent minor infection e.g. almost
  healed pressure sores 1
- current/recent major infection, recent stroke,
  major surgery, fractures, active pressure ulcers,
  active inflammatory Bowel Disease, depression
  and dementia 2
- multiple/deep pressure ulcers, burns,
  malignant disease 3

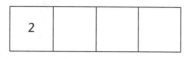

Section 6: Recent weight history e.g. 2–3 months

- no unintentional weight change 0
- decreased gradually e.g. up to 3kg 1
- decreased rapidly e.g. 3–6kg 2
- considerable weight loss >6kg 3

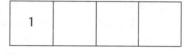

Section 7: Swallowing ability

- normal swallow 0
- poor dentition 1
- swallowing difficulties e.g. modified diets and
  fluids/increased time to eat/oral infection 2
- severe swallowing difficulties e.g. not managing
  modified diet and increased risk of aspiration..........3

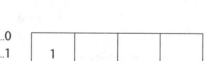

TOTAL SCORE:

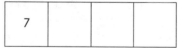

ACTION PLAN

Dietician:

Score

0–3 LOW RISK
- Weigh in one week and rescore. Arrange special diets e.g. soft, puree, diabetic order from the menu as appropriate

4+   AT RISK
- Weigh in one week and rescore. Order High Protein diet and encourage 2–3 nutritional supplements (e.g. Ensure Plus, Enlive, Build Up) between meals, e.g. 10 a.m., 3 p.m., and 7 p.m.
- Monitor intake using Food Record Charts. Refer if intake still poor

Table 10.6 (continued)

Occupational Therapist:

Score

1+   (on Section 3)   ● Check sitting posture – consider seeking PT/OT advice
                      ● Consider using non-slip mats and plate guards
                      ● Consider using adapted feeding equipment if not already being used
                      ● Consider referral to OT:
                        ● if difficulty lifting hands to mouth
                        ● consistently dropping cutlery
                        ● spilling food
                        ● leaving food on half of the plate

Speech and Language Therapy:

Score

1–2 (on Section 7)   ● Check sitting/upright position for eating/drinking. Consider seeking PT/OT advice
                      ● Check dentition and oral hygiene
2+   (on Section 7)   ● Refer to Speech and Language Therapy
                      ● Continue oral intake by giving Grade II thickened fluids and pureed diet
                      ● If unable to manage above OR at high risk of aspiration – place NBM and discuss with medical team regarding alternative hydration and nutrition. Await SALT assessment

(Reproduced by kind permission of the Medical and Elderly Care Directorate, Southampton University Hospital Trust)

> Using the nutritional risk assessment tool, Jack scored 7 out of a possible 21, on admission. This places him in the at-risk category.

  What strategies can be used to increase Jack's nutrient intake and reduce his level of risk?

Nutritional support

Jack is underweight, and malnourished. He is therefore in need of building up, rather than trying to adhere to healthy eating principles. However, he is elderly and has a small appetite. Look for ways of fortifying the food a patient like this eats, and making every mouthful count. Examples:

- Encourage fluids with calories rather than just water, tea or squash, for example milky drinks with added milk powder, 'sip feeds', high calorie drinks and thickened soups.
- Add protein or fat such as grated cheese over potatoes/soup, extra margarine on vegetables, cream/ice-cream with puddings.
- Add sugar, for example jam or honey in puddings, sugar in drinks.
- Use neutral or vanilla flavour 'sip feeds' in place of milk on cereals.

> **_Activity 10.10_**
>
> For more ideas, read Section 6.1 'Small is beautiful' in _Eating Matters_ (Bond 1997).

? How will you monitor Jack to ensure that he is gaining weight? (Refer to the action plan accompanying the risk assessment tool in Table 10.6.)

? What are the potential consequences of malnutrition for Jack?

Consequences of malnutrition

There are a wide variety of complications associated with the development of malnutrition, which may lead to increased mortality:

- Reduced mobility, leading to increased risk of deep vein thrombosis and pressure ulcers (see Chapter 12 on rehabilitation for more discussion).

> On admission, Jack was found to have developed a Grade 2 pressure ulcer over his left trocanter.

- Protein, vitamin and mineral deficiency, leading to increased risk of delayed wound healing.
- Reduced immunocompetence, leading to increased risk of infection.
- Muscle atrophy and weakness, causing reduced respiratory function, reduced cardiac function and fatigue. This can lead to a chest infection or heart failure.
- Atrophy of the intestinal mucosa, leading to reduced absorption of nutrients.
- Apathy and depression.
- Increased drug toxicity.

This will result in delayed recovery and prolonged hospital stay. All these factors have cost implications, both for the individual and for the health service.

? What are the factors that have led to Jack developing a pressure ulcer?

What is meant by the term Grade 2 pressure ulcer? (See Reid and Morison, 1994; and Table 10.7 below.)

Table 10.7 Grading of pressure ulcers

Pressure ulcers are graded according to severity, and there is now an internationally agreed classification

Grade 1 Discoloration of intact skin – either non-blanching erythema, or blue/black (bruising)

Grade 2 Partial thickness skin loss involving epidermis/dermis

Grade 3 Full thickness skin loss involving damage to subcutaneous tissue

Grade 4 Full thickness, with extensive destruction extending to underlying bone or tendon
(Reid and Morison 1994)

Pressure ulcers

The factors that have put Jack particularly at risk are malnutrition and loss of body weight, age and immobility. See below for factors affecting development of pressure ulcers and for a more detailed discussion of the importance of nutrition in wound healing, see either Green and McLaren, (1998) or Russell, (2001).

Evidence-based practice

Assessment and management of pressure ulcers

The critical determinants of pressure ulcers are believed to be the intensity and duration of applied pressure (Cullum and Clark 1992). There are a number of extrinsic and intrinsic factors that influence tissue tolerance:

- Intrinsic factors, such as age, nutritional status, increase or decrease in body weight, immobility, incontinence, neurological factors, vascular factors, concurrent disease or infection.
- Extrinsic factors, such as inadequate support surfaces, poor hygiene, poor positioning, poor moving and handling technique of carers or prolonged sitting without adequate support.

A pressure ulcer can be defined as an area of tissue death caused by pressure distorting the capillaries and cutting off the blood supply for a critical length of time (Bliss 1990). Pressure ulcers are unlikely to heal unless the pressure is removed, and as many as possible of the predisposing factors alleviated. Nutrition is one of the most important factors to address (Green and McLaren 1998). Jack should be assessed on admission for risk of developing further pressure ulcers. A validated risk-assessment tool could be used as part of that assessment.

 As the named nurse responsible for Jack's care, how would you select an assessment tool that identifies patients at risk of developing pressure ulcers? What factors are considered?

A number of scales have been developed that try to take risk factors into account in assessing the risk to an individual of developing a pressure ulcer. Most of these scales are based on the first one developed by Norton, McLaren and Exton-Smith in 1962. They attach a numerical score to each factor assessed, depending on the level of dependence or severity. The total score is an indication of the level of risk that person has, for developing a pressure ulcer.

 Activity 10.11

Find out if a pressure ulcer risk assessment scale is used in the practice area where you are working. Are all patients assessed? If so, how often are they reassessed? Find out if there is a protocol to follow for patients identified at risk? How suitable would it be for assessing Jack's level of risk? How valid and reliable is it? (See Ratcliffe 1998.)

Jack was assessed using the Waterlow Pressure ulcer risk assessment scale and scored 13, which puts him at moderate risk of developing another pressure ulcer. He already has an existing Grade 2 pressure ulcer on his trocanter (see Waterlow 1985 for more details about this particular risk assessment scale).

What strategies would you, as the named nurse, use to reduce the risk of Jack developing further pressure ulcers?

Strategies to reduce risk of pressure ulcer development

Royle (1992) recommends the following strategies:

- Assess the patient for risk factors.
- Ensure regular changes of position to relieve pressure on vulnerable areas such as the heels, sacrum, elbows, or shoulders.
- Maintain good standards of hygiene.
- Prevent mechanical, physical or chemical injury.
- Ensure adequate nutrition and hydration.

- Promote continence.
- Careful positioning.
- Use devices to equalise pressure over pressure points.
- Inspect the skin several times a day.
- Promote mental alertness and orientation.
- Educate the patient, family and care givers in skin care measures.

It would be appropriate for him to be nursed on an alternating pressure overlay or mattress, which ensures that no part of his skin is subjected to constant pressure. He should be encouraged to be as mobile and active as possible or otherwise turned regularly, using the 30° tilt, to relieve pressure on his ulcer. There are internationally agreed guidelines for the prevention and treatment of pressure ulcers, based on the available research evidence (European Pressure Ulcer Advisory Panel, 1998). The existing ulcer should be assessed in order that the most appropriate wound dressing can be applied.

Activity 10.12

A See Thomas 1997 for a review of current wound dressings. See also Chapter 9 on older people.

B Find out how pressure ulcer prevention is managed in the practice area where you are working. Is there a pressure ulcer prevention policy?

 What types of support surfaces are available, to reduce the risk of pressure ulcers?

There are two main types of support surfaces: conforming and alternating. Conforming mattresses/overlays and static air overlays conform to body contours, and thus spread the load. This type of support surface has a higher contact pressure than alternating pressure air mattresses (APAM), and is thus more suitable for low and moderate risk patients. APAMs systematically vary the areas of skin through which the weight of the body is transmitted, and thus high risk areas of the body are relieved of pressure for a given length of time in each cycle. For example, zero pressure for two minutes, every 7.5 minutes. There are many different types available, either overlays or replacement mattresses. Low air loss beds, and air-fluidised beds, provide uniform low pressure on the maximum body surface area, and are therefore suitable for patients at high risk of pressure ulcer development. Each patient needs to be assessed for his or her risk of developing a pressure ulcer, and then nursed on the appropriate support surface.

What is the evidence to support pressure ulcer prevention policies? (See *Effective Health Care Bulletin* (1995) on the prevention and treatment of pressure sores.)

A high-protein and high-energy diet was ordered for Jack. This included increasing the calorific content of his food and nutritional supplements. The majority of patients receive their nutrition from the Catering Department. It is important that all the different agencies that have any responsibility for patient nutrition work together to ensure optimum nutritional care.

Activity 10.13

Study some hospital menu cards and find out how the needs of different patients are catered for. Consider how flexible you could be over dietary choice if Jack was being cared for in a practice area where you have recently had experience.

> Jack has a poor appetite and needs encouragement to take an adequate diet.

? Would it be possible for Jack to receive 5 small meals/snacks a day, with added butter/cheese to vegetables and added ice cream to puddings? If not, then how else could his dietary needs be met? (See the Nutritional Guidelines for Hospital Catering, DoH 1995; and Millar 1998.)

? In what other ways can Jack's appetite be promoted during his stay in hospital?

Promoting appetite in the elderly

- **Presentation of food** Is the portion size appropriate? Does the food look attractive? Is it served at the correct temperature? Are meal times appropriate?
- **Variety and choice of food** Are familiar foods served? Are they an appropriate type/consistency? Have the needs of ethnic minority groups and individual food preferences been acknowledged?
- **Frequency** The elderly often prefer smaller meals with snacks between meals.
- **Time** Are meals rushed? Is assistance provided, if needed?
- **Oral hygiene** Are dentures well fitting? Is the mouth clean, fresh and without infection?
- **Positioning** Are patients positioned comfortably, and supported if necessary, to allow them to manage their meal?
- **Exercise** Appetite depends partly on the body's demand for energy. How active/mobile are the clients?

- **Social event** Do clients eat alone or do they have company during mealtimes?
- **Distractions** Are there other activities going on at mealtimes? Are there any smells/sounds/sights and so on that may be off-putting?

Activity 10.14

Reflect on possible ways in which mealtimes in your practice area could be better managed to give a higher priority to patient nutrition. See also the last paragraph of the professional conversation below.

Professional conversation

Anne, sister on an elderly care unit

'Jack is strong enough to feed himself whilst in hospital, but a number of our patients are not. Various ideas have been promoted in the 'Eating Matters' pack, such as inviting visitors and friends in at mealtimes to help, or using volunteers. Several trusts have reverted to a bulk food delivery system, so that patients can choose, at the time of each meal, what food they want and how much they wish to eat. Others have employed a unit cook for long-stay wards, so that patients' individual needs and preferences can be more easily met. We have a responsibility to ensure that our patients receive the food they need, and to monitor their intake (RCN guidelines 1996).

Nutrition needs to be given the priority it deserves and the ward organisation needs to reflect this. Nursing staff need to be available to help with mealtimes rather than completing administration, taking our own lunch-break or handing over to nurses on the next shift. Patients need to be on the ward at mealtimes, and investigations, physiotherapy and other essential activities, should be planned around mealtimes, whenever possible. For patients who are not on the ward when meals are served, there should be provision to ensure that they do not miss their meal. Similarly, there needs to be a procedure for newly admitted patients, or for patients whose surgery has been postponed, to receive a meal. This is especially important now that food can no longer be prepared on the Unit, because of the Health and Safety regulations.

Mealtimes are not just the main source of nutrition; they are also a social event for most people. We must try to ensure that patients have the opportunity to socialise over meals if their condition allows. Many wards were not designed with communal meals in mind, and nurses need to be imaginative to try and create an atmosphere conducive to eating. This is especially true on long-stay wards and elderly care units such as this one.'

Jack was admitted to a four-bedded bay. In the bed next to him was a rather confused, elderly man, who frequently refused to eat. He was already malnourished, and at risk of becoming dehydrated.

Nurses tried to persuade him and coax him to eat and drink, but often to no avail.

What are the signs of dehydration? (See Chapter 11 on hydration needs; and Bond (1997, Section 6.9).

 If you were the nurse giving care, what would be your response to this man? (You may wish to discuss this with your peers and with practitioners and teachers, in relation to ethical considerations. Read Clibbens 1996 pp. 29–30.)

> The man in the bed opposite was friendly and always keen to come over and talk to Jack. He regaled Jack with stories of his youth in the Punjab region of India. He was a Hindu and a vegetarian, and he found hospital food generally tasteless and unappetising.

 ### Activity 10.15

Find out about the nutrition provision for ethnic minority groups in the hospital or institution where you are working.

Check out which nutrients are most likely to be deficient in people who are vegetarian or vegan. (See HEA 1991 and Nestle and British Dietetic Association 1998), Section B9, B10).

> Jack's food and fluid intake was monitored for four days. His nutrition score was reassessed after one week, and was found to have reduced to four. This still places him in the at-risk category, and therefore he was referred to the dietician. His scores for 'ability to eat and drink', and 'swallowing ability' were both low, so he did not require a visit from either the Speech and Language Therapist or the Occupational Therapist.

 What role can these therapists and others play in nutrition? (See Chapter 12 on rehabilitation and Chapter 9 on older people for more extensive discussions of the roles of different members of the interprofessional team; see also professional conversation with a dietician below.)

 ## Professional conversation

Jane, a hospital dietician

'Nurses and dieticians do not have the same role in the management of patient nutrition, but have complementary skills that can be used together in a useful partnership. Many people think dieticians are only interested in patients who need special diets, such as patients with liver or renal disease, but dieticians want to be involved in the management of any patient who is at high risk of malnutrition, so that we can make a full nutritional assessment. We can then try and calculate the exact nutritional needs of an individual. We work closely with occupational therapists and speech and language therapists, especially in the management of patients with swallowing or other eating difficulties, to ensure that the patient receives the optimum nutrition. There is also a dietician in the nutrition support team, where her role is particularly with patients requiring enteral feeding.

We spend a lot of time talking to patients about their diet and giving information and advice, especially if the nutrition problems are multiple or complex. This could be teaching a group of newly diagnosed diabetic patients the importance of healthy eating, or helping the parents of children with coeliac disease to explore the world of gluten-free diets, or giving one-to-one advice to a patient with diabetes mellitus who has just been diagnosed with coronary heart disease. We see a lot of our patients in outpatient clinics as well as on the wards. We also consider that teaching nurses and other health professionals is important, so that consistent messages are given to patients. It is important that nurses understand our role, so that they can make appropriate referrals to us.

We rely on nurses to identify the patients at risk and deal with straightforward nutrition-related problems, reinforcing the nutritional advice given by a dietician. There are only a few dieticians working in each trust, so it's vital that our expertise is used as effectively as possible. Ideally, we should be involved in all cases where the diagnosis or the nutritional advice is complicated, and where nutritional support is required. We are also happy to see anyone that does not seem to be making progress.

In Jack's case, we were asked to advise after he had been in a few days. The nurses had carried out an initial nutritional assessment and identified him as at risk. We carried out a more detailed assessment and were then able to give them advice about increasing the calories of Jack's food and helping them work out what nutritional advice he needed before going home. It's important that dietary advice is given as practical guidance and not just theoretical principles, with the patient involved in the decisions about his eating patterns.'

Nutrition support

Nutritional assessment is a more in-depth investigation to identify the extent and nature of malnutrition. This may include anthropometric measurements, such as skin-fold thickness and mid-arm circumference, biochemical measures, such as plasma albumin and plasma transferrin, physical examination, dietary history, or recorded intake of food. A member of the nutrition support

Activity 10.16

Find out if there is a nutrition support team, or a nutrition nurse specialist in the trust where you are working. What do they do?

team, such as the dietitian or nutrition nurse specialist would normally carry this out. (See Bond 1997, chapter 3.4 for further details of nutritional assessment.)

 In summary, what are Jack's problems on admission to hospital? Consider your response before reading on.

Problems on admission to hospital

- Dehydration, leading to fluid and electrolyte imbalance.
- Malnutrition, leading to increased risk of morbidity. (Check out the section on the consequences of malnutrition above.)
- Immobility, leading to pressure ulcer development. (Have you read the section on development of pressure ulcers above?)
- Possible trauma, from fall.
- Fear of falling again (see Askham et al 1990; and NSF for older people web page).
- Mild confusion, possibly due to dehydration or vitamin deficiency.

 What nutrition-related actions would you consider to be appropriate?

Appropriate nutrition-related actions

- **Nutritional support** Reduces malnutrition and increases appetite. As Jack is able to swallow and has no known digestive/absorption difficulties, then oral nutrition should be sufficient. (Review the sections above on nutritional support and promoting appetite in the elderly.)
- **Maintenance of fluid and electrolyte balance** Monitor intake and output, oral/intravenous fluids (if given), check blood levels of electrolytes regularly.
- **Pressure ulcer prevention and management** Pressure-relieving mattress, regular turning, mobilisation and wound care. (Revisit the section above on prevention and management of pressure ulcers.)
- **Mobilisation** To reduce muscle atrophy, increase circulation, increase appetite and energy requirements, and increase confidence and independence.

> Jack is keen to return home as soon as possible.

What would you include in your discharge planning?

Discharge planning

Health education on meal planning and healthy eating (review the section above on what constitutes a healthy, balanced diet) should be included along with:

- Community support: community nutrition, such as meals on wheels or luncheon clubs, home help, bereavement counselling
- Investigate alternative living arrangements, such as residential home or warden-assisted flats, or enabling Jack to live more safely in his own home; for example installation of personal alarm or telephone.

 Who will be responsible for Jack's care when he returns to the community?

 Activity 10.17

Find out who this might be in the community where you are placed. What role would they play in maintaining Jack's health?

Conclusion

In this chapter you have considered what constitutes a healthy, balanced diet and the factors that might affect it. There have been opportunities to identify the need for a nutritional assessment which can be used in both community and hospital settings, and to consider how nutritional needs can be met. Some of the health issues related to poor nutrition, such as development of pressure ulcers and constipation, have been explored and you have examined suitable interventions to prevent and manage these problems. You should now be equipped to go out and contribute to meeting the nutritional needs both of your clients and yourself.

References

Arrowsmith, H. (1997) Malnutrition in Hospitals. *British Journal of Nursing* 6 (19), pp1131–6.

Association of Community Health Councils for England and Wales (1997) *Hungry in Hospital?* Health news briefing. London: ACHC.

Buttriss, J., Wynne, A., Stanner, S. (2001) *Nutrition: A Handbook for Community Nurses.* London: Whurr Publishers.

Caroline Walker Trust (1995) *Eating Well for Older People:Practical and Nutritional Guidelines for Food in Residential and Nursing Homes and for Community Meals.* London: Caroline Walker Trust.

Clibbens, R. (1996) Eating, ethics and alzheimers. *Nursing Times* 92 (50), pp. 29–30.

Cotton, E., Zinober, B., Jessop, J. (1996) A nutritional assessment tool for older patients. *Professional Nurse* 11 (9), pp. 609–12.

Department of Health (1992) *The nutrition of elderly people. Committee on Medical Aspects of Food Policy (COMA) Report on Health and Social Subjects* 48. London: HMSO.

Department of Health (1992) *Health of the Nation: A Strategy for Health in England.* London: HMSO.

Department of Health (1991) *Dietary Reference Values for Food, Energy and Nutrients for the UK: A Guide.* (RHSS 41). London: HMSO.

Department of Health (1994) *Nutrition: Core Curriculum Guidelines for Nutrition, in the Education of Health Professionals.* London: HMSO.

Department of Health (1994) *Eat Well: An Action Plan from the Nutrition Task Force to Achieve the Health of the Nation Targets on Diet and Nutrition.* London: HMSO.

Department of Health (1995a) *Nutrition Guidelines for Hospital Catering.* Nutrition Task Force Hospital Catering Project Team. London: HMSO.

Department of Health (1995b). *Balance of Good Health: Nutrition Task Force.* London: HMSO.

Department of Health (1996) *Eat Well II: A Progress Report from the Nutrition Task Force on the Action Plan to Achieve the Health of the Nation Targets on Diet and Nutrition.* London: HMSO.

Department of Health (1998) *Our Healthier Nation – A Contract for Health. Consultation Paper.* London: HMSO.

Department of Health (2001) *The Essence of Care: Patient Focused Benchmarking for Healthcare Professionals.* London: HMSO.

Dickerson, J.(1995). The problem of hospital-induced malnutrition. *Nursing Times* 91 (4), pp. 44–5.

Dudek, S. (1993) *Nutrition Handbook for Nursing Practice.* Philadelphia, PA: Lippincott.

English National Board for Nursing, Midwifery and Health Visiting (1995) *Nutrition for Life: Issues for Debate in the Development of Education Programmes.* London: ENB.

Gilford, A., Khun, R. K. (1996). Development of nutritional risk screening in the community. *British Journal of Community Health Nursing* 1 (6), pp. 335–9.

Health Education Authority, in association with the Ministry for Agriculture, Fishery and Food and the Department of Health (1997) *8 Guidelines for a Healthy Diet: A Guide for Nutrition Educators.* London: HEA.

Holmes, H. S. (1998) Food for thought. *Nursing Standard* 12 (46), pp. 23–7.

Lennard-Jones, J. E. (1992) *A Positive Approach to Nutrition as Treatment.* London: King's Fund.

Lennard-Jones, J. E. (1998) *Ethical and Legal Aspects of Clinical Hydration and Nutritional Support.* Report. Maidenhead: BAPEN.

Ministry of Agriculture Fishery and Food (1994) *The Dietary and Nutritional Survey of British Adults.* London: HMSO.

Ministry of Agriculture Fishery and Food (1995) *Manual of Nutrition.* 10th Edition. London: HMSO.

McLaren, S. (1998) Undernutrition in older adults living in the community. *British Journal of Community Nursing* 3 (6), pp. 290–6.

McWhirter, J. P, Pennington, C. K. (1994) Incidence and recognition of malnutrition in hospital. *British Medical Journal* 308, pp. 945–8.

Millar, B. (1998) Dying for a good meal? *Health Service Journal* 23 April, pp. 24–7.

Monaghan, H. (1998) Meeting the nutritional needs of the older adult. *Professional Nurse* 14 (3), pp. 186–90.

Pattison, R., Ogilvie, M., Corr, J. et al (1995) Validation of a subjective nutritional scoring system used in the elderly. *Clinical Nutrition* 14 (Supplement 2), pp. 54–5.

Potter, J., Klipstein, K., Reilly, J. J., Roberts, M. (1995) The Nutritional status and clinical course of acute admissions to a geriatric unit. *Age and Ageing* 24, pp. 131–6.

Royal College of Nursing Dynamic Quality Improvement Programme (1993) *Nutrition Standards and the Older Adult.* London: RCN.

Royal College of Nursing (1996) *Statement on Feeding and Nutrition in Hospitals.* London: RCN.

Reilly, H. M., Matineau, J. K., Moran, A., Kennedy, H. (1995) Nutritional screening – evaluation and implementation of a simple nutrition risk score. *Clinical Nutrition* 14, pp. 269–73.

Scanlan, F., Dunne, J., Toyne, K. (1994) No more cause for neglect: introducing a nutritional assessment tool and action plan. *Professional Nurse* 9 (6), pp. 382–5.

Scott, J. (1995) Dietary guidelines for adults. *Primary Health Care* 5 (5), pp. 41–5.

Sizer, T. (1996) *Standards and Guidelines for Nutritional Support of Patients in Hospital.* A Report by a BAPEN Working Party. Maidenhead: BAPEN.

Taylor, S., Goodinson-McLaren, S. (1992) *Nutritional Support: A Team Approach.* London: Wolfe Publishing.

Thomas, B. (1996) *Nutrition in Primary Care: A Handbook for GPs, Nurses and Primary Health Care Professionals.* Oxford: Blackwell Science.

Constipation

Brocklehurst, J. (1990) Constipation and faecal incontinence. *Nursing the Elderly* February, pp. 17–18.

Pressure ulcer

Bliss, M. (1990) Geriatric medicine. In: Bader, D. L. (ed.). *Pressure Sores: Clinical Practice, a Scientific Approach.* London: Macmillan.

Cullum, N., Clark, M. (1992) Matching patient need for pressure sore prevention with the supply of pressure redistributing mattresses. *Journal of Advanced Nursing* 17, pp. 310–6.

Cullum, N., Dickson, R., Eastwood, A. (1996) Prevention and treatment of pressure sores. *Nursing Standard* 10 (26), pp. 32–3.

European Pressure Ulcer Advisory Panel (1998) A policy statement on the prevention of pressure ulcers. *British Journal of Nursing* 7 (15), pp. 888–90.

Fletcher, J. (1996). Types of pressure-relieving equipment available. *British Journal of Nursing* 5 (11), pp. 694–701.

NHS Centre for Research and Dissemination and University of York 1995. The prevention and treatment of pressure sores. *Effective Health Care Bulletin* 2 (1).

Norton, D., McLaren, R., Exton-Smith, A. (1962) *Investigation of Geriatric Nursing Problems in Hospital*. Reissued 1975. Edinburgh: Churchill Livingstone.

Pendleton, S. (1998) Relieving the pressure. RCN Nursing Update 81. *Nursing Standard* 12 (36).

Reid, J., Morison, M. (1994) Towards a consensus: classification of pressure sores. *Journal of Wound Care* 3 (3), pp. 157–60.

Rollins, H. (1997) Nutrition and wound healing. *Nursing Standard* 11 (51), pp. 49–52.

Royle, J. (1992) Caring for the patient with a disorder of the skin. In: Royle, J., Walsh, M. (eds) *Watson's Medical-Surgical Nursing and Related Physiology*. London: Ballière Tindall.

Resources

📖 Further reading

Barasi, M. E. (1997) *Human Nutrition: A Health Perspective*. London: Arnold.

Bond, S. (1997) (ed.) *Eating Matters.* Centre for Health Services Research University of Newcastle: Newcastle-upon-Tyne.

Garrow, J. S., James, W. P. T. (1999) *Human Nutrition and Dietetics.* 10th Edition. Edinburgh: Churchill Livingstone.

Health Education Authority (1991) *Nutrition in Minority Ethnic Groups: Asians and Afro-Caribbeans the UK*. London: HEA.

Holmes, H. S. (1996) Nursing management of oral care in older patients. *Nursing Times* 92 (9), pp. 37–9.

Nestlé and British Dietetic Association (1998) *Practical Nutrition in Primary Care – A Resource for Nurses*. Croydon: Nestlé UK.

NHS Centre for Research and Dissemination and University of York (2001) Effectiveness of laxatives in adults. *Effective Health Care Bulletin* 7 (1).

Winney, J. (1998) Constipation. *Nursing Standard* 13 (11), pp. 49–53.

Askham, J., Gluckman, E., Owens, P. (1990) *A Review of Research on Falls among Elderly People*. London: DTI.

Green, S., McLaren, S. (1998) Nutrition and wound healing. *Community Nursing* 4 (7), pp. 29–32.

Ratcliffe, P. (1998) Under pressure to update research. *Nursing Times* 94 (16), pp. 59–61.

Russell, L. (2001) The importance of patients' nutritional status in wound healing. *British Journal of Nursing* 10 (6), S42–S49.

Thomas, S. (1997) Update: a guide to dressing selection. *Journal of Wound Care* 6 (10), pp. 479–82.

Waterlow, J. (1985) Pressure sores: a risk assessment card. *Nursing Times* 81 (48), pp. 49–55.

Annotated bibliography

Bond, S. (1997) *Eating Matters*. (ed.) Newcastle: University of Newcastle-upon-Tyne Centre for Health Service Research.

Developed in response to the Association of Community Health Councils' report, this pack brings together the research and expertise of many of the leading nurses in this field. It aims to offer a valuable resource to help nurses provide good nutritional care in hospital. It is full of examples of good practice and advice, as well as including detailed information on topics such as the causes of malnutrition, nutritional assessment and the management of feeding difficulties. It includes suggestions for action and detailed case studies.

British Association for Parenteral and Enteral Nutrition (1996) Sizer, T. (ed.). *Standards and Guidelines for Nutritional Support of Patients in Hospital*. Maidenhead: BAPEN.

BAPEN was formed in 1992, following the recommendations made by Lennard-Jones in the King's Fund report. It recommends the development of nutritional guidelines, regular nutritional assessment and records of nutrition intakes. It sets standards for use with hospital patients, and outlines a protocol for nutritional assessment.

Buttriss, J., Wynne, A., Stanner, S. (2001) *Nutrition: A Handbook for Community Nurses*. London: Whurr Publishers.

This book provides a wealth of information on various aspects of nutrition for community nurses and others working in public health. The authors are renowned experts in the field of public health nutrition and have written the text in a question and answer format that facilitates ease of access and responds to many of the questions commonly asked by patients. It addresses the issues of nutrition in health and illness, nutrition through the lifespan and nutrition issues in the media. An example question is 'are people living alone in the community worse off nutritionally than those being cared for in institutions?' Each answer draws on recent research and directs readers to other resources.

Lennard-Jones, J. E. (1992) *A Positive Approach to Nutrition as Treatment*. London: King's Fund.

This is an influential report that identifies a number of ways in which nutritional care could be improved. It recommends that heights and weights should be monitored in adults, and that growth and development be recorded in children. The report emphasises the need for assessing nutritional status and suggests that this should include recent diet history and changes, as well as physical examination. This report stimulated a number of hospitals to develop their own nutritional assessment tools, for identifying patients at risk of malnutrition. For example Scanlan, Dunne and Toyne in 1994 published the first nutrition assessment tool.

National Dairy Council Nutrition Service. *Fact Files.*

These useful booklets are full of information from a variety of sources. They are well referenced and cover a wide range of topics from nutrients to needs of different age groups and client groups to nutrition-related diseases.

Nestlé and British Dietetic Association (1998) *Practical Nutrition in Primary Care – A resource for nurses.* Croydon: Nestlé UK.

This up-to-date resource pack is aimed at all practitioners who require accessible, practical information about the nutritional needs of a wide range of client groups in the community. It contains comprehensive material related to healthy eating, nutritional assessment and practical guidance. This latter section focuses on the needs of specific groups, such as children, teenagers and the elderly, as well as those with particular nutrition-related problems, such as coronary heart disease, cancer and those with swallowing difficulties. This pack has been written by a range of specialists in nutrition and nursing, with the support and approval of the British Dietetic Association.

Royal College of Nursing Dynamic Quality Improvement Programme (1993) *Nutrition Standards and the Older Adult.* London: RCN.

This report outlines standards for the nutritional care of older adults. It recommends nutritional assessment, to include dietary intake, food patterns, height and weight and their changes. It highlights the need for monitoring and evaluating nutritional care, and emphasises the benefits of a multi-disciplinary approach.

@ Web pages

British Dietetic Association: **www.bda.uk.com**
British Nutrition Foundation: **www.nutrition.org.uk**
Centre for Research and Dissemination: **www.york.ac.uk/inst/crd/ehcb.htm**
Clinical Guidelines for Pressure Ulcer Prevention and Risk Assessment:
   www.rcn. org.uk/home/home.html
Essence of Care: **www.doh.gov.uk/essenceofcare/intro.htm**
Index of Food and Nutrition Internet Resources:
   www.nal.usda.gov/fnic/etext/ fnic.html
National Dairy Council: **www.milk.co.uk**
National Service Framework for Older People:
   www.doh.gov.uk/nsf/older-people. htm
Online Diet Analysis Programme: **www.ag.uiuc.edu/~food-lab/nat/**
World Health Organisation Nutrition Programme: **www.who.int/nut/index.htm**

⌨ Videos

Clinical Enteral Nutrition (1992) RCN Update, Unit 1. Discusses malnutrition and options available to establish good nutrition.

Fats of life (1993) RCN Update, Unit 34. Discusses the role of fats in the diet and sources of different types of fat.

Food in the Balance: The Nurse's Role (1997) RCN Nursing Update, Unit 69. Considers factors influencing food choices and Government initiatives.

Guess Who's Coming to Dinner, Part 1 and Part 2 (1986) Boulton-Hawker Films. A very simple introduction to nutrients.

The Meal Ticket (1992) National Dairy Council. Introduces a simple method of constructing a diet.

Constipation: The Hard Facts (1991) RCN. Examines the nurse's role in prevention and treatment of constipation.

Relieving the Pressure: Important Points (1998) RCN Update, Unit 81. Looks at aetiology and grading of pressure sores and risk assessment.

Insights into Meeting Hydration Needs

Vanessa Lockyer-Stevens and
Anne Francis

This chapter is arranged in two parts. The first part explores hydration in relation to children, introducing Sophie who has severe vomiting and diarrhoea. The second part considers adult issues in relation to hydration with the story of Peter who has sustained serious burns.

Part 1 Child perspectives in relation to hydration

Introduction

The care of children and their families is receiving increasing attention. Changes to social policy in the UK and the wider global community are at last encouraging the peoples of the world to acknowledge children as unique individuals. The increased visibility of children means that nurses from all disciplines may come into contact with children in different ways, from being young parents themselves to providing intensive and community care.

Advances in scientific research, notably improvements in the survival of premature babies and those with chronic illnesses, are changing the way hospital and community services are utilised (Edwards 1996). Ambulatory care services and an increase in community nursing teams are changing the admission pattern for a large number of children. Care of this group makes demands on a range of professionals, including those who may not specialise in children's nursing. However, the central tenet for the care of all children, irrespective of the arena in which they are cared for, remains one of nursing's guiding principles. It is the Children Act (1989) which clearly states that

'The welfare of the child is of paramount consideration.'

The following learning outcomes reflect this ethos of care and focus on the care of a sick child admitted to hospital with dehydration.

This section will examine factors that give rise to, and the epidemiology and incidence of, diarrhoea and vomiting in young children that account for 16 per cent of medical attendees at Accident and Emergency departments and for an estimated 526,000 consultations with GPs annually (Armon et al 2001). It will focus on how to assess the type and degree of dehydration, calculate fluid replacement, and discuss the child's care in partnership with their family. Finally, it will explore how health professionals can best support primary carers in reducing the incidence of diarrhoea and vomiting.

Aim

The aim of this section is to explore the role of the nurse in the care of a 2-year-old child admitted to hospital with dehydration following a severe bout of diarrhoea and vomiting.

Learning outcomes

By the end of this section of the chapter students will be able to:

- Describe fluid compartments of the body.
- Discuss a range of clinical conditions that give rise to a compromised physiological status as a result of diarrhoea and vomiting.
- Outline socioeconomic and cultural factors that may contribute to the incidence of diarrhoea and vomiting.
- Explore the nurse's role in the assessment and care of a child requiring therapeutic interventions that restore homeostasis.
- Identify the therapeutic interventions required to restore homeostasis.
- Examine evidence-based literature that supports the notion of 'best practice' in the care of the child and family.
- Discuss contemporary issues in health care that impact upon health education programmes for the child and family.
- Discuss the role of the multi-professional team in the care of the sick child and family.
- Explore the role of support agencies in the care of the child and family following discharge.

Concepts

- Growth and development
- Safety in hospital
- Evidence based practice
- Dehydration
- Fluid resuscitation
- Physiological derangement

- Homeostasis
- Health education
- Continuity of care
- Record keeping
- Primary health care services
- Multi-disciplinary team

Activity 11.1

There are many other themes that you may have already decided that you would like to explore. Note these down before you start reading. As you work through the text, more may arise.

As you work through this section refer to a dictionary to check your understanding of technical words and phrases.

The following scenario has been developed to help you to gain theoretical knowledge underpinning the care this child and their family will require.

Scenario *Introducing Sophie*

Sophie, a normally active and healthy 2-year-old girl, is admitted to your ward at 6 a.m. with a history of severe diarrhoea and vomiting. On arrival she has sunken eyes, inelastic skin, is irritable and lethargic, and complains of a 'tummy ache'. She is accompanied by her parents Susan and Tom. Her older brother Matthew, aged 6, and baby Georgia, 13 months, are being cared for by a neighbour. You are assigned to Sophie's care.

Activity 11.2

A The care of any child requires an understanding of growth and development. Discuss with your peers what factors influence normal growth and development of a healthy child using the following headings: physical, environmental, socioeconomic and emotional.

For more detail, a supporting text such as *The Developing Child* (Bee 1994) will help.

B Now think about those factors which might affect Sophie's growth and development as a result of her illness.

How illness may impact on normal growth and development

> ### *Evidence-based practice*
>
> The care of children of all ages requires knowledge of normal growth and development, as this will underpin nursing practice. As discussed in the scenario, Sophie is normally a fit and healthy 2-year-old girl. Her safety following admission is paramount and is best met by understanding normal growth and development for a toddler her age. For the purpose of this activity, you may therefore want to consider 'growth' in terms of 'quantitative' change for example determining expected height and weight for a 2-year-old child, taking account of the sociocultural context and ethnic background of the child and family. Ways of monitoring these changes include measuring the child's height, weight, head circumference and length, which are plotted on growth (percentile) charts and give a guide to the child's rate of growth. Development may be reflected in 'qualitative' changes using, for example, Swanwick's work which studied children's understanding of the 'concept' of illness at various ages (Swanwick 1990).

Table 11.1 Impact examples of illness on normal growth and development

- **Physical changes** Sophie is still growing rapidly and at 2 years old is normally very active. Indeed, toddlers rarely rest unless they are unwell or asleep. Sophie's body has undergone several major physiological changes since birth, all of which will make her less vulnerable to illness as she grows up. For example, rapid growth of lung tissue and structures of the chest wall takes place before the age of 2, making Sophie less vulnerable to respiratory disorders in childhood than in infancy. Other systems are maturing also. Of note are changes in the distribution of total body water (TBW) which in children is approximately 10 per cent higher than in adulthood, which as Sophie grows will make her less vulnerable to dehydration. Also, it is well documented that illness and starvation slow down growth and it is not until recovery begins that the unique phenomenon of 'catch-up growth' takes place (Rudolf and Levene, 1999).
- **Psychological factors** Sophie is dependent upon her parents and siblings for love, a sense of security and emotional well-being. 'Separation distress' is not uncommon in this age group (Davenport 1991, p. 73).
- **Socio-economic factors** Sophie is dependent on her parents to provide sufficient food, warmth, clothing and education (UNICEF 1990).
- **Cultural factors** Sophie relies on the daily routines within her life in order to ensure that she feels secure. Admission to hospital may make her feel vulnerable and distressed.

- **Cognitive factors** Sophie's language and comprehension is developing. Children of this age often use 'horographic' or 'telegraphic speech' in which key content words are used all the time; for example 'Daddy gone work' (Campbell and Glasper 1995, p. 147). Knowledge of the development of speech and language provides important cues for carers of the unwell child, as toddlers in particular appear sensitive to a change of environment.

  Admission to hospital can be particularly stressful for both child and parents. Young children, sensitive to parental stress, may respond by becoming stressed themselves. This phenomenon known as 'social referencing', and described by Lewandowski (1992 cited Hazinski 1992a) takes account of the child's immature coping strategies. In recognising such stresses the nurse is in a unique position to support the child and family at such a vulnerable time (White 1992 cited in Carter and Dearmun 1995; see also Chapter 3 on insights into child and family health.

- **Psychomotor ability** Sophie has reached her expected milestones for running and walking.
- **Health and disease** As we already mentioned, Sophie is normally a fit, healthy little girl.
- **Resources available** The health visitor helps to promote the health of children. Together with other community services such as play groups, Sophie will have access to environments that help to promote normal growth and development.

Plus, in hospital, there may be other factors

- **Environmental factors** Strange surroundings are likely to exacerbate Sophie's distress.
- **Disruption of routine** Sophie's sleep pattern and eating habits have been disrupted by her illness and hospital admission.
- **Effect on parents** Sophie has become lethargic which will frighten her parents. Tom and Susan now rely on skilled practitioners to provide the care Sophie requires. Information that is clear, understandable and consistent will help reduce their anxiety.
- **Institutional factors** The changes to Sophie's routine such as eating and drinking, sleep, noise pollution in the ward, missing siblings and dealing with strangers are likely to heighten her anxiety.
- **Increased nutritional requirements** Sophie will probably have lost weight as a result of her illness. Early referral to the dietician may be necessary.

Admission to hospital

On admission a child health history is taken. Assessment of Sophie's care will take account of both her past and current health status. This requires health professionals to acknowledge the unique knowledge carers often have of their child's needs in health and when they are sick (Sidley 1995 cited in Carter and Dearmun 1995). The context of this view should not be underestimated, as evidence suggests conflict can arise between professional and maternal knowledge. Indeed, a study by Callery (1997) suggests that primary carers sometimes found it difficult to 'convince health professionals that their concerns were justified' about their child's illness.

Practice tip

One way of sharing information about Sophie's health status is through the use of her 'Personal Child Health Record'. This record, which is kept by all families of pre-school children, enables parents and the primary health care team to share information about the child's growth and development pattern, and take account of any concerns parents may have about their child.

The Personal Child Health Record is often used by health visitors when a newborn child is taken on to their case load. In general these records are kept within the family home, giving parents 'ownership' of important information about their child's progress. Moreover parents are encouraged to share this information by documenting personal accounts of their child's achievements or concerns that are then shared between themselves and key professionals such the health visitor.

> ### Activity 11.3
>
> Look through a copy of a Personal Child Health Record and make notes about how growth and development is assessed and monitored. *Do ask permission first.*

However, ways in which health visitors offer advice is changing. New services are being offered via telephone helplines, not dissimilar to NHS Direct, a 24-hour nurse-led health advice line. Against this background, it must be remembered that children's health needs are unique and require skilled professionals in this distinct area of practice (Hawley and Howkins 1999).

> Sophie had been unwell since attending her playmate Melanie's second-birthday party that afternoon. She vomited once since returning home, but continued to play unperturbed. At 6 p.m. Sophie asked to go bed complaining that she had a 'tummy ache', was hot and tired. Susan gave Calpol (children's paracetamol) and telephoned NHS Direct for some help. The nurse suggested that Calpol and clear fluids be given regularly and Susan observe for any further vomiting.
>
> Sophie continued to vomit and had bouts of diarrhoea. The GP was contacted who also suggested regular Calpol, keeping her cool to alleviate a further rise in temperature, and giving clear fluids only to drink. Instructions were left to ring the 'out of hours' doctor service should Sophie remain unwell.

How can new ways of accessing health care services help Sophie? Before reading on consider methods of accessing services.

Evidence-based practice

Health care services – a review of what's new

In response to the White Paper *The New NHS: Modern, Dependable* (1997) several nurse-led 24-hour health advice services have been introduced throughout the UK. The largest of these services, called NHS Direct, went 'live' nationally in 2000.

Its introduction has encouraged professionals with specialist skills in child health to develop additional telephone helplines. For example Hawley and Howkins (1999) describe how health visitor-run helplines offer information and advice, particularly in instances of meningitis or immunisation scares.

The service is available to all, but estimates are that the 'highest level of use will be from mothers of young children, particularly with parents of children under five' (NHS Executive 1998a). Indeed Kenally and Dale (1998) confirm these findings in their study which indicated that of the 50 per cent of calls which were for children aged 15 years and under, 68 per cent were for children under 5 years. Early evidence does suggest that the service is 'saving lives' because callers who have not necessarily appreciated the gravity of their illness are contacting the helpline (NHS Executive 1998b). Whether this evidence applies to identifying sick children is unclear.

There is, however, some concern, notably from GPs, that the service is increasing the workload of family doctors rather than reducing it. Their view is that nurses are over cautious in managing telephone enquires, and refer patients to GPs 'just in case'. This advice, GPs say, is making demands on the service that for many turn out to be a minor clinical complaint.

Activity 11.4

Visit your nearest GP surgery or library and find out what primary health care services are available to Sophie and her family.

Overnight Sophie continued to vomit with profuse bouts of diarrhoea and was admitted to hospital following a visit by the GP at 5 a.m. Tom and Susan mentioned to their doctor that other children from the party had also been unwell with diarrhoea and vomiting (D and V) which the GP noted in the admission letter.

What is diarrhoea and vomiting? Consider what you currently know before reading on.

Evidence-based practice

Diarrhoea and vomiting: friend or foe?

Diarrhoea is defined by Rudolf and Levene (1999) as 'an increase in the frequency, fluidity and volume of faeces' and they comment that as many as three acute/severe episodes may be experienced by the child before the age of 3. Bacterial or viral pathogens are commonly responsible for infection, although causes extrinsic to the gastrointestinal tract, such as antibiotic induced diarrhoea, can be a problem in all age groups. Armon et al (2001) state that acute diarrhoea often results from infectious intestinal disease (IID) and describes how as many as 1 in 6 children visit their GP with an episode of IID. Care of this group may therefore pose difficulties for health care professionals in terms of identifying children at risk of dehydration which, in severe cases, can be a life-threatening consequence of diarrhoea and vomiting.

Campbell and Glasper (1995) state that vomiting is generally regarded as 'forceful ejection' of stomach contents through the mouth, which arises as a result of stimulation to the vomiting centre in the medulla oblongata (Green 1987). Vomiting is not uncommon in infancy and early childhood. The degree and severity of vomiting can vary from a single episode to a precursor of more life-threatening disease such as meningitis or pyloric stenosis (Rudolf and Levene 1999).

Use your knowledge of growth and development to help you to think through your answer. For example, some young babies develop projectile vomiting within the first 4–6 weeks of life as a result of a condition known as pyloric stenosis. The effect of age on physiological processes influences the child's susceptibility to different causes of diarrhoea and vomiting. Here are some more ideas.

Children of Sophie's age are active and industrious. Regarded as toddlers (age 1–3 years), they rarely rest unless asleep. This period, like infancy, is one of rapid growth during which many developmental milestones are achieved. Among these milestones is a child's insatiable desire to explore the world around them. This potentially leaves them exposed to environments that pose a

Activity 11.5

Find out what are the common causes of diarrhoea and vomiting in childhood.

Activity 11.6

Now consider the signs and symptoms of each – diarrhoea and vomiting. For a further description of causes of diarrhoea and vomiting refer to a major child health text such as Hazinski (1992) Rudolf and Levene (1999).

risk to their health such as dirty floors, a fascination for toilets! Sharing food and sweets, and ingesting poisonous substances. Ingestion of bacteria and foreign bodies is therefore not uncommon in young children.

 Did your answers include looking for signs and symptoms which might indicate infection other than in the gastrointestinal tract and which cause episodes of diarrhoea and vomiting? For example a common cold, respiratory syncytial virus (RSV) or otitis media or otitis externa (inner- or outer-ear infection).

Following examination Sophie is diagnosed with gastroenteritis probably caused through food contamination. Susan and Tom are clearly anxious about Sophie and ask if their other children are at risk of similar infection.

 Which common organisms give rise to vomiting and diarrhoea in childhood? See McVerry and Collin. 1998 pp. 31–3 for more help.

 What help and advice do Sophie's parents require in order to reduce the risk of cross infection to the family?

 What is the role of the infection control nurse at this time?

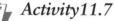 *Activity 11.7*

A Find out what types of infective organisms causing diarrhoea require notification to Public Health Service and how is this process undertaken.

B Find out if there is an opportunity to spend some of your time in practice 'shadowing' members of the infection control team. The experience would be invaluable.

Dehydration and its effect on the body

Fluid losses from diarrhoea and vomiting can result in varying degrees of dehydration, particularly if losses are persistent or the child is unable to tolerate oral fluids.

 What is dehydration?

Evidence-based practice

Dehydration is a term used when salts and water are lost from the fluid compartments of the body. It is apparent in clinical conditions in which the total output of fluid exceeds that of its total intake irrespective of underlying pathophysiology (Campbell and Glasper 1995). Disturbances to the 'finely tuned' balance of water and electrolytes disrupt homeostasis resulting in significant morbidity and in severe cases, early mortality.

As early as 1832 a physician called Latta treated patients suffering severe dehydration from Cholera with intravenous saline. Yet over a century later it was estimated that in 1999 about 3 million children died as a result of dehydration caused by diarrhoea alone, 80 per cent in the first two years of life (Rehydration Project 2002). Chameides and Hazinski (1994) further state that hypovolaemia still remains 'the commonest cause of shock in children worldwide'.

Dehydration is often a common complication of diarrhoea and vomiting. Babies and young children are more vulnerable, particularly in the developing world where poor access to oral and intravenous fluid-replacement therapy is apparent.

Charities and organisations across the world play a key role in the delivery and administration of these often life-saving treatments for children most in need. But even in the developed world, there appears to be a lack of knowledge and training in the use of oral replacement solutions (ORS), the increased use of which may reduce currently high admission rates for children. Conway and Newport's study in 1994 confirms this view by stating that only 29% of children received ORS treatment of this kind at home. There may however be an increasing move towards self-medication and self-referral as the growth of telephone helplines, direct access services and the internet provide information for families within the home. Irrespective of any health care advice service, early recognition and treatment of dehydration is the key to both prevention and reduction of the child's susceptibility to critical illness.

Activity 11.8

Find out about oral rehydration therapy.
The following resources may be helpful:

Walker-Smith et al (1997) for recommendations on feeding in childhood gastroenteritis. www.rehydrate.org/html/deh010.htm for further reading on the use of ORS.

The Sleep Tight Video #169; Help for sleepless parents. 'Dehydration in children always happens as a complication of diarrhoea and vomiting, especially if combined with fever – most commonly gastroenteritis'. For further information: <u>www.drhull.com/Ency/Master/D/dehydration.html</u>.

Armon et al (2001) for guidelines on acute diarrhoea management: <u>www.archdischild.com</u>.

What do you understand by the term *'fluid compartments'* of the body? What is the *function* of each?

Use a text such as Tortora and Anagnostakos (1997) to help you.

Activity 11.9

Name the key electrolytes involved in maintaining normal homeostasis.
Explain the function of each, particularly Sodium and Potassium.
Find out what the normal blood plasma levels of Sodium and Potassium are.
Identify the role of water (H_2O) in maintaining homeostasis.
Consider what you know about each of these aspects before reading on.

The role of water and electrolytes

Evidence-based practice

Pathophysiology perspective

Water and electrolytes are key players in the maintenance of homeostasis, their distribution being dependant on the age of the child. For example, the amount of total body water (TBW) in a full-term infant is approximately 75%, of which 53% is found in the extracellular compartment (outside the cell, and divided into two further compartments; intravascular and interstitial spaces). Forty-six per cent of water is found in the intracellular ICC (within the cell) compartment (Lam 1999). As the child grows TBW is replaced by an increase in total body fat (Lam 1998) and by the age of 3 years, the proportion of water is reduced by 10% to about 65% (Rudolf and Levene 1999).

Any disturbance to the balance between the intake and output mechanisms such as:

- Sweating
- Fluid intake
- Urine output
- Insensible loss (water vapour in breath and skin)
- Stool volume

can cause significant morbidity as the integrity of the meticulous salt and water balance is disrupted.

Excessive loss of water and electrolytes results in varying degrees of dehydration, its **cause**, **type** and **severity** dependant upon the movement and concentration of water and electrolytes during illness. As a complication of diarrhoea and vomiting, fever may exacerbate the degree of dehydration through increased insensible water loss (IWL) from sweating and mouth-breathing. Normal IWL through the skin and lungs is, for example, 1/2ml/kg/hour which, during fever, increases by 12% for every degree rise in temperature (Lam 1998). Energy requirements also increase exponentially by 12% for every degree rise above 37° Celsius (Hazinski 1992b). Thus the younger the child is, the more vulnerable they become because of the differences in total water distribution, which in illness is lost more readily from the extravascular space.

Lastly, the loss of key electrolytes, such as sodium through vomiting and potassium from diarrhoea, disrupt the balance of water in both intracellular and extracellular compartments causing what is known as a metabolic acidosis.

An understanding therefore of the fluid compartments of the body is essential as fluid replacement therapy can be safely utilised using this principle (Lam 1998).

Activity11.10

With reference to Rudolf and Levene (1999) or Hazinski (1992a and 1992b) answer the following questions about the *causes, types* and *severity* of dehydration. Remember to look up unfamiliar words as you read through and add them to your personal glossary, increasing both your knowledge and understanding of the subject.

What is the probable *cause* of Sophie's diarrhoea and vomiting? Refer to the McVerry and Collin (1998) article, p. 30 for examples of common types of infection.

What *type* of dehydration is it? For example, is it likely to be *Isotonic, Hyponatraemic* or *Hypernatraemic* dehydration? See Hazinski (1992a, pp. 723–7) for further explanation and also refer to the section above on the role of water and electrolytes to support your answer.

How is the *severity* of Sophie's dehydration estimated? See below.

Dehydration: calculating the risk?

Evidence-based practice

The percentage of dehydration is assessed in two ways:

- First, by observation criteria of clinical features of dehydration (such as shown in Table 11.2 below.
- Second, by measuring the estimated or actual weight loss against that of a recent weight of the child pre illness.

Armon et al (2001) argue that this is the 'gold standard' by which treatments are calculated and tested. For example, **1g** body weight is equal to **1ml** of water lost therefore a 10kg child with 10% dehydration would now weigh 9kg = 1000ml fluid loss. An easy formula (APLS 1997) to remember for calculating the percentage fluid is

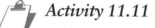

10 × body weight in kg × percentage dehydration = fluid lost (deficit)

Example: 10 × 10kg × 10% = 1000mls or 1kg.

But first ask yourself some key questions when assessing any child. Think ABC everytime!

Is this child awake, rousable, irritable, lethargic, conscious!?

1 Is there any obstruction to their airway?
2 Is there any difficulty with breathing?
3 Is the pulse rate normal or absent?

Activity 11.11

Sophie is admitted to a side room and as part of your assessment of her you look to see how dehydrated she is. Write down what you need to look for and why.

See Hampton-Evans and Bingham (1998, pp. 188–93) for further reading. Also see Chapter 3 in this volume on child and family health.

Assessment for dehydration

Now think about your assessment of Sophie using the following headings:

Find out

- Child's age
- Normal physiological parameters for that age group
- Temperature, pulse, respirations, blood pressure
- Naked weight

- Length of illness prior to admission
- Advice and treatments given prior to admission
- The normal plasma sodium level

Table 11.2 Clinical features of dehydration

Mild dehydration <5 per cent: 50ml/kg fluid lost

The child will demonstrate the following:

- Thirsty
- May tolerate oral fluids
- Urine output normal or slightly reduced, i.e. dark yellow but passed at least three times in 24 hours
- Dry mouth
- Sleepy or irritable as dehydration progresses to 5%
- Normal capillary refill time is <2 seconds (APLS 1997)

Moderate dehydration 5–10 per cent: 50–100ml/kg fluid lost

The child demonstrates all the above plus:

- Cannot tolerate oral fluids
- Dry uncomfortable mouth and tongue
- Oliguria <1/2 ml/kg/hour occurs in response to an increased secretion of anti-diuretic hormone (ADH) in an attempt to preserve circulating volume. Urine may be dark and offensive
- Sunken eyes due to loss of intra-occular fat from fluid loss
- Tachycardia and corresponding tachypnoea
- Crying with few or no tears
- Lethargy or confusion
- Inelastic skin; for example, when skin is gently lifted, it remains folded for some time

Severe dehydration >10 per cent: 100–150ml/kg fluid lost

The child will demonstrate the following:

- Very confused, semi-conscious or comatosed
- Very sunken eyes or fontanelle in children under 18 months old
- Very dry mucus membranes
- Acute tachycardia with poor volume (rapid and thready pulse)
- Acute tachypnoea caused by lactic acidosis and loss of oxygen carrying circulating volume
- Hypotension – a late and very life threatening sign
- Anuric – no urine output
- Prolonged capillary refill time >2secs

Child is in a 'shocked' state and requires early resuscitation with intravenous fluid therapy.

Ask about

- Normal diet and eating habits
- Is she thirsty?
- How many drinks has Sophie tolerated? And, if so, how much and what type?
- How many times per day has the child passed urine? Less than three times in 24 hours probably means there is a degree of dehydration (Rudolf and Levene 1999
- Vomiting – how often? How much? Colour and characteristics?
- Stools – colour, frequency, smell, consistency?

Look at

- Sophie's conscious level – is she irritable, lethargic, listless, confused, reluctant to maintain eye contact with close carers (gaze aversion)?

> Looking at Sophie, you see that she remains lethargic and irritable and that her eyes remain sunken. She has inelastic skin and very dry mucous membranes.

- Her breathing – is she tachypnoeic in an attempt to compensate for any acidosis and adequate oxygen delivery to the tissues?
- Her eyes – are they sunken due to the loss of peri-orbital fat from fluid loss?
- Signs of inelastic skin – for example, does Sophie's skin remain in a pinched position following gently lifting together of skin folds over the abdomen? This physiological response occurs when water is lost from within the cells into the extravascular space in order to maintain adequate circulating blood volume and is called the 'pinch test'. Normal recoil is present in the well child, recoil within 1–2 seconds indicates mild to moderate dehydration and longer than 2 seconds, severe dehydration exists (Armon et al 2001).
- Moistness of her mouth and the presence of tears.

Complete your assessment of Sophie by taking her pulse, blood pressure, respirations, temperature and naked weight and send off a stool and urine specimen for microscopy, culture and sensitivity (M, C and S). Chart and report her observations.

Scenario *Sophie's observations*

Temperature 39° Celsius
Pulse 130 beats per minute
Respirations 35 breaths per minute
Blood pressure 90/60mmHg
Naked weight 12.6kg. Normally weighs 14kg
Sophie's urea and electrolyte (U and Es) results show plasma sodium result is Na$^+$ 125mmol/L.
Urine sample (clean catch) report shows no 'bacterial growth' on microscopy.
Stool specimen shows heavy growth of Rotavirus.

Activity 11.12

A Find out what the normal temperature, pulse and respirations should be for a 2-year-old child.

B Using the following formula, work out what Sophie's approximate systolic blood pressure should be for her age, e.g. 80 + (age in years × 2) (APLS 1997 p. 16) and weight:

> **(kg) = 2 (age + 4)** (APLS 1997, p. 7) or
> **(kg) = 8 + (age in years × 2)** (Stillwell 1994, p. 56)

C Using the information in Table 11.2 (pp. 346–7) work out what percentage dehydration Sophie is suffering from.

So how did you get on answering the questions above p. 344? Lets work through them together:

Question 1 *Cause*
Rotavirus is common to ingestion of contaminated food.

Question 2 *Type*
Sophie has *Hyponatraemic* dehydration caused by her low sodium levels.

Question 3 *Severity*
Sophie is suffering from *10% dehydration* which has been calculated in 2 ways:
First, by weight; Sophie has lost 1400 grams which is equivalent to 10% of her body weight.
Second, by the clinical features that Sophie presents with on admission.

Fluid replacement

Sophie's rehydration therapy

Sophie requires intravenous (IV) fluid therapy to replace lost fluid and sodium electrolytes. She is lethargic and experiences 'gaze aversion' whilst the doctor inserts an intravenous cannula into her left arm. Once the IV site is secured, Sophie receives a bolus of 20ml/kg of normal saline, followed by a regime of intravenous fluids including sodium replacements. These are written up on the prescription chart and commenced at 108mls per hour over 24 hours. Sophie complains of being thirsty and is encouraged to drink 'little' and 'often', with further instructions left to supplement any additional diarrhoea or vomiting with 10ml/kg oral replacement therapy where possible.

Sophie makes progress over the following 12 hours but has several more watery stools. Susan stays with her and is careful having been shown how to minimise cross-infection when caring for Sophie. Both later 'cat nap' as they are exhausted.

Activity 11.13

Consider how you know that Sophie is receiving the correct amount of intravenous fluids before reading on.

Evidence-based practice

Getting the right balance

Children receiving intravenous fluids:

- Must receive the correct type of solution
- Rate per hour must reflect the normal fluid requirements for the weight of the child
- Total amount prescribed must be given.

In general doctors calculate the child's fluid requirements, including volume and rate required. The nurse can confirm the prescription is correct using the following fluid requirement formula.

Normal fluid requirements

Body weight	Fluid requirements per day	Fluid requirements per hour
First 10kg	100ml/kg	4ml/kg
Second 10kg	50ml/kg	2ml/kg
Subsequent kg	20ml/kg	1ml/kg

Children with dehydration require two lots of replacement fluid. The first will replace the percentage of water and salts lost through illness, and the second provides normal maintenance fluid requirements based on the weight of the child until they can tolerate oral fluids.

The **severity** and **type** of dehydration governs the rate at which replacement fluid is given. For example children with hypernatraemic dehydration can suffer severe cerebral oedema or haemorrhage following rapid infusion of IV replacement fluid (Hazinski 1992a, p. 729; APLS 1997, p. 249), whereas those with severe isotonic dehydration will require rapid fluid replacement. Lastly, regular measurement of sodium electrolytes provide a continuous evaluation of Sophie's clinical state.

Activity 11.14

Sophie is receiving 108ml per hour over 24 hours. Using the formula above, work out if that amount is correct.

How did you get on? Let's do it together:

We know that Sophie has lost 1400 grams in weight. By using the fluid requirement formula shown above it was calculated as fluid lost in the following way:

$$10 \times 14\text{kg} \times 10 \text{ per cent} = 1400\text{mls}$$

Sophie's fluid deficit is therefore 1400mls.

Her maintenance fluid requirements are calculated using the APLS formula:

$$100\text{ml/kg for the first 10kg} = 1000\text{mls}$$

$$50\text{mls/kg for the second 10kg} = 200\text{mls}$$

Sophie's maintenance fluid requirements are therefore 1200mls per 24 hours.

So now add the two together and divide by 24 hours, giving the hourly rate required, e.g.

$$1400\text{mls} + 1200\text{mls} = 2600\text{mls} \div 24 \text{ hours} = 108.3\text{mls per hour}$$

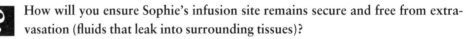 How will you ensure Sophie's infusion site remains secure and free from extravasation (fluids that leak into surrounding tissues)?

Activity 11.15

Find out which types of infusion pumps are used for children of different ages and which types of giving sets are required for different fluids, for example blood products.

By mid-afternoon Sophie is looking a little brighter. She has not vomited for a few hours, she feels thirsty and has a very wet nappy. Intravenous fluids have been running for seven hours. She has woken up from her 'nap' and points to the television.

Activity 11.16

A List, with rationale, what you will reassess now that Sophie is awake.

B Find out what kinds of oral fluids will aid the absorption of water and electrolytes through the bowel wall. Contact your children's dietician to help you.

What would be the normal urine output for a child of this age? Refer to Hazinski's text (1992a) to help you.

Activity 11.17

A In partnership with Tom, Sue and Matthew plan how Sophie might be encouraged to drink.

B Find out what types of oral rehydration therapy can be bought 'over the counter' and are also used in your practice areas.

How can the children's dietician help at this time?

The role of the children's dietician

The role of the children's dietician is unique. They often have solutions to the 'fussy eating habits' that most families complain about in their children at some time or another, be it the tantrum 2-year-old or the adolescent with complex eating disorders.

Dieticians also have considerable knowledge in the management of children with a range of complex dietary needs, and work in partnership with families and other specialists such as occupational therapists, health visitors, and speech and language therapists in achieving healthy children in acute and community settings.

The special relationship between the nurse and dietician must not be underestimated either. In hospital settings the dietician relies upon the nurse for accurate information about the child's condition and, in particular, comment on the child's progress. Good record keeping is therefore essential not only from a legal perspective, but in enhancing relationships between the dietician, family and nurse.

Professional conversation

Heather, the children's dietician

'I visited Sophie and her Mum soon after admission, having first looked through her medical admission notes, and then I talked to the nurse caring for her. I was asked to advise on the most appropriate kind of oral rehydration therapy and estimate a time when foods could be reintroduced. So, following a detailed assessment of Sophie's likes and dislikes, I was able to give both mum and the nurses some practical guidance relating to Sophie's nutritional needs now, and when she is beginning to feel better.'

Activity 11.18

A Find out how you would contact the dietician.

B Find out if you can 'shadow' a dietician as part of your clinical placement.

Sophie's progress continued and over the following days she began to eat and drink. Her diarrhoea subsided and the last specimen sent to the laboratory yielded no bacterial growth. Intravenous fluids were discontinued. Sophie was discharged after four days.

Activity 11.19

Identify members of the multi-disciplinary team who need to be involved in Sophie's discharge planning.

 What discharge advice will Tom and Sue require?

 In summary, what were Sophie's main problems on admission to hospital? Make your list before reading the review below.

Problems on admission

- **Diarrhoea and vomiting** Leading to malnutrition and weight loss. Review the sections on the effects of illness on growth and development (p. 337) and on diarrhoea and vomiting (pp. 340–1).
- **Moderate Dehydration** Leading to fluid and electrolyte imbalance. Review the sections on the effects of dehydration on the body (pp. 341–2), and on the role of water and electrolytes from a pathophysiological perspective (pp. 343–4).
- **Disruption to activity levels** Leading to anxiety and fear. Loss of energy to play.

 What actions would you consider to be appropriate?

Appropriate actions

- **Checking for severity of dehydration** Review the section on dehydration and calculating the risk (pp. 345–6).

- **Maintenance of fluid in electrolyte balance** Monitor, record and report intake and output of oral and intravenous fluids. Blood taken to evaluate serum sodium levels. Review the section on getting the balance right (p. 349).
- **Diversion therapy** To help protect against accidental disconnection of Sophie's intravenous fluids. The ways in which illness can impact upon normal growth and development (p. 337) are relevant here, review that section again.
- **Preservation of skin integrity** Watch out for skin excoriation caused by profuse diarrhoea.
- **Risk of cross infection** Leading to other family members becoming ill.

? What would you include in your discharge planning?

Discharge Planning

- **Hospital support** From the dietician. See the professional conversation with the dietician (p. 351).
- **Community support** From the health visitor and practice nurse. Review McVerry and Collin 1998, pp. 31–3.
- **Open access arrangements** Leading to immediate self-referral if required. Review the evidence-based practice section on health care services (p. 339).

References

Advanced Paediatric Life Support Group (1997) *Advanced Paediatric Life Support: The Practical Approach.* 2nd Edition. London: BMJ Publishing Group.

Armon, K., Stephenson, T., MacFaul, R., Eccleston, P., Wernerke, U. (2001) An evidence- and consensus-based guideline for acute diarrhoea management. *Archives Diseases in Childhood* 85, pp. 132–42.

Bee, H. (1994) *The Developing Child.* 7th Edition. New York: Harper Collins.

Callery, P. (1997) Maternal knowledge and professional knowledge: co-operation and conflict in the care of sick children. *International Journal of Nursing Studies* 34 (1), pp. 27–34.

Campbell, S., Glasper, E. A. (1995) *Whaley & Wong's Children's Nursing.* New York: Mosby Year Books.

Carter, B., Dearmun, A. K. (eds) (1995) *Child Health Care Nursing: Concepts, Theory and Practice.* Oxford: Blackwell Science.

Chameides, L., Hazinski, M. F. (1994) Fluid therapy and medications. In: *Paediatric Advanced Life Support.* New York: American Heart Association, Sections 6.1–6.18.

Conway, S. P., Newport, S. P. (1994) Are all hospital admissions for acute gastroenteritis necessary? *Journal of Infection* 29, pp. 5–8.

Dale, J., Crouch, R., Lloyd, D. (1998) Primary care: nurse-led telephone triage and advice out of hours. *Nursing Standard* 12 (47), pp. 41–5.

Davenport, G. C. (1991) *An Introduction to Child Development*. London: Collins Educational.

Davenport, M. (1996) Paediatric fluid balance. *Care of the Critically Ill* 12 (1), pp. 26–31.

Dearmun, A. K., Campbell, S., Barlow, J. (1995) Nursing support and care: meeting the needs of the child and family with altered gastro-intestinal function. In: Carter, B., Dearmun, A. K. (eds) *Child Health Care Nursing*.

Department of Health (1989) *Children Act*. London: HMSO.

Edwards, N. (1996) Temperature rising for paediatrics. *Health Service Journal* 1 February, pp. 24–5.

Green, J. H. (1976) *An Introduction to Human Physiology*. 4th Edition. Oxford: Oxford University Press.

Harms, D., Scharf, J. (1997) *Memorix: Paediatrics*. Edinburgh: Chapman & Hall Medical.

Hawley, N., Howkins, E. (1999) A health visitor-run helpline: meeting family health needs. *Community Practitioner* 72 (7), pp. 208–11.

Kennally, C., Dale, J. (1998) Direct enquiries. *Health Service Journal* 30 July, pp. 24–5.

Lam, Hui, W. (1998) Fluids in paediatric patients. *Care of the Critically Ill* 14 (3), pp. 93–6.

Lam, Hui W. (1999) Mechanism and management of paediatric head injury. *Care of the Critically Ill* 15 (3), pp. 95–8.

Lewandowski, L. A. (1992) Psychosocial aspects of paediatric critical care. In: Hazinski, M. F. (ed) *Nursing Care of the Critically Ill Child*.

NHS Executive (1998a) *Developing NHS Direct. A Scoping Study Commissioned by the Operational Research Branch of the NHS Executive HQ and supported by Coopers & Lybrand and South West Thames Regional HIS Consortium*. London: DoH.

NHS Executive (1998b) NHS Direct press announcement. NHS Direct to cover 40 per cent of England by 1999. UK: www.open.gov.uk/doh/nhsexec/direct.htm.

Nursing and Midwifery Council (2002) *Code of Professional Conduct*. London: NMC.

Rehydration Project (1996–2002) P.O. Box 1, Samara 5235, Costa Rica: www. rehydrate.org.

Sidley, A. (1995) Community nursing perspectives. In: Carter, B., Dearmun, A. K. (eds) *Child Health Care Nursing*.

Stillwell, S. B. (1994) *Quick Critical Care Reference*. 2nd Edition. New York: Mosby.

Swanwick, M. (1990) Knowledge and control. *Paediatric Nursing* 2 (5), pp.18–20.

Tortora, G. J., Anagnostakos, N. P. (1997) 7th Edition. *Principles of Anatomy and Physiology*. London: HarperCollins Publishers.

United Kingdom Central Council for Nursing, Midwifery and Health Visiting (1993) *Standards for Records and Record Keeping*. London: UKCC.

United Nations Children's Fund (1990) *First Call for Children: World Declaration Plan of Action from the World Summit for Children Convention: The Rights of the Child*. New York: UNICEF.

Whaley, L. F., Wong, D. L. (1997) *Essentials of Pediatric Nursing*. 5th Edition. New York: Mosby Year Books.

White, C. J. (1995) Life crisis for children and their families. In: Carter, B., Dearmun, A. K. (eds) *Child Health Care Nursing*.

World Health Organisation (WHO/CDD) (1990) *A Manual for Treatment of Diarrhoea*. Geneva: WHO.

Resources

📖 Further reading

Bee, H. (1994) *The Developing Child*. 7th Edition. New York: Harper Collins.

Hampton-Evans, D. C., Bingham, R. M. (1998) Paediatric resuscitation: the European resuscitation guidelines (1998). *Care of the Critically Ill* 14 (6), pp. 188–93.

Hazinski, M. F. (ed.) (1992a) *Nursing Care of the Critically Ill Child*. New York: Mosby Year Books.

Hazinski, M. F. (1992b) Common clinical conditions. Cited in Kennedy, J., Renal disorders. In: Hazinski, M. F. (ed.) *Nursing Care of the Critically Ill Child*, pp. 652–9.

McVerry, M., Collin, J. (1998) Managing the child with gastroenteritis. *Paediatric Nursing* 10 (8), pp. 31–3.

Rudolf, M. C. J., Levene, M. I. (1999) *Paediatrics and Child Health*. Oxford: Blackwell Science.

Walker-Smith, J. A. Sandhu, B. K., Isolauri, E., Banchini, G., Van Caillie-Bertrand, M., Dias, J. A., Fasano, A., Guandalini, S., Hoekstra, J. H., Juntunen, M., Kolacek, S., Marx, D., Micetic-Turk, D., Razenberg, M. C., Szajewska, H., Taminiau, J., Weizman, Z., Zanacca, C., Zetterström, R. (1997). Recommendations for feeding in childhood gastroenteritis. Medical position paper: guidelines prepared by the ESPGAN working group on acute diarrhoea. *Journal of Pediatric Gastroenterology and Nutrition* 24, pp. 522–7.

Annotated bibliography

Advanced Paediatric Life Support Group (1997) *Advanced Paediatric Life Support: The Practical Approach*. 2nd Edition. London: BMJ Publishing Group.

This book focuses on the emergency care of children and is the core text accompanying the APLS (UK) course. The text acknowledges that sick children generate considerable anxiety to those who care for them thus this easy to read book reflects assessment skills that can be utilised by a range of practitioners.

Rudolf, M. C. J., Levene, M. I. (1999) *Paediatrics and Child Health*. Oxford: Blackwell Science.

This excellent book is easy to read and understand, and examines a range of childhood illnesses including a section on the causes of diarrhoea and dehydration. Rudolf and Levene have published several times, including on neonatal medicine and the causes of diarrhoea in infancy.

Walker-Smith, J. A. et al (1997) Recommendations for feeding in childhood gastroenteritis: medical position paper – guidelines prepared by the ESPGAN working group on acute diarrhoea. *Journal of Pediatric Gastroenterology and Nutrition* 24, pp. 522–7).

This work looks at recommendations for feeding children with childhood gastroenteritis. It makes specific reference to the care of children with acute diarrhoea and has developed guidelines and standards for children of all ages.

World Health Organisation (1990) *A Manual for Treatment of Diarrhoea.* Geneva: (WHO/CDD).

This work sets out the guidelines for treatment of diarrhoea and dehydration notably that which arises in the developed world. Its publication is set against powerful evidence that morbidity and mortality can be reduced particularly when ORT is used. Shamsul Hag, Minister of Health and Population Control, Government of Bangladesh comments: 'ORT holds the promise of healthier childhoods and more productive adult lives.' The key role of professionals is also explored.

@ Web pages

Diarrhoearal diseases: **www.rehydrate.org/resources**
Oral replacement solutions: **www.rehydrate.org/html/deh010.htm**
Professional information: **www.rehydrate.org/support_health_professional_health.**
Treatment plans using oral rehydration therapy to prevent and treat dehydration: **www.rehydrate.org.dehydration**
www.drhull.com/Ency/Master/D/dehydration.html
www.archdischild.com

Videos

The SleepTight Video#169. Help for sleepless parents, 'Dehydration in children always happens as a complication of diarrhoea and vomiting, especially if combined with fever – most commonly gastroenteritis.' For further information.

Part 2 Adult perspectives on fluid loss using burn management as the example.

This is the second part of a chapter on fluid loss. This part focuses on an adult with a significant burn injury, leading to hypovolaemia.

Introduction

A burn is one of the most devastating injuries that can happen to a person and affects them, their family and society. Not only is the individual with a significant burn likely to be critically ill, but they will possibly need reconstructive surgery. They will experience itching, disfigurement and psychological consequences, sometimes for the remainder of their lives. The role of the interprofessional team is of paramount importance in caring for a burn-injured individual. The nurse plays a vital role in caring for and supporting the individual and their family and coordinating the interprofessional team.

There are in excess of 10,000 burn injuries which occur in the UK per annum (Lawrence 1991). A decrease in mortality over the past 40 years has been linked to the introduction of topical silver salts for antibiotic prophylaxis, improved infection control, greater frequency of successful early surgery, and improved intensive care procedures, particularly of renal failure (Lawrence 1996). Nurses may care for burn-injured individuals both in the hospital and community setting.

Learning outcomes

- To identify the population at risk of burn injury.
- To recognise the types and causes of burn injury.
- To explore evidence-based literature to inform the management of the burn-injured individual.
- To explore the nurse's role in the assessment, planning, implementation and evaluation of the care of a burn-injured individual.
- To identify the factors contributing to maintaining fluid balance in the burn-injured individual.
- To discuss the ethical and legal aspects of caring for a burn injured individual.
- To discuss the role of the nurse within the interprofessional team when caring for a burn-injured individual and their family.

Concepts

- Burn types
- Causes of burns
- Fluid resuscitation
- Hypovolaemic shock
- Dehydration
- Assessment
- Burn management
- Inhalation injury

- Pain nutrition
- Wound care
- Patient education
- Interprofessional team
- Evidence based practice
- Skin grafts
- Body image
- Disfigurement

Activity 11.19

There may be other concepts that you have already decided you would like to explore. As you work through the text yet more may arise. As you work through the chapter, refer to a dictionary to check your understanding of technical words and phrases.

Scenario Introducing Peter

Peter is a 38-year-old accountant, weighing 70kg, whose hobby is sailing, and he was involved in an explosion on board his yacht. His clothing caught alight and he was thrown overboard by the force of the blast.

The aims of first aid are to:

1 Maintain the safety of the rescuer, who should not place himself in any danger. For example, if the victim had electrocuted himself, the rescuer should ensure that the electricity supply is disabled before attending to the victim, otherwise he could find himself a victim.

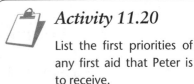

Activity 11.20

List the first priorities of any first aid that Peter is to receive.

2 Stop the burning process.
3 Ensure that the victim has a patent airway, is breathing and has a circulatory output.
4 Relieve pain.
5 Cover the burn wound.
6 Seek appropriate medical aid or transport to hospital.

Can you think of other examples that relate to the safety of the rescuer(s)?

? Have you ever treated anyone who has suffered from a burn injury? If so, what first aid treatment was given?

Activity 11.21

A Refer to a current first aid manual, such as St John Ambulance (2002) for more detailed coverage of first aid management.

B Consider what is meant by a burn injury, and how it can be caused.

Burn injuries

A burn is an injury resulting in tissue loss or damage. Injury can be caused by exposure to thermal, electrical, chemical or radiation sources. Injury to the tissue is determined by:

1 The temperature or causticity of the burning agent; and
2 Duration of tissue contact with the source.

At a cellular level, the burning produces a dilatation of the capillaries and small vessels, thus increasing the cellular permeability. Plasma seeps out into the surrounding tissue, producing blisters and oedema. The type, duration and depth of the burn affect the amount of tissue loss. This fluid loss becomes reduced over time although this results in a decrease in circulation blood volume which, if not replaced, can progress. In major burns this can result in death. This primary cause of death from major burns in the past was due to fluid loss. This will be discussed in more depth later when describing hypovolaemic shock.

The three main stages of a significant burn injury are resuscitation (which refers to fluid resuscitation), the acute phase and the rehabilitative phase.

Some authors suggest that some groups are more susceptible than others to burn injury. These include the very young and the elderly, those suffering from alcohol and substance misuse, those with diabetes, epilepsy or other medical problems such as transient ischaemic attacks, those with mental health problems, and the socially deprived.

Activity 11.22

Find out which individuals are more at risk of a burn injury. Burn injury is the most common form of accident in many parts of Africa. Consider why this is true.

> Peter was taken to an accident and emergency department for assessment. Peter is single, with a girlfriend who lives 250 miles from the burns unit to which he is admitted. He has a history of alcohol abuse, and drinks two bottles of wine a day and more at weekends. He has, in the past, been treated for depression with antidepressants. He has a medical history of hypertension and mild asthma.

Airway and cervical spine management

1 Clear Peter's airway and open the airway if necessary with a chin lift and/or jaw thrust.
2 Ensure that cervical spine movement is kept to a minimum in case a cervical spine injury has occurred.

> **Activity 11.23**
>
> List the priorities of Peter's assessment.

The history of the incident is significant; for example, a person may have had to jump from a building to escape a house fire. Therefore that person is more likely to have had a cervical spine injury than an individual with a scald as a result of spilling boiling water over themselves.

Breathing

1 Expose Peter's chest to ensure that chest expansion is equal and not compromised. Assist ventilation if necessary.
2 Administer oxygen.
3 Observe his respiratory rate, rhythm and depth of ventilation.
4 Be aware that circumferential burns to the chest could compromise ventilation and require immediate medical attention.

> In Peter's case, it is likely that he could have sustained an inhalation injury as his accident occurred in a confined space.

An accurate history is vital and may differ. It is important to obtain a history from a number of people including the paramedics, if they were the first on the scene.

? What signs would you expect to see if there is inhalation injury?

Signs of inhalation injury include:

● Burns around the mouth and /or nose
● Intraoral burns
● Intraoral oedema
● Hoarseness of voice

- Soot in nostrils, mouth, singed nasal hair
- Pharyngeal oedema (visible on examination)
- Inspiratory stridor
- Laryngeal oedema (visible on examination)

> On initial assessment, Peter did not have an inhalation injury.

If inspiratory stridor and/or laryngeal oedema are present then intubation will be necessary (Judkins 1996).

Activity 11.24

Refer to Settle (1996) chs 9 and 26, for a more in-depth discussion of the types, signs and symptoms and management of inhalation injuries.

Practice tip

An inhalation injury can become evident up to several days post-injury and it is vital that nurses caring for the patient observe them for signs and symptoms and contact the doctor if they are present.

Circulation

- Assess Peter's circulation by observing and recording his blood pressure, pulse and temperature (peripheral and core).
- Arrest any bleeding by applying direct pressure.
- Observe peripheral circulation. Where there is a circumferential burn to a limb, a capillary blanch test should be performed. The normal return is two seconds. A longer return may indicate circulatory compromise due to a deep burn or hypovolaemia. The doctor should be informed.

Neurological status

Assess Peter's level of consciousness. Is Peter:

- Alert?
- Responding to vocal stimuli?
- Responding to painful stimuli?
- Unresponsive?
- Are the pupils equal and responding to light?

Again, the history might indicate the potential for the patient to have a head injury.

Extent of burn injury

Expose the burn wounds, remove jewellery and observe the depth and percentage. Once the burn has been assessed and following first aid, it is important to protect Peter from the environment by keeping him warm.

> Peter sustained flame burns to 40% of his body: his face, chest, arms and legs. His burns are mainly partial thickness with deeper areas on his anterior thighs.

Practice tip

Cling film can be applied directly on to the burn tissue and acts as a temporary dressing.

How is the percentage burn surface area (BSA) estimated? Find out if there is more than one way to work this out.

Various charts exist as a guide to assessing the percentage of the body burned, for example, Rule of Nines and the Lund and Browder chart shown in Figure 11.1 documenting Peter's burns. In all cases, erythema should be disregarded when calculating the percentage BSA, although if the area blisters in the first 16 or so hours, it should then be included when assessing percentage BSA.

Evidence-based practice

Assessing the percentage of the burn surface area

It is widely accepted practice that the patient's hand represents approximately 1 per cent BSA. There is debate as to whether 1 per cent BSA is the palm minus digits or the whole hand with closed fingers.

Rossiter et al (1996) reviewed the use of the hand when estimating the percentage BSA of adults with burns; they concluded that if the hand alone is used to estimate the percentage BSA, the burn could be overestimated. They therefore stress the importance of accurately monitoring the burn-injured patient during the shock period of resuscitation.

Why is it important to assess the percentage burn that Peter has sustained?

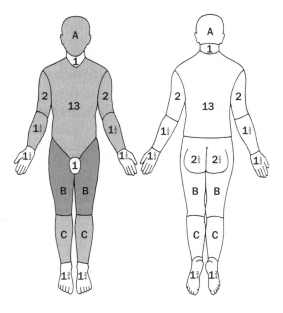

Ignore simple erythema

Partial thickness loss (PTL)

Full thickness loss (FTL)

REGION	% PTL	FTL
Head	$3\frac{1}{2}$	
Neck		
Ant. trunk	13	
Post. trunk		
Right arm	$3\frac{1}{2}$	
Left arm	$3\frac{1}{2}$	
Buttocks		
Genitalia		
Right leg	$3\frac{1}{2}$	$4\frac{3}{4}$
Left leg	$3\frac{1}{2}$	$4\frac{3}{4}$
TOTAL BURN	$30\frac{1}{2}$	$9\frac{1}{4}$
	40	

Relative percentage of body surface area affected by growth

AREA	AGE 0	1	5	10	15	ADULT
A = $\frac{1}{2}$ of head	$9\frac{1}{2}$	$8\frac{1}{2}$	$6\frac{1}{2}$	$5\frac{1}{2}$	$4\frac{1}{2}$	$3\frac{1}{2}$
B = $\frac{1}{2}$ of one thigh	$2\frac{3}{4}$	$3\frac{1}{4}$	4	$4\frac{1}{2}$	$4\frac{1}{2}$	$4\frac{3}{4}$
C = $\frac{1}{2}$ of one leg	$2\frac{1}{2}$	$2\frac{1}{2}$	$2\frac{3}{4}$	3	$3\frac{1}{4}$	$3\frac{1}{2}$

Figure 11.1 Lund and Browder burn assessment chart

Activity 11.25

Find out what assessment tool is used to estimate percentage BSA in the trust where you are currently working.

Adults with greater than 10% burns to their body surface have a reduced circulating blood volume and require intravenous fluid replacement. Body weight is important to assess the normal circulating blood volume.

Fluid assessment

Fluids are the final aspect that requires assessment:

- Assess the amount of fluid replacement necessary and administer that prescribed if the burn surface area (BSA) is greater than 15% in an adult.
- Assess urinary output by passing a urinary catheter.

- Obtain blood for full blood count, urea and electrolytes, coagulation, amylase and carboxyhaemoglobin via wide-bore cannulae.
- Assess nutritional status, using a nutritional assessment tool. (See Chapter 10 on nutritional needs for discussion of nutritional assessment tools.) A naso-gastric tube may be required.
- Tetanus status should be ascertained. Tetanus is a rare complication following a burn injury, but prophylaxis should be offered.

Mortality can be described as the likelihood of survival or death following an injury or disease.

> ### Activity 11.26
>
> **A** Revise homeostasis and fluid balance in a physiology textbook.
>
> **B** List the factors that influence the mortality of the burn injured individual.

Factors affecting survival

Tools exist as a guide to possible mortality rate. It must be remembered that they are simply an empirical guide, and as such they are developed retrospectively. They consider the age of the patient, an important factor as the old and young have a poorer prognosis than a young fit person. They do not consider an individual's past medical history or the involvement of inhalation injury, both of which can considerably affect the individual's outcome.

?   **What types of shock may result from a significant burn injury?**

> ### Activity 11.27
>
> Define hypovolaemic shock (you may wish to refer to a critical care text, such as Urden et al 1996.

Hypovolaemic shock

Hypovolaemic shock develops when there is a shift in volume from the cardiovascular compartment to another internal compartment or the external environment, following a burn injury of more than 10% BSA; the shift in volume is both external and internal. This drop in circulating blood volume results in reduced blood flow, and therefore tissue perfusion. A shift of fluid to the external environment leads to hypovolaemia if there is insufficient volume replacement. Vasodilatation and increased permeability of the capillaries leads to localised oedema and a shift of fluid internally.

Physiologically, the events leading to hypovolaemic shock are a reduction of intravascular volume leading to reduced venous return. This leads to a decrease in ventricular filling and accompanying reduced cardiac output.

Burn shock differs from normal hypovolemic shock as chemical mediators are also involved resulting in disruptions at cellular level.

Initial phase

As cardiac output falls so also the blood pressure falls, reducing the blood flow and oxygenation through the capillary networks. This includes the kidneys, where urine output may be inadequate. There are no detectable signs that this clinical process is occurring, but blood analysis shows raised lactic acid levels. If the shock phase is allowed to progress, the body moves into compensatory phase.

Compensatory phase

This process consists of neural, hormonal and chemical responses, which adapt the cardiovascular system in order to maintain adequate oxygenation of essential tissues. Each individual may differ in the degree of compensation. The elderly are less able to compensate than a young fit individual like Peter.

Progressive phase

If the compensatory mechanisms start to fail, the perfusion of the vital organs is grossly inadequate and these organ systems also begin to fail. When one system starts to fail, it accelerates the failure rate of the other organs, hence the term multi-organ failure. Loss of auto-regulation and increased permeability of the capillary beds affect blood flow through the coronary artery, and results in myocardial function depression, ischaemia and infarct. The decreased oxygen transport affects other organ systems such as the gastrointestinal tract, liver, pancreas, lungs, kidneys and brain.

Fluid resuscitation

Controversy exists about the type of fluid that is most effective in maintaining the circulatory blood volume with the least harm to the patient. Discussion around this argument can be found in Settle (1996).

Various formulae exist to assist in the calculation of the amount of fluid replacement that a patient requires. Care should be taken to ascertain whether the formula is based on crystalloid or colloid fluid replacement.

There are numerous fluid resuscitation formulae that are used. Care must be used when selecting a formula to administer the type of fluid for which the formula was developed, for example crystalloid and colloid.

In Peter's case we will use the fluid resuscitation formula detailed below, otherwise known as the Muir and Barclay formula:

$$\frac{\text{Total percentage area of burn} \times \text{weight in kg}}{2}$$

(i.e. 0.5ml/kg/% burn).

The fluid is given in 'periods' of time, the aim being to replace the fluid lost as soon as possible.

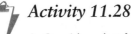

Activity 11.28

A Consider what factors need to be taken into account when choosing the type of fluid with which Peter is transfused.

B Consider what factors are included to calculate the amount of fluid that Peter requires.

Activity 11.29

Based on the information presented about Peter, calculate the amount of fluid he will require in each fluid replacement period.

In Peter's case:

$$\frac{40\% \times 70\text{kg}}{2}$$

$$= 1400 \text{ ml per period}$$

Hartman's solution is the fluid of choice prescribed using this formula. This equates to the following (refer to Figure 11.2 below):

From the time of injury to 4 hours post-injury = 350ml per hour

4–8 hours post-injury = 350ml per hour

8–12 hours post-injury = 350ml per hour

12–18 hours post-injury = 233ml per hour

18–24 hours post-injury = 233ml per hour

24–36 hours post-injury = 117ml per hour

A maintenance fluid may need to be administered.

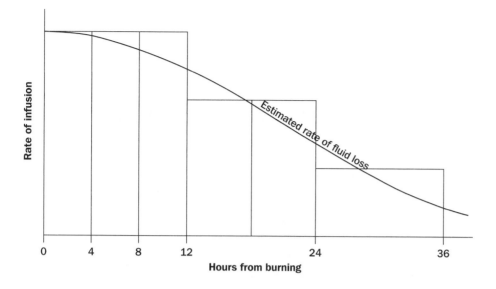

Figure 11.2 Fluid replacement regime

? How does this compare to patients receiving intravenous fluids in your clinical area? Suggest reasons why there is a difference.

It must be remembered that the calculated fluid requirements are only a guideline. The quantity and type of fluid required depends on the individual's response and can be observed by careful monitoring and observation. Peter should be observed for signs of over- and under-transfusion. Under-transfusion can result in under-perfusion and a potential for conversion of a burn wound to a greater depth and renal failure. Too much fluid can result in pulmonary oedema.

> **Activity 11.30**
>
> Plan the care that a patient with an intravenous infusion (IVI) requires, giving rationale.

Blood should be given at the end of the third period as haemolysis occurs with a large full thickness burn, due to the heat of the burning agent. Other factors which are largely uncertain also contribute, although it is thought that chemical mediators may be responsible. Blood is usually prescribed towards the end of the resuscitation phase. It is usually given for full thickness burns over 10%, at 1% of the patient's normal volume for 1% BSA affected.

It is important that Peter's condition is accurately monitored during the fluid resuscitation period.

> **Activity 11.31**
>
> Identify what the nurses should monitor Peter for during the resuscitation period. Consider what other monitoring may be required.

These observations include:

- **Blood pressure and pulse** The frequency should depend on the clinical condition of patient and be either half-hourly or hourly. Patients may compensate and other factors may affect these, for example pain. Therefore trends in the rate are more important than fluctuations.

- **Respiratory rate** This is usually raised due to an increased metabolic rate, although an increase in the rate and depth could be an indication of shock.

- **Temperature** Both peripheral and core. A difference between the two can indicate the degree of vasoconstriction and thus shock.

- **Skin colour** Perfusion can be demonstrated and is again an indicator of shock. With adequate circulation the patient is pink. A pale appearance could indicate constricted arterioles, and a bluish tinge could indicate stagnation of blood in the capillaries that are dilated.

- **Urine output** This is an indicator of renal function. The stress response will affect the output. In an adult the expected output is 1ml/kg body weight per hour. The concentration is also of note. A low urine output with concentrated urine suggests under-transfusion and a high output with dilute urine over-transfusion during the resuscitation phase. Urine concentration can be measured with osmolality. The osmolality should decrease after the first 24 hours. A careful record of fluid balance should be kept.

> ### Activity 11.32
>
> Remember to keep checking out your understanding of the technical terms, e.g. osmolality.

- **Orientation** This is of significance as a disorientated patient may be showing signs of sepsis. Other causes may be drugs or previous alcohol intake, although these factors should not be assumed to be the cause and the patient should be monitored closely for other causes.

- **Blood samples** These are usually taken during each 'period' to provide an indication of the adequacy of the fluid replacement. It is normal to have disturbed electrolyte levels at this time.

- **Haematocrit** This is recorded as a percentage. Haematocrit is the proportion of red blood cells to plasma and it rises with a low plasma volume. It is a useful adjunct to monitoring, although a normal haematocrit is not an indicator of adequate fluid resuscitation. The patient may require a central venous line to monitor the central venous pressure.

 How much urine should we expect Peter to produce per hour? (Remember that his weight on admission was 70kg.)

A fluid challenge may need to be administered. In Peter's case this may be an extra 500ml of crystalloid given over a one-hour period. He will need to be monitored closely for a rise in blood pressure, tachycardia and increased respiratory rate. The doctor will advise on how much urine volume is expected, usually greater than 50ml per hour. The nurse needs to communicate the outcome to the doctor.

Burns are usually defined as flame, flash, chemical, electrical, contact or explosion. The cause of the burn affects the depth and an accurate history will guide the clinician to the possible forms of treatment for the patient.

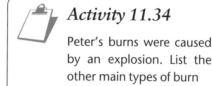

> ### Activity 11.33
> Consider what steps might be made to correct Peter's fluid balance if it is higher or lower than expected.

> ### Activity 11.34
> Peter's burns were caused by an explosion. List the other main types of burn

? **What are the main ways of categorising burn depth?**

Categories such as first-, second- and third-degree burns tend not to be used now. They are largely replaced by the following:

Erythema
Superficial
Deep dermal } Partial thickness
Full thickness

See Table 11.3 (below) for a more in-depth classification and for a more thorough discussion of causes and types of burn, see Herndon 2001 or Settle 1996.

> ### Activity 11.35
> **A** From Table 11.3, identify what type of recovery Peter might make.
>
> **B** Consider the term 'septic shock'. What signs and symptoms would you expect and why are they of significance in Peter's case?

Septic shock

Because the burn wound provides an ideal environment for the proliferation of bacteria, and the burn-injured individual is immunocompromised as a result of a major burn injury, the individual is at risk of developing septic shock.

Table 11.3 Classification and clinical appearance of burn injury and depth

| | Erythema | Depth of burn | | |
		Partial thickness Superficial	Partial thickness Deep dermal	Full thickness
Usual history	Sunburn	Scalds of limited duration	Scalds of long duration, contact with high temperature, eg; hot fat	Contact with high temperature eg; flame burn, chemicals, electrical injury
Appearance	Red	Red or pink with capillary return	Red without capillary return	Charred, white, dry with thrombosed vessels
Sensation	Painful	Painful	Often painful around the margins with altered pain sensation in deeper areas	Initially insensate but painful at a later stage
Hairs	Present	Present	Present and easily removed or absent	Absent
Blister formation	Absent	Present	Absent	Absent
Results	Heals within days, no dressings necessary	Heals within 14 days if infection free	Heals in months therefore surgery indicated	Granulated therefore surgery indicated
Scan formation	No scar	Can remain red and become hypertrophic	Often becomes hypertrophic	Becomes hypertrophic

There are many signs and symptoms of septic shock and their discussion is beyond the scope of this chapter. For a more detailed explanation, see Herndon 2001.

Partial thickness burns heal by regeneration of new skin from epithelial calls at the periphery of the wound, and from structures such as the hair follicles and sweat glands. Full thickness burns destroy all the skin structure, and therefore healing will occur by repair with scar-tissue formation. Peter's burns are mainly partial thickness.

Activity 11.36

Check in an anatomy and physiology text to see why this occurs.

Peter required surgery to repair the integrity of 50% of his burned skin. The remainder healed with conservative treatment using dressings.

Wound care

The aim of wound care in burns is to maintain a moist, clean environment, protect from infection and further injury, and promote healing and comfort.

In the immediate period after burning, the wounds should be cooled by applying cold water for 10–20 minutes to reduce pain and tissue damage.

Dressings should be chosen that allow passage of fluid from the wound bed, do not adhere and are not painful or damaging to remove. Silicone dressings are an example of such a dressing. The simpler the dressing the better when choosing dressings for burn wounds. The nurse should have a clear rationale for selecting dressing types and for frequency of changing. Nurses often remove dressings more often than is necessary, thus causing damage to delicate epithelial tissue of the superficial burn. Silicone dressings can remain *in situ* for several days without disturbing, and the secondary dressing changed as frequently as required. Debate about the deroofing of blisters and debridement is ongoing and the nurse should consider the site, size of blisters, stage of healing and depth of the injury when deciding how to manage the wound.

Most burn wounds are covered with dressings as opposed to being left exposed. The burn wound should be gently cleansed with warmed normal saline before redressing. Photographing the wound can give clinicians

Activity 11.37

Consider what factors you would use to choose the wound care products with which to dress Peter's burn wounds.

Activity 11.38

For further reading and exploration, see Flanagan and Graham 2001; or Hartford 2001; or Rockwell and Ehrlich 1990; or Swain and Azadia 1987.

Activity 11.38

For further discussion of wound dressings used in burns, see Fowler 1999.

and the patient an indication of the rate of healing and can, if taken by the hospital photography department, be useful in medico-legal cases.

 How likely is it that Peter's burn wounds will heal?

As Peter has some areas of partial thickness burn, it is possible he may need surgery. The first stage of surgery usually involves debridement of the necrotic tissue and harvesting of a split-thickness skin graft, this area is known as the donor site. The harvested skin is then positioned on the recipient site and fixed in position. Various processes occur which, it is hoped, result in skin 'taking'. Factors affecting the 'non-take' of

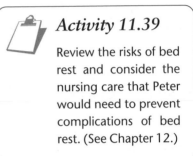

Activity 11.39

Review the risks of bed rest and consider the nursing care that Peter would need to prevent complications of bed rest. (See Chapter 12.)

the skin graft include infection, friction and unsuitable recipient site. Care must be taken when caring for Peter if he requires a split skin graft on his legs, as he may need to be on bed rest and need to be prescribed anticoagulants.

The depth, site and rate of healing of the burn wound inform the management process. If a superficial wound, which has been treated in a conservative manner, is not healed by three weeks, referral to a specialist should be considered as surgery may be indicated.

Nutrition

Nutrition is an important factor in wound healing and recovery following a burn injury of >15% BSA. In adults, a person enters a catabolic state. This results in the utilisation of proteins for metabolism leading to a reduction of lean body mass and poor wound healing. With-

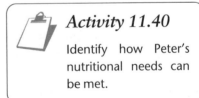

Activity 11.40

Identify how Peter's nutritional needs can be met.

out adequate nutritional support, this can prove to be fatal.

 Why is it important to begin feeding Peter as soon as possible? Check out your answer in the information below.

Nutrition and the burn injured patient

- Peter's nutritional risk should be identified and various tools have been developed for this. Risk factors include age, size and depth of injury, nutritional status, and drug and alcohol abuse among others (see Chapter 10 on nutritional needs).

- Based on the nutritional risk score, consult with the dietician who will prescribe supplements or enteral feeds to meet the energy requirements of the individual.

- Metabolic demand for protein and energy will be considerably increased. Peter will need approximately 25 kcal per kg body weight + 40 kcal × % BSA plus 1g protein per kg body weight, + 3g × % BSA (Pape 2001).

- Peter may need to be fed enterally, either via a naso-gastric or naso-jejunal tube or, if required for more than 30 days, a percutaneous endoscopic gastrostomy (PEG) may need to be considered.

Activity 11.41

Work out how many kcals and grams of protein Peter needs per day. Which vitamins and minerals are important for wound healing? (See Chapter 10 on nutritional needs.)

- Peter may develop deficiencies in micronutrients, as well as energy and protein, as losses may be high and demands are higher during wound healing.

- The nurse will have a large part to play in supporting, monitoring and feeding Peter so that the best outcome can be achieved. Eating is a social activity and patients often have an improved appetite when eating together. However, it should be acknowledged that the odour of the burn wound could affect the appetite.

- Studies have shown that the earlier feeding is started the better. This protects the gut mucosal lining. Bacterial translocation has been identified as a potential cause of septic shock in patients who are not fed (see Settle 1996 for a more in-depth explanation).

- It is essential to monitor Peter's nutritional status. This includes recording the nutritional intake, body weight (usually weekly), blood samples for urea, iron, trace elements, electrolyte levels and liver function, in addition to considering and evaluating the rate of healing and need for general anaesthesia.

Peter was in quite a lot of pain and he was very anxious.

How can pain resulting from a burn be assessed, managed and evaluated?

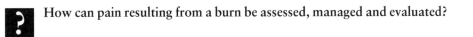

Professional conversation:

Alan, the staff nurse caring for Peter

Pain control

'Peter may not need as much analgesia as expected in the early period, as many of his burns were deep dermal burns, where many of the nerve endings have been destroyed. However, the superficial burns were painful and he was also very anxious. The paramedics at the scene may have given him Entonox and small doses of IV morphine once he arrived at the burns unit. Intravenous morphine is not given immediately, as it is not able to be absorbed until the circulation improves an hour or two later.

When asked, most people would imagine that a burn is one of the most painful injuries that can occur to a person. The cause of the pain is multi-factorial and can differ depending on the time of the day and the treatment being carried out. The burn-injured patient will almost inevitably experience background pain, pain on dressing changes, physiotherapy, and post-operatively after skin grafting. Each cause may require a different form of treatment. The individual's psychological state plays a significant role in the experience of pain; anxiety and depression will also heighten the person's awareness of pain. According to Charlton, (1983), approximately one-third of severely burn-injured patients will exhibit signs of clinical depression. As Peter has already suffered from depression he will be very vulnerable. As a burn wound is rarely uniform in depth, any burn is painful. It is important to assess the patient's pain, administer prescribed analgesia and introduce measures that aim to reduce pain, including listening and believing the patient, giving information, evaluating the treatment and altering the interventions accordingly. The support of a clinical psychologist or psychiatrist may assist the patient.'

Activity 11.42

A See Chapter 13 on pain and Chapter 6 on mental health for more detail on many of the aspects mentioned here.

B Consider how you perceive yourself: what is your image of yourself? Now imagine you are Peter. In what ways might you perceive yourself differently after the accident? How might this affect your relationships with others?

An individual's body image is personal to them and has been defined in many ways. Inevitably, Peter will experience a change in his body image, which is often referred to as an altered body image or disfigurement. Price (1990) offers a good introduction to the concept of body image, he suggests that body image has three essential components: body reality, body ideal, body presentation. Following a burn injury, the individual will need to make adjustments to all of them.

Rehabilitation should begin at the time of injury and be supported with explanations to the patient and family. Rehabilitation should involve reintegration into society and the multi-disciplinary team plays a large role.

Activity 11.43

Write down your current definition of rehabilitation.

Factors that could adversely affect Peter's psychological recovery include his pre-injury depression, altered body image, a possible negative reaction from his girlfriend and alcohol dependency. Alcohol dependency needs to be considered, as a person who is dependent on alcohol and abruptly stops drinking can enter a stage of withdrawal.

Activity 11.44

Identify the other healthcare professionals that nurses caring for burn injured individuals need to work with.

Professional conversation

Chris, a nurse in a burns unit

Role of the multi-disciplinary team in treating the burn-injured individual

'As a nurse in a Burns Unit I really appreciate working in a team with many health care professionals who are involved in caring for the burn-injured individual. These include: Plastic surgeons and other doctors, dieticians, physiotherapists, social workers, occupational therapists, clinical psychologists, psychiatrists, specialist nurses, such as the tissue viability nurse, diabetes nurse specialist, palliative care nurse. It is important that the multi-disciplinary team work together in a collaborative way, with a joint aim to treat the patient in a holistic manner.'

Communication is a fundamental part of the multi-disciplinary team's role. On both an individual basis and group basis, they play a vital role in communicating to other members of the multi-disciplinary team. Nurses have a particular role in empowering the patient and acting as patient advocate.

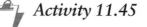

Activity 11.45

If any of the roles above are unfamiliar, check out what are their main functions.

Accountability is an important consideration when treating burn-injured individuals and health care professionals should practice evidence based care. The clinical governance agenda should inform this process and nurses should ensure that their practice is supported by lifelong learning in order to facilitate best practice for patients.

Accident prevention and health promotion are a fundamental part of the nurse's role. On both an individual basis and a group basis, the nurse is in a prime position to positively influence the health behaviour of patients. The public can be empowered through the attainment of knowledge and information to enable them to make choices and decisions regarding their safety and that of others.

Post-burn education

The nurse caring for Peter needs to inform him about the following, ensuring that he understands and is therefore likely to concord with the advice:

- Importance of cleansing the newly healed skin with unperfumed soap, rinsing it, drying and reapplying moisturising cream and massaging the area twice per day.
- Importance of daily shower/bath when burnt areas are healed.
- Explanation of cold/heat injury.
- Information on what to expect regarding scar formation and management, and altered body image.
- Advice on diet.
- Advice on sun protection.
- Advice on managing itching and ongoing pain.
- Information on follow-up appointments.
- Information on swimming, exercise and rest.

Conclusion

This two-part chapter has considered the hydration needs of children and adults during a health care crisis. Although their relatively small total blood volume exacerbates fluid loss in children, the principles of care and management are common to both groups. A decrease in circulation blood volume can result in death, and were Sophie to develop a diarrhoeal illness in certain countries this might be the natural course of events. Similarly, in the second scenario Peter, a burns victim, reflects one of the commonest forms of accidents in the third world. Fluid resuscitation is therefore key to the management of all patients who, for whatever reason, develop hypovolaemic shock. The role of the nurse in the management of such patients and their families is of paramount importance and considerable acumen is required to ensure that evidence-based protocols are adhered to during the period when fluid replacement is the major facet of treatment.

References

Bosworth, C. (ed.) (1997) *Burns Trauma Management and Nursing Care.* London: Prentice Hall.

Carolan, J. M. (1984) *Shock: A Nursing Guide.* Bristol: John Wright and Son.

Charlton, J., et al (1983) Factors affecting pain in burned patients – a preliminary report. *Post Graduate Medical Journal* 59, pp. 604–7.

Judkins, K. (1996) Inhalation injury. In: Settle, J. (ed.) *Principles and Practice of Burns Management.* London: Churchill Livingstone.

Lawrence, J. C. (1991) *Burn and Scald Injuries.* Topic Briefing HS40. Birmingham: The Royal Society for the Prevention of Accidents.

Lawrence, J. C. (1996) Burns and scalds: aetiology and prevention. In Settle, J. (ed.) *Principles and Practice of Burns Management.* London: Churchill Livingstone.

Muir, I. F. K., Barclay, T. L. (1962) *Burns and Their Treatment.* London: Lloyd-Luke.

Pape, S., Judkins, K., Settle, J. (2001) *Burns: The First Five Days.* 2nd Edition. Hull: Smith and Nephew.

Price, B. (1990) *Body Image: Nursing Concepts and Care.* London: Prentice Hall.

Rossiter, N. D., Chapman, P., Haywood, I. A. (1996) How big is a hand? *Burns* 22 (3), pp. 230–1.

Resources

📖 Further reading

Flanagan, M., Graham, J. (2001) Should burn blisters be left intact or debrided? *Journal of Wound Care* 10 (1), pp. 41–5.

Fowler, A. (1999) Burns. In: Miller, M., Glover, D. (eds) *Wound Management.* London:Nursing Times Books.

Hartford, C. (2001) In: Herndon, D. (ed.) *Total Burn Care.* 2nd Edition. Philadelphia, PA: W. B. Saunders.

Herndon, D. (ed.) (2001) *Total Burn Care.* 2nd Edition. Philadelphia, PA: W. B. Saunders.

St. John Ambulance (2000) *First Aid Manual.* 8th Edition. London: Dorling Kindersley.

Rockwell, Ehrlich, H. (1990) Should burn blister fluid be evacuated? *British Journal of Rehabilitation* 11, pp. 93–5.

Settle, J. (ed.) (1996) *Principles and Practice of Burns Management.* London: Churchill Livingstone.

Swain, A., Azadia, B. (1987) Management of blisters in minor burns. *British Medical Journal* (Clin Res) 285, p. 181.

Urden, L., Lough, M., Stacey, K. (1996) *Critical Care Nursing.* London: Mosby.

Annotated Bibliography

Bosworth, C. (ed.) (1997) *Burns Trauma Management and Nursing Care.* London: Prentice Hall.
An edited book, with contributions from health care professionals, of value mainly to nurses who are new to the speciality. It acknowledges the unique nature of burn injury discussing the pathophysiology of burns, their presentation, management, psychological consequences and reintegration of the patient into society.

Pape, S., Judkins, K., Settle, J. (2001) *Burns: The First Five Days.* 2nd Edition. Hull: Smith and Nephew.
This slim volume provides concise, readable and practical guidance for those faced with managing and supporting patients, following a major burn injury. This booklet is only concerned with major burns in the first few days after injury and does not pretend to be a comprehensive text. It is aimed at all health professionals involved in the care of these patients.

Settle, J. (1996) *Principles and Practice of Burns Management.* London: Churchill Livingstone.

This is an edited book written specifically for health care professionals. It has contributions from experts in burns care. It is separated into principles and practice to divide the underpinning scientific facts from practical management of the burn-injured individual. As an edited book some areas are duplicated, although this often serves to emphasise important points.

@ Web pages

www.health.nsw.gov.au/public-health/burns/burnsmgt.html

A site is currently being developed for healthcare professionals specifically on burn injury management.

Insights into Rehabilitation

12

Stephen O'Connor and Bernard Gibbon

Introduction

The care and management of patients at all points on the health illness continuum incorporates the notion of caring for patients through complete episodes of illness, from the acute presentation through into post-acute care and rehabilitation.

The care and management of the stroke patient is representative of the challenge to the multi-professional team in caring for patients who have complex needs. Significant durations of inpatient care require the services of many health care professionals and frequently require post-hospital care and management.

Aim

To understand the experience of stroke.

Learning outcomes

- Identification of the physical, psychological and social needs of the patient and his carers following stroke and an awareness of the values and concepts of individual care.
- Application of the principles of problem solving to the planning of care, its implementation and evaluation.
- Familiarity with the terminology associated with stroke care and management.
- Appreciation of the incidence and prevalence of stroke.
- Understanding of the pathophysiological basis of stroke, predisposing factors and preventative measures.
- Identification of appropriate forms of assessment for patients following stroke and of those which can be used to monitor progress.
- Identification of the complications of stroke and measures to prevent complications arising.
- Understanding of the impact of stroke on the person and his/her family,
- Understanding of the roles and responsibilities of the different members of the multiprofessional team.

- Understanding of the different approaches to the managerial organisation of stroke services.
- Identification of evidence to support clinical practices.

Concepts

- Rehabilitation nursing
- The nurse's role
- Stroke

- Individualised care
- Problem solving
- Multi-professional working

This chapter will provide an insight into rehabilitation nursing focusing on Frank Sargeant and his family who have recently experienced stroke.

Scenario *Frank Sargeant's experiences*

Frank Sargeant collapses at his social club and on his return home appears rather incoherent. He is seen by his GP.

Activity 12.1

Frank's GP undertakes a full medical assessment, which includes the following. What significance might these have and why?

1 Take a full history
2 Full physical examination
3 Determine any loss of consciousness
4 Take blood pressure
5 Discuss plan of action

Frank is found to be hypertensive with a blood pressure recording of 190/100mmHg. Following further examination and the responses to questions, the GP strongly suspects that Frank has experienced a 'transient ischaemic attack' (TIA).

What is hypertension and what is a TIA? Before reading on think about what you already know about the way that blood pressure is controlled and why hypertension might rise. Think about how oxygenated blood reaches the brain and consider what might happen if this flow is obstructed in any way. As a starting point you may wish to access a physiology textbook and map out the cerebral circulation, determining both the origin and destination of the internal and external carotid arteries.

Transient ischaemic attack (TIA)

A 'TIA' is a stroke where the neurological deficits clear spontaneously within 24 hours. This may result from emboli. Emboli that give rise to stroke have their origin in the left side of the heart or in the arteries between the heart and the brain.

Emboli formation is often associated with either valvular damage of the mitral (bicuspid) valve in the heart, which separates the left atria from the left ventricle, or damage to the semi-lunar valves at the opening of the aorta. This thrombotic clot known as a mural thrombus has formed on the inner wall of the ventricle, usually following a myocardial infarction. If the mural thrombus breaks away, it then becomes an embolus flowing towards the brain, until it becomes lodged as the blood vessels get smaller. The amount of damage caused will depend upon the size of the vessel, the degree of obstruction and what part of the brain is denied oxygen. Sometimes emboli can be very small and the resulting effects may be only transient. Frank Sargeant is thought to have experienced such a 'transient ischaemic attack'.

Emboli can also form in damaged arteries, especially where arteries bifurcate, and this is frequently associated with artherosclerotic changes in which the lumen of arteries becomes reduced. When the carotid arteries are affected in this way, there is a high risk of stroke. However, an understanding of the predisposing factors leading to stroke can facilitate the development of preventative strategies.

Activity 12.2

Refer to a nursing or medical textbook. Consider those causes of heart disease, which might give rise to mitral valve damage.

Activity 12.3

It would seem that Frank might well have experienced a TIA. Reflect on Frank's lifestyle and identify potential factors that may have given rise to this.

Frank Sargeant considered himself to be a fit and well 67-year-old. Frank retired two years ago from the light engineering factory where he started work as an apprentice tool-maker at the age of 14, 53 years before. He knows he was lucky to have stayed in work all his adult life, and puts this down to his own hard work and ability to 'fit in'; he is well aware that his children may not be so lucky, but feels strongly that they must work hard to succeed.

Frank is married. His wife Joan is 55 and is still working at the local supermarket, doing shift work as a garage receptionist. They live in their own home, which they now own after paying off the mortgage on Frank's retirement.

Frank and Joan have three children. Ken the eldest is 37, married with two children, and lives away in London. Frank and Joan are extremely proud that Ken is a successful professional; however, he rarely visits and when he does, it tends to be whilst on business trips and he does not bring his family. Mary is now 33, divorced, with one child. She lives locally and works shifts in a local factory, and relies on her mother for childminding. This is difficult as they both work shifts and is a cause of ongoing friction between father and daughter. Barry is 30 and lives at home. He is unemployed at present, having followed his father into engineering. Barry is in a long-term relationship and plans to marry, but feels that he should not until he has a job that is secure and has prospects.

Frank's social life rotates around his local CIA social club where he has a part-time job as barman. He is also vice-chairman of the 'old folks' entertainment committee and captain of the club's first division cribbage team. Frank prides himself on the fact that he has never had a day off sick in his life and does not even know who his GP is. However, Frank smokes 40 cigarettes a day, drinks at least 50 units of alcohol a week (mainly beer), and even he accepts his wife's opinion that he is overweight. He will also admit to easily 'losing his breath', often getting headaches and feeling 'flushed'.

In Frank's case a number of predisposing factors could have influenced his stroke. These might include; stress, obesity, high alcohol consumption and cigarette smoking which may have contributed to an increased risk of hypertension or heart disease.

Reduction in the incidence of stroke is a government Health of the Nation target (DoH 1992). Stroke preventative strategies include:

- Discouraging smoking
- Screening for and treating high blood pressure
- Screening for abnormal lipids and treating as appropriate
- Ensuring the optimal control of diabetes where appropriate. (See also Chapter 8 on community care).

Smoking

Cigarette smoking is a major cause of ill health and is implicated in a range of respiratory and circulatory disorders. Public health messages have been attempting to discourage people from smoking and encourage people to give up smoking for a number of years with only limited success. Frank describes himself as addicted, having tried to give up several times but failed. The addictive nature of smoking has been recognised in addition to the habitual element.

Activity 12.4

A. Consider the smoking behaviour of people and reflect on 'anti smoking' campaigns.

B. Consider strategies that could be deployed to reduce the number of people who smoke and the number of cigarettes that people smoke.

C. Reflect on the use of nicotine replacement therapy as a method to reduce the number of people who smoke.

(See also Chapter 5 on nursing adults.)

Frank suddenly collapses at home and loses consciousness. Joan accompanies him in the ambulance to the accident and emergency department at the local general hospital. As Frank arrives he regains consciousness and is seen immediately by the Registrar and transferred to the admissions ward. It is strongly suspected that Frank has experienced a major stroke.

What is a stroke and how does this differ from a TIA? (Consider what you may already know before reading on.)

Stroke

A stroke is defined as the rapid onset of neurological deficits that persist for at least 24 hours and are caused by either haemorrhage or partial or complete blockage of a blood vessel supplying or draining a part of the brain, leading to infarction of brain tissue.

'Cerebrovascular accident' is a term often used to refer to a stroke, frequently shortened to CVA. This term, whilst accurately describing the notion of damage to the part of the brain, the cerebrum, and that the cause is vascular, is now not commonly used. A stroke is a collective term for a syndrome. Additionally, a stroke is not an accident in the 'normal' meaning of this word.

Activity 12.5

If unsure check out the meaning of the word 'syndrome'.

Stroke is commonly caused by cerebral thrombosis or embolism, and less commonly by cerebral haemorrhage. The most common underlying pathology in these conditions is arterial damage, often associated with hypertension. The type of stroke often gives some indication of the prognosis and the onset of stroke can *suggest* the underlying type. For Frank Sargeant, it is important for investigations to be undertaken as a matter of urgency and this will be discussed later under 'Assessments'.

Types of stroke

The most common pattern of the onset and prognosis for stroke is set out below:

Table 12.1 Typical pattern of onset and prognosis according to type

Type	Onset	Prognosis
Thrombotic	Slow	Variable: from good to very poor
Embolic	Sudden	
Haemorrhagic	Sudden	Usually poor

Thrombosis refers to the formation of a blood clot within the blood vessels during life. Blood clotting within the body depends upon the same factors as in clotting outside the body, such as following a laceration. The rough edges of a wound or rough surface in the lining of a blood vessel will have similar effects, both trigger the blood clotting mechanism.

> ### Activity 12.6
>
> Refer to a physiology textbook and study 'blood clotting mechanism'. You may wish to draw a diagram to show the cascade theory of blood clotting.

Therefore an indirect cause of thrombosis is usually some damage to the smooth lining of the blood vessels brought about by inflammation, or most typically in stroke, the result of atheroma, a chronic disease of vessel walls.

Embolism refers to the plugging of a small blood vessel by material which has been carried through the larger vessels in the blood stream.

> ### Activity 12.7
>
> Reflect back on what you have already learnt about embolism in relation to transient ischaemic attacks (TIA). You may wish to access a clinical nursing or clinical medicine text book and study 'embolism' in more depth. Think about the different substances that form emboli and where emboli can lodge in relation to their origin.

Haemorrhage means any escape of blood from the vessels which naturally contain it. It may occur from a wound on the skin, in which case it escapes externally, or into some internal cavity such as the stomach, or it may simply escape into the tissues surrounding the site of blood loss. In the case of cerebral haemorrhage the skull acts to contain all blood lost through haemorrhage, and hence any intracerebral haemorrhage not only irritates the neurological cells, but also acts to exert pressure on the brain.

Therefore, in summary, Frank Sergeant's stroke may have resulted from:

- *Atheroma* (associated with cigarette smoking, high blood pressure, diabetes and hyperlipidaemia)
- *Micro-aneurisms* (associated with high blood pressure)
- *Emboli* (associated with a range of heart disorders)
- *Thrombus* (associated with other conditions such as severe dehydration)

An understanding of the pathology of stroke gives some understanding on how to embark on prevention, including secondary prevention and, following a stroke, provides the basis for the range of investigations. As yet no specific treatment exists for stroke, but an understanding of the pathology provides the basis for considering treatment options.

? How common are strokes?
Key resource: *National Service Framework for Older People* (DoH 2001, ch. 5).

Evidence-based practice

Incidence of stroke – making use of statistics

Incidence refers to the number of *new* cases in a particular time frame, say one year, whereas prevalence is number of *existing* cases. Stroke is a common problem, being the third most common cause of death in the UK. and at any one time 25–35 patients with stroke will occupy beds in an average district general hospital (Wolfe et al 1996).

There are about 100,000–120,000 people who have their first strokes in any one year in the United Kingdom, and additionally, about a further 30,000 people have a recurrence or subsequent stroke in any one year. Stroke carries a high mortality of somewhere around 80,000 people per year dying following a stroke. The consequence of these figures means that the prevalence of people with stroke is between 55,000–70,000 in the UK. It is noteworthy that men and women are equally affected, though a slight rise in the number of elderly women is noted, probably attributable to the greater proportion of elderly women than men in the older elderly sector of the population (Rudd et al 1999). An average Health District with a population of 250,000 can expect to see about 500–650 new patients following a stroke per year. Many patients survive the initial stroke, but have a degree of residual disability. At a local level you could expect about 900–1200 people who have survived a stroke with some degree of disability (Wolfe et al 1996).

> ### Activity 12.8
>
> There are clear implications for stroke prevention. Reflect back on the issues identified previously in relation to Frank's lifestyle and that of his family. How much at risk of stroke are Frank's children and grandchildren, and are they at any greater risk than the rest of the population?

Giving advice is an important role for all health practitioners. However, enabling individuals to understand and to concord with health advice is a key skill that all nurses have to develop.

> ### Activity 12.9
>
> When you are next in a practice setting (in the community or elsewhere) try to observe a health education activity. Consider such issues as:
>
> - Who takes the initiative in providing health education?
> - How are health needs assessed?
> - What format is used; for example, verbal information, leaflets, videos, one-to-one or group activities?
> - How is the activity evaluated?
>
> You may like to begin to find out more about health education models and ascertain which model may be most effective in providing health advice for Frank, his wife, their children and grandchildren.

Nurses work as members of the multi-professional team which is essential in relation to the rehabilitation of patients following stroke, and to their family. Communication is key and nurses need to be able to not only converse with patients and relatives to enable clear understanding, but also to thoroughly understand the medical terminology.

Practice tips

Using key terms in relation to stroke

Stroke, which affects a major control system like the nervous system, gives rise to a number of clinical features, such as loss of consciousness, difficulty with mobility, difficulty with speech or swallowing, difficulty with understanding or perception. Many of these clinical features are described by the following terms.

- *Hemiplegia* – refers to paralysis of one side of the body. It is due to cerebral disease. The lesion (damage to the brain) is in the side of the brain opposite to the side paralysed.
- *Hemiparesis* is a similar term, which refers to a partial paralysis of one side of the body.

- *Aphagia* refers to the loss of swallowing ability, and *aphasia* refers to the loss of speech, or the loss of power to understand the written or spoken word. The prefix 'a' meaning 'lacking' or 'loss of'.
- *Apraxia* refers to the inability to recognise common articles or perform correct movements because of a brain lesion, and not because of sensory impairment or loss of muscle power in the limbs. *Agnosia* is an inability to recognise sensory objects, as the sensory stimulus cannot be interpreted in spite of a normal sense organ.
- *Dysphagia* means difficulty in swallowing and *dysphasia* means difficulty in speaking. 'Dys' is used as a prefix meaning 'difficult'. *Dysphasia* may be receptive or expressive. Receptive dysphasia refers to difficulty in understanding. Expressive dysphasia means difficulty in speaking.

Activity 12.10

Having been introduced to some of the medical terminology associated with stroke, you may like to confirm the meaning of: *dysarthria; dyspraxia; neglect syndrome; homonymous hemianopia;* and *apoplexy.*

Initial admission and assessment

Frank's wife had decided to go home to collect some night-clothes so did not accompany Frank to the ward. Once Frank was settled in bed on the emergency medical assessment ward, Staff Nurse Jenny Jones had a brief discussion with the nurse responsible for Frank's care in the accident and emergency department. She then made an immediate assessment of his condition, decided on a number of priorities and instigated a plan of action. This she then handed quickly to a colleague, as she wanted to be off duty by 3 p.m

Table 12.2 Care Plan

Immediate Care Plan for: Mr Frank Sargeant Admitted to Ward: Aug 2nd, 14.30hrs

Named Nurse: Jenny Jones

ADL	Normal state	On admission	Actions
Breathing	SC	Semi-conscious	GCS hourly TPR\BP hourly
Body temperature	SC	Semi-conscious	Keep warm
Eating and drinking	SC	Semi-conscious	Offer fluids
Elimination	SC	Semi-conscious, incontinent of urine in casualty	Observe for incontinence Offer bottle.

Table 12.2 (continued)

ADL	Normal state	On admission	Actions
Skin	INTACT	Semi-conscious	Turn hourly
Mobility	SC	Semi-conscious ? Rt hemiparesis	Bed rest
Rest and sleep	SC		
Communications	SC	Semi-conscious ? some difficulty with speech	Answer patient and relatives questions
Sexuality			
Work and leisure	Retired		
Hygiene and grooming	SC		

Practice tip

Abbreviations

In the above chart you will see several examples of abbreviations: ADL = activity of daily living; SC = self-caring; GCS = Glasgow Coma Scale.

Many abbreviations are used in health care and especially in nursing and medical notes. It is a legal requirement that documentation is clearly written and understood by all so it is very important that only accepted abbreviations are used. In your general reading, notice what accepted abbreviations are used and try to ascertain which are commonly accepted (e.g. TPR) and which are more doubtful (e.g. Rt). There is a need to avoid risk of confusion, for example what does MI mean? Consider how such confusion might be avoided.

Activity 12.11

Now put yourself in the shoes of Staff Nurse Jenny Jones. What might you have done differently over the first 24 hours and why? Consider the merits and shortcomings of Frank Sergeant's immediate plan of care with a colleague. How well does it:

- address Frank Sergeant's immediate needs and those of his family?
- reflect on the function of an emergency assessment ward?

Frank Sargeant is shortly due for transfer to the acute stroke unit, so try finding out about the purpose of such a unit, consider possible benefits and limitations.

Evidence-based practice

The nature and purpose of stroke units

The quality of care received by stroke patients in acute wards has been questioned by a number of authors over a long period of time (Stockwell 1972; Patrick 1972; Hamrin 1982; and Gibbon 1991). Studies in community nursing by Kratz (1978) and Gibbon (1993) describe a similar picture, contrasting it with the care available in stroke units. There have been a large number of randomised controlled trials comparing care provided in stroke units with that in acute medical and care of the elderly units. These trials demonstrate that patients who are cared for in a stroke unit have a lower rate of mortality and morbidity than those who are cared for in acute medical and care of the elderly units (Stroke Unit Trialists' Collaboration 1995).

Rehabilitation

The next day Frank Sargeant is transferred to the hospital's acute stroke unit. His rehabilitation needs will have to be assessed by the multi-disciplinary team.

Activity 12.12

Many rehabilitation activities require specialist input from different members of the multi-disciplinary team. Frank Sargeant may well need a range of specialist interventions built into his plan of care. Some of these might include compensatory training, managing cognitive and perceptual deficits, and managing speech and language disorders; you may like to look out for opportunities in practice to learn more about these. Try to arrange visits to rehabilitation areas and negotiate opportunities to work alongside members of the multi-disciplinary team.

Working in a multi-disciplinary team

Waters and Luker (1996) suggest that multi-disciplinary teamwork is central to the policy and practice of care of the elderly, and further suggest that it is this notion of multi-disciplinary teamwork which distinguishes care of the elderly from other medical specialities. Multi-professional teamwork is recognised as the approach to complex problems where the services of more than one occupational group are necessary ʳ improve patient outcomes. It has to be recognised, however, that each of the occupational groups have their own unique contribution to make in addition to the contribution to the team.

Recognising that the needs of Frank Sargeant might be best met by the services of more than one professional group goes some way to encouraging the development of a multi-professional team, and it follows that there must be some understanding of how that team will work together. It is evident, however, that tensions can exist between team members and efforts have to be made by all parties to ensure that the work of the team is towards the common good.

The factors promoting interdisciplinary teams can be conceptualised as gains for the recipients of care and the organisation, that is third-party gains, rather than for the individual profession (first-party gains); hence the *raison d'être* of rehabilitation teams is to improve patient outcomes. Forbes and Fitzsimons (1993) propose that the individual's professional autonomy, and hence their claim to professionalism, is not eclipsed by the development of an interdisciplinary team, but is enhanced in concert with the other disciplines. The notion of the whole being greater than the sum of its parts is consistent with a high value being placed on an interdisciplinary team in rehabilitative care.

An interdisciplinary approach requires, at least, that the members of the team collaborate with other colleagues and other professional groups. Forbes and Fitzsimons (1993) refer to education as being the key to interdisciplinary collaboration. Their exploration of the term 'collaborate' brings together two connotations: first working together *especially in a joint intellectual effort*; and second *cooperating reasonably, as with an enemy occupying one's own country*. The second interpretation of the word is interesting in that it raises issues of territory and domains of practice. This is of particular interest in the context of a rehabilitation team, where individual disciplines lay claim to specific areas of practice (territory), yet are requested to collaborate (work cooperatively) with other disciplines who may or may not have the skills or knowledge.

A review of the literature does not provide encouraging reading for those wishing to develop and sustain an interdisciplinary team in practice. The issues which appear to drive a team together include a shared desire to provide optimal patient care (Mullins et al 1994), allowing the patient to achieve maximum potential in terms of independence (Pearson 1983), and some recognition that complex problems require services of more than one occupational group (Mariano 1989). Other reasons for a team approach are organisational imperatives (McEwen 1994).

Factors militating against interdisciplinary teams include professional jealousies, role boundaries (distinct and indistinct) (Brunning and Huffington 1985; Strasser et al 1994), ignorance/lack of education, loss of autonomy, threat to professional status, role specialisation, staff turnover, physical rehabilitation territory (Forbes and Fitzsimons 1993); unequal social proximity, high value placed on own role (Pearson 1983); time of referral/access to patient, organisation management, lack of team learning, role perceptions, expectations of others, lack of respect for others (Fried and Leatt 1986, Strasser et al 1994); and perceived poor problem solving in others, and increased defensiveness when 'pushed' to work as a team (Fried and Leatt 1986; Mariano 1989).

Activity 12.13

Research would suggest that there is much to gain from a multi-disciplinary approach to rehabilitation and yet the realities are that when any group gets together there are challenges that have to be addressed. Think of your own experiences of working in a group, or as a team, can you relate to the commentary above? Identify the specific factors and behaviours, which made it a comfortable and enabling, experience and think about how this could be applied in practice to promote holistic care and the achievement of agreed patient outcomes. If you have worked in a team where there were tensions, how were these addressed and remedied?

Frank Sargeant has arrived in the acute stroke unit accompanied by his wife. He still has a right sided hemiparesis and some difficulty with communication although he is now fully conscious and continent. Frank is feeling very depressed about the future.

Ongoing assessment

It is imperative to undertake a thorough assessment of the patient, initially to confirm the diagnosis of stroke, and second, to prescribe a patient management plan. The complex nature of stroke necessitates the use of numerous assessments and these assessments are completed by the respective members of the multi-professional team. As we have acknowledged, each member of the team has a unique contribution to make in addition to the core aspects of care and patient management.

Professional conversation

Jennifer Shepherd, nurse practitioner

'Although the initial assessment is undertaken on admission to hospital, I always see this as an on-going process which informs the patient management plan. This in turn informs discharge planning and post inpatient care. In addition to the physical examination, which will be made by the doctor, assessments will be needed relating to Frank Sergeant's psychosocial status as well as detailed assessments of his functional ability. The multi-professional nature of stroke care requires team work and we use single patient documentation (team notes) to facilitate this. It is working very well, as it avoids unnecessary duplication of records and everybody is kept updated on progress.'

The use of scales to assess progress by measurement offers a tangible way to monitor patient progress. A number of different assessment tools are available which are appropriate for assessing disability following stroke. These include, amongst others: the Activity of Daily Living Scales; Barthel Index; Rivermead ADL Scale; and the Nottingham 10-Point ADL Scale. In the acute stroke unit the team constantly review existing tools and seek out new developments. Some of these tools are discussed below.

Practice Tips

Measurement tools

Measurement tools have long been established to quantify aspects of patient care and this is no less true for disabled people, including scales specifically designed for stroke patients (Gibbon 1991). The battery of measurement tools includes those measuring impairment, the physiological consequences of pathology, disability, the functional consequences and handicap, and the social consequences. It is therefore important to consider what domain is to be assessed prior to employing an assessment tool.

Activity 12.14

Find some examples in practice of different assessment tools and consider what aspects of assessment are amenable to measurement. Think about the form of assessment tool that could be used as part of Frank Sergeant's rehabilitation in assessing progress in the biological, psychological and social domains. (Refer also to Chapters 10, 11 and 13 on nutrition, hydration and pain respectively).

A range of assessment tools

Activity of Daily Living Scales are commonly used measurement scales, which are based upon activities of daily living (ADLs). This concept will be reasonably familiar to most nurses although it should not be confused with Activities of Living (ALs) as commonly associated with the Activities of Living Model (Roper et al 1985). ADLs have become the mainstay of disability measurement.

A number of these scales are general measures of disability which can be used for a range of client groups, whereas others have been specifically designed for the stroke patient. The commonly used scales include the *Barthel Index* (Mahoney and Barthel 1965) which is a summed index (1–3 points per item), validated for assessing self-care, continence and mobility, and can be administered through formal testing, interview or informal assessment.

The Rivermead ADL Scale (Whiting and Lincoln 1980) was devised for use with stroke and head-injury patients and includes additional domestic items. It is a hierarchical scale and is administered as a formal assessment. It was revalidated for use with elderly stroke patients, which resulted in some re-ordering of items (Lincoln and Edmans 1990).

The Nottingham 10-Point ADL Scale (Ebrahim et al 1985) was designed for use with stroke inpatients and, like the Rivermead Scale, is hierarchical but does not include additional domestic items. The Nottingham 10-Point Scale can, however, be administered by observation, interview or by post.

Using tools would appear to be helpful to facilitate speed of assessment, ensuring that the same things are measured in the same way by each member of the multi-professional team. They also facilitate effective communication. However, they need to have been proven to be effective before they are implemented in practice.

Evidence-based practice

Accurate assessment tools

Assessment tools need to demonstrate **validity**; that is, they test what they are intended to test. They must also be **reliable**; that is, the same score is attained when applied to the same patient on two separate occasions unless a real change has occurred. The issue of **sensitivity** is closely related to reliability in that a measure of change is only useful if it can detect change relevant to the user (Wade 1988). Tools used in clinical practice must be simple, but not at the expense of reliability or sensitivity. It is unlikely that a single tool will be developed that can usefully address all areas of disability.

Practitioners require tools that, in addition to their length, simplicity and sensitivity, can be used effectively and that facilitate communication between disciplines. The sensitivity of a tool may be compromised for the sake of simplicity. A single summary score which conveys the level of functional ability from one practitioner to another lends weight to the adoption of a hierarchical (Guttman) scale such as the Nottingham 10-Point Scale or Rivermead ADL Scale. The Barthel Index, whilst recognised to be a good measure of physical disability and requiring only a few minutes to complete, is not hierarchical and therefore does not end up with a summated score which gives a clear indication of the level of disability. That is, the overall score can be gained by a variety of abilities. The completed assessment could, however, be communicated either verbally or in writing in a matter of seconds.

Frank Sargeant has experienced quite severe depression following his stroke, symptoms which are distressing, but not unusual following such a devastating event. Assessment of mental state is of great importance and assessment tools have been developed to assess anxiety, mood and other psychological traits. These tools are useful when used as an adjunct to clinical decision making; they can provide objective data on patient progress and give early warning of possible complications.

Investigations

These are required to confirm the diagnosis, to check for further pathology (e.g. has Frank also had a myocardial infarction?) and to establish base lines against which to measure change. In Frank's case the medical staff decided to request:

- Full blood count
- Erythrocyte sedimentation rate (ESR)
- Carotid doppler examination
- Electrocardiogram (ECG)
- Computerised Tomography (CT) Scan
- Magnetic resonance imaging (MRI) scan
- Cerebral angiography

Activity 12.15

Put yourself in the role of the staff nurse caring for Frank Sargeant. How would you go about providing Frank and his wife with a clear explanation of the meaning and purpose of these investigations? What would the nurse's role be in preparing Frank for these investigations and caring for him during and after the investigation?

Following the initial multi-disciplinary assessment on admission to the stroke unit a plan of care was developed for the first 24 hours. The assessment was conducted by different members of the multi-disciplinary team who communicated with each other to avoid duplication and repetition. The team now regularly meets together, involving Frank and his wife to review the care and treatment plan, check progress and adjust goals. Over the first 24 hours it was decided to:

- Monitor temperature, pulse, respiration and blood pressure
- Continue with neurological assessment
- Action swallowing assessment and request special diet if needed
- Monitor continence and elimination
- Carry out moving and handling assessment
- Commence fluid balance recordings
- Estimate tissue viability rating
- Apply TED stockings

- Mr and Mrs Sargeant:
  - give introductory ward information
  - assess level of understanding of the situation
  - instigate initial planning regarding discharge
- Set date for first interdisciplinary meeting with Mr and Mrs Sargeant

In addition the medical staff included:

- Prescribe if required:
  - intravenous (IV) fluid
  - subcutaneous heparin
  - dexamethazone

These interventions were incorporated into Frank Sergeant's plan of care.

The evolving care plan

Assessment is ongoing and documentation is kept updated and the care plan amended as Frank's condition changes. Members of the multi-professional team communicate changes in his condition, and consequent changes in care, to each other. This is effectively cascaded to others through written and verbal reports.

Activity 12.16

Reflect on the above action points, what information would you expect Mr and Mrs Sargeant would want regarding:

- The type of diet most suitable now and as the condition improves.
- Why IV fluids may be required.
- The function of heparin and why this might help Mr Sargeant.

One of the main concerns of the team is to avoid the potential of complications that follow stroke. A number of preventative strategies have therefore been introduced into the care plan. Stroke is a major illness which can kill at the time of onset. A large number of people do, however, survive the stroke, but are at risk of developing complications. Some of these are as a direct consequence of reduced mobility or bed rest. These include: depression; deep vein thrombosis (DVT) which can lead to pulmonary embolus; pneumonia/aspiration pneumonia; pressure ulcers; urinary incontinence; spasticity; contractures; shoulder pain/dislocation; and malnutrition.

Activity 12.17

Before reading on you may like to consider what you know about each of these complications and the effects that they would have on Frank Sargeant. Find out why they occur and what actions might be taken to prevent them.

Depression is frequently seen following stroke and there is little doubt that stroke can give rise to considerable feelings of misery. Depression can act as a barrier to rehabilitation in that the patient lacks motivation to seek independence. Frank and his family will need time and space to grieve and adjust to the change in body image and any longer term residual disability that there might be. Being listened to and acknowledged, involved and empowered to make decisions helps preserve self-esteem. The poor handling of the grieving process is therefore seen as the predominant cause of the common problem of post-stroke depression. (Kirkevold 1997). The nurse's task therefore is to be instrumental in the reduction of the incidence of depression by the level of emotional support that they deliver. (See Chapter 9 on nursing older people, which explores the grieving process.)

Frank has retained his cognitive and perceptual function and can engage in conversation. However, where there is significant cognitive and perceptual dysfunction it can be challenging to provide interventions which can lift mood. Company, the use of communication aids, and sensitive use of distraction through, for example, the radio or television can all help to lift the mood. Medication in the form of antidepressants may sometimes be required.

> ### Activity 12.18
>
> You may wish to check out how you can best recognise the characteristics of depression, especially in patients who have difficulty communicating. Access a textbook on mental health nursing.

> ### Care Plan
> - Frank and his family will need time and space to adjust to the change in body image and any longer term residual disability. Set aside time for listening to their needs and concerns, keeping them informed and involved in all decisions.
> - Monitor mood through sleep pattern, appetite, activity and Frank's desire to communicate.

Deep vein thrombosis refers to the development of a blood clot in one of the large veins usually in the lower limb. This may go undetected as Frank may have a loss of sensation in the leg as a consequence of his stroke. Careful observation for signs associated with deep vein thrombosis have been instigated. Preventative measures to reduce the likelihood of deep vein thrombosis have included the use of elasticated stockings to reduce the risk of thrombus formation. These 'thrombo-embolic deterrent' (TED) stockings should be carefully fitted as they work by exerting an external pressure on the legs, and subsequently the veins which force the blood back towards the heart. The stockings are designed to compensate for the loss of the 'muscle pump' which occurs in normal activity thereby assisting venous return. The one-way valves in the veins ensure that blood travels to the heart. Early mobilisation and regular and frequent passive limb exercises help to reduce the risk of developing deep vein thrombosis.

> ### Care plan
> - Application of TED stockings
> - Observe for redness, tenderness/pain in calf
> - Early mobilisation and regular and frequent passive limb exercises

Pneumonia is a risk in all patients with reduced mobility and a particular problem in a person like Frank, following stroke, as a high proportion of patients have swallowing difficulties and lose their swallowing reflex. Saliva and aspirate fluid can more easily enter the lungs and create an environment rich for micro-organism growth and subsequent chest infection and pneumonia.

> ### Activity 12.19
> Find out about swallowing deficit and the appropriate interventions used to maintain hydration and nutrition. Who can undertake a swallowing assessment?

> ### Care plan
> - Frequent positional change and chest physiotherapy to reduce the risk of pneumonia;
> - Assess for swallowing deficit.
> - Assist with choice of appropriate foods
> - Help to regain independence with feeding

Pressure ulcers can result from inadequate perfusion of the tissues as a result of reduced mobility and loss of sensation, for example by being confined to bed or chair. Risk increases due to a variety of factors including: debilitation confusion incontinence, poor diet and inadequate nutrition. Regular changes of position, the use of pressure relieving aids, and interventions that address the risk factors will help to prevent pressure ulcers occurring. (See chapter 10 on Nutrition.)

> ### Care plan
> - Assess for pressure ulcer risk
> - Assist with frequent change of position (at least 2-hourly)
> - Assist with washing and choice of clothing to reduce accumulation of sweat

> ### Activity 12.20
>
> Use a pressure sore risk assessment tool to determine whether Frank Sargeant is at high or low risk of developing pressure ulcers. Identify those areas of the body most at risk and consider the actions the multi-professional team may take to reduce the risk of pressure ulcer development.

Urinary tract infection and incontinence can be distressing symptoms resulting from the stroke or its effects; thankfully, Frank Sargeant quickly regained continence following his stroke. Around 23% to 51% of stroke patients experience alterations in their urinary continence to some degree. These alterations usually occur during the acute phase and over the following sub-acute and rehabilitative phases, a significant number of these patients will recover their normal function with no interventions being required. Problems that may remain include urinary frequency, dysuria, urge incontinence and urinary retention.

Urinary tract infection is common in patients with reduced mobility and particularly with those who are incontinent of urine. High standards of nursing care, paying particular attention to adequate hydration, positioning and hygiene, can help prevent urinary tract infection.

> ### Care plan
> - Encourage fluids and initially monitor fluid intake and output
> - Monitor pattern of elimination for signs of urgency, dysuria, and constipation
> - Discreetly place urinal within easy reach, assess level of independence and assist if required

Practice tip

Always assess the patient's level of pre-stroke continence. In their study Borrie et al (1996) noted that 17% of patients had pre-stroke urinary incontinence to some degree.

Contractures can be a distressing complication following stroke when the limbs contract towards the body, resulting in deformity and loss of functional ability. Contractures can be painful and once a limb is contracted, it is difficult to extend it again.

Evidence-based Practice

Consensus regarding positioning which maintains 'reflex inhibiting patterns' (Carr and Kenney 1992)

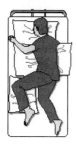

The following positions have been advocated following stroke in order to reduce the risk of spasticity and contractures.

These result from a consensus of opinion reached by Carr and Kenney taken from commonly used texts relating to recom-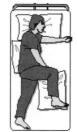mended postures to be adopted following stroke. You may need to use a dictionary to identify the meaning of the anatomical terms used.

(Reproduced by kind permission of Peter Gardiner, medical illustrator)

Position	Lying on unaffected side	Lying on affected side	Supine-lying	Sitting-up in bed	Sitting in a chair
Part of Body					
Head and neck	Neutral, symmetrical position	Neutral, symmetrical position	Support on pillow in 'slight' flexion	Midline position	Midline position
Affected upper limb	Shoulder protracted and arm forward on pillow. Wrist in neutral position. Fingers extended. Thumb abducted.	Shoulder protracted to 90° of body if possible. Arm forward. Elbow extended. Forearm, hand supinated. Wrist neutral. Fingers extended. Thumb abducted.	Shoulder protracted and arm forward on pillow. Wrist in neutral position. Fingers extended. Thumb abducted.	Shoulder protracted and arm forward. Elbow flexed. Hand pronated. Wrist in neutral position. Fingers extended. Thumb abducted.	Shoulder protracted and arm forward. Hand pronated. Wrist in neutral position. Fingers extended. Thumb abducted.
Trunk	Straight	Straight	Straight	Straight and supported by pillows.	Straight and supported.
Affected lower limb	Hip forward, flexed, supported. Knee forward, flexed supported.	Knee flexed.	Hip forward on pillow. Nothing against soles of feet.	Legs straight out in front.	Hips flexed at 90° to trunk. Knees flexed at 90° to hips. Equal weight through both hips. Feet flat on floor.
Unaffected lower limb(s)	Behind affected limb.	Knee flexed? Supporting pillow.			

Strategic positioning will reduce the risk of contracture formation, whilst additionally ensuring the optimum functional position which will assist those who have the potential to make a full or near full recovery.

Key positioning enables the patient to adopt a neutral or normal posture. The aim is to reduce spasticity and contractures by maintaining 'reflex inhibiting patterns of posture.

Care plan

- Adhere to positioning guidelines which maintain reflex inhibiting patterns.

Activity 12.21

Check the meaning of the word 'spasticity'.

Shoulder pain is one consequence of the affected arm not being positioned or supported appropriately. The weight of the arm has the tendency to allow the head of the humerus to dislocate or 'subluxate' from the ball and socket joint formed with the scapula. Inappropriate moving and handling, such as repositioning the patient by using the arm as a lever, or raising the patient by gripping them either by the arm or under the arm, can cause or exacerbate the problem of shoulder pain and dislocation. Correct moving and handling techniques and correct positioning as described in the box above can help reduce the risk of these complications.

Care plan

- Apply moving and handling strategies that minimise risk of shoulder injury.
- Particular care to be observed when assisting with bathing, dressing and walking practice.

Activity 12.22

Find out what is the latest local guidance for moving and handling, applied to the care of a person following stroke; and when in the practice setting, observe if these recommendations are followed. Discuss with colleagues the challenges of encouraging patient independence, whilst being responsible for their safety. Find out how each member of the multi-professional team maintains their skill and keeps up to date with evidence-based practice in relation to moving and handling.

Practice tip

Throughout your nursing career it is essential that you always keep up to date with the recommendations about moving and handling. Being appropriately assertive is an essential nursing skill, which will also enable you to ensure that those around you are also following recommendations which provide safe and effective practice in this area.

Activity 12.23

You may like to consider how Mrs Sargeant and other family members can be directly involved to help prevent complications of stroke. Also, what about Frank's friends? What support might they need to be able to be involved? In practice observe if relatives and friends are actively encouraged to play a part in rehabilitation. Consider the benefits and challenges.

Five days after his admission to hospital Frank Sargeant is transferred to the stroke rehabilitation unit in a community hospital nearer his home, where his planned rehabilitation continues. Frank is making excellent progress, with sensation and power returning to his affected limbs. He is mobile, although he does require the use of a walking aid. He is eating well, generally caring for himself and much more optimistic about the future.

Activity 12.24

There is now an opportunity to reflect back on the specific role of the nurse in Frank's rehabilitation. Look back at the different interventions which were included in his care plan. How many of these do you consider Frank's named nurse might be responsible for directly managing and evaluating?

The role of the nurse in stroke rehabilitation

Whilst some research has identified specific nursing roles, others have shown some nurses to be less clear of their rehabilitation role. With an increasing emphasis on interprofessional and multi-disciplinary working, it is essential that all nurses are helped to clarify and develop a clear understanding of their specific contribution to the team.

Researchers such as Gibbons (1993); O'Connor (1997); and Kirkevold (1997) have identified emerging and developing roles of nurses working in rehabilitation. Other findings have tended to support the perception of the nurse as the natural manager or coordinator of patient care with a 24-hour presence rather than having more specific role definitions (Waters (1991, 1996); Myco (1984); Nolan (1998a, 1998b, 1998c).

By the early 1990s, O'Connor (1993) had noted the development of a role for the nurse within stroke rehabilitation that was non-therapeutic and managerial in emphasis. This managerial role was reinforced by the importance of the 'understudy' role, a function of this 24-hour presence, which was portrayed as central to the nurse's standing in the multi-disciplinary team. There was, however, an emerging category of specialised care noted by others (Waters 1991, 1996; Gibbon 1993).

Waters (1991, 1996), who had studied nurses working in elderly care rehabilitation wards, found that they did not consider themselves to have a major contribution in the rehabilitation process. The areas of work she identified, although important for the patient's overall well-being, were seen as 'maintaining the patient' so that others, namely the therapists, could undertake rehabilitation. At that time, Waters considered nursing as an under-utilised resource which nursing managers had to develop.

Nolan (1998a, 1998b and 1998c) also found that whilst activities were clearly defined for the nurse in the acute setting, it is the acute orientated physical activities that are more visibly being carried out, with the psychological, emotional and 'family' orientated aspects being less well addressed. This was partly supported by O'Connor (1997) who identified that specific care in rehabilitation was care in which the nurses believed that they had particular skills, above and beyond the remit of the 'average' nurse. Interventions required for caring for relatives; giving psychological care; continence care; and handling and positioning skills were areas in which they needed additional skills. However, in 1997 Kirkevold identified four specific nursing functions directly related to the nurses role in rehabilitation, and these are set out in the box below.

Evidence-based practice

Rehabilitation nursing: four integrated nursing functions

- **Interpretative Function** Educating and supporting the patient and their carer through the delivery of the information required to understand, comprehend and make sense of the changes that have come about so suddenly due to their stroke. Information giving concerning stroke itself, its treatment and prognosis are seen as central to the nurse's role in this function.

- **Consoling Function** The support of the patient and their family through the emotional trauma of the stroke experience. The ability of the nurse to facilitate the patients' and their carers' normal grieving process in the maintenance of hope and the prevention of depression is central to this function. The grieving to be experienced after the loss of the previously known self and loved one due to the stroke is to be expected and appropriate emotional care has to be planned.

- **Conserving Function** a dynamic delivery of essential care that prepares and maintains the patient in as fit a state as possible to fully partake in their rehabilitation programme. The patient can only fully partake in rehabilitation if they are as fit as possible to do so.
- **Integrative Function** Nurses translate the skills relearned in the therapy sessions, which usually take place in different distinct areas to the every-day situations that patients experience. Hence patients and their carers rehearse skills in 'real' situations so that skills have a purpose; they become meaningful activities in that they can be related to the future lived experience and, if possible, integrated with a social focus.

(Kirkevold 1997)

It is suggested by Myco (1984) that where nurses have lacked role clarity, this may have resulted from a lack of research, a superficial view of the nurse's role presented within the literature and a failure of nurse educators to adequately integrate rehabilitation into the nursing curriculum.

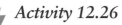

Activity 12.25

Having considered the above empirical studies, reflect again on the role of the nurse in stroke rehabilitation. Consider the relationship between the picture of stroke rehabilitation that you have, and that which would adequately describe rehabilitation in general.

Frank is offered the opportunity to be assessed at home by the occupational therapist, to see how he might cope and to see whether any specific equipment might need to be installed before it is safe for him to be discharged home. A convenient time is arranged with Frank's wife and you (as the student) have an opportunity to go along.

Activity 12.26

- Consider the purpose of the home visit: what assessments may be undertaken, what recommendations made and outcomes achieved?
- Consider what anxieties the progress from hospital to home may create for Frank and his family: what services may be available to alleviate some if not all of these concerns?
- What is intermediate care, how relevant is this to Mr and Mrs Sargeant?

Read National Service Framework for Older People (DoH 2001, ch. 3).

Frank demonstrated his ability to be quite independent in most activities of living. He had, however, agreed to have his bed moved downstairs temporarily and a grab rail fitted in the downstairs shower and toilet. Luckily, there is level access to the property so no ramps or other alterations would be required. Frank returned home and although he has been discharged from hospital, the policy of the stroke unit is to visit the patient and their family one month after discharge to see how things are going.

Both Frank's nurse and the occupational therapist (OT) arranged to meet Frank and his wife about a month after discharge. After the visit they recorded the following in Frank Sergeant's notes:

20/10 4:30 p.m.
Mr Sargeant was very pleased to see us both and quickly commented that he missed the unit, especially the company of the other patients. While his wife was in the room he was cheerful and repeatedly said that things were going well. When his wife and Sarah (OT) went out to the kitchen, his mood changed and he was visibly upset. Whilst he appreciated that his wife was doing her best, he complained that she did too much for him and that he felt that he had 'gone backwards' since he left the unit. He also mentioned that he thought his wife was tired and worried but would not say why.

Additional note by OT:
In the kitchen Mrs Sargeant burst into tears and said that she did not know how much longer she would be able to cope. She had hurt her back lifting her husband out of his chair, even though she knew that he was quite capable of getting up himself. Also, she was dreadfully worried by the pressures on the rest of the family created by her having to care 24 hours a day for her husband.
Both the Nurse and OT independently recorded Mr Sergeant's Barthel Index as 18

Activity 12.27

- List the problems that may well have arisen since Mr Sargeant's discharge.
- Reflect back on his care and think about how these problems might have been prevented.
- Consider the role of intermediate care services, would this be an appropriate resource for Mr and Mrs Sargeant to access?

Your list may have included issues which relate to:

- caregiver burden
- caregiver burnout
- family overcompensation
- family role conflict

Activity 12.28

Think about what each of these terms mean. Try coming up with a definition.

The last six months have been difficult as Frank and his wife have adjusted to the fact that life has to be different. Whilst Frank has continued with many of his interests, he finds the residual weakness in his arm and leg frustrating. Sometimes he vents his anger on the family, but they have all developed their own coping strategies. Mrs Sargeant has found particular support from the local branch of the Stroke Association, and although Frank is reluctant to attend she often helps out at the day centre. Frank has eventually given up smoking, which to him is a great achievement. They have also turned the downstairs dining-room into a proper bedroom; one of the things that the Sergeant's were reluctant to talk about was their sexual needs. It transpired that one of the reasons for the initial lack of progress following discharge had been the need for Frank and his wife to sleep in separate rooms, they have always been sexually active and they are now happily reunited.

Within this chapter you have been introduced to a large number of concepts. Now that we have concluded our look at the experiences of Mr and Mrs Sargeant, in the final activity it is timely to invite you to reflect on the positive and negative impact that terminology has on client care.

Activity 12.29

- Consider the two sets of WHO definitions below, why might there have been a need to update these definitions between 1980 and 1999?
- Are there still short-comings in the later definitions?

Rehabilitation and the World Health Organisation (WHO 1980) definitions

Impairment

Any loss or abnormality of psychological, physiological or anatomical structure or function.

Disability

Any restriction or lack (resulting from an impairment) of ability to perform an activity in the manner or within the range considered normal for a human being.

Handicap

A disturbance for a given individual, resulting from an impairment or disability, that limits or prevents the fulfilment of a role that is normal (depending on age, sex, social and cultural factors) for that individual.

WHO International Committee on Impairment, Disability and Handicap (ICIDH) (WHO 1999) definitions

Impairment

A loss or abnormality of body structure or of psychological function.

Activity

The nature and extent of functioning at the level of the person. Activities may be limited in nature, duration and quality.

Participation

The nature and extent of a person's involvement in life situations in relationship to impairments, activities, health conditions and contextual factors. Participation may be restricted in nature, duration and quality.

Disablement

An umbrella term that covers all the negative dimensions (impairment, activity limitations and participation restrictions) either together or separately.

Conclusion

Through the scenario you will have experienced some of the challenges and identified some of the essential skills which nurses and other professionals utilise in the challenging field of rehabilitation following stroke. Many of these will be to do with effective communication throughout assessment, the planning of care and its delivery. Ask any patient, or their family, what is most important to them and many will tell you that their needs are best met when professionals communicate with each other and actually work together. It will have been important to reflect on research about working in teams and how we can work together even more effectively (Davis and O'Connor 1999).

Frank Sargeant and his family found it difficult to come to terms and adjust to the major changes to their routine following Frank's stroke. You will see the distress this caused not only in the early stages, but also later when everything seemed to be improving. This is a lesson for us all: the importance of long-term support which someone must arrange and be responsible for. It can be very convenient for planned care to just cease and, with it, all support to the client and their family. Thankfully, in Frank's case this did not happen.

We have posed many questions but by no means have we provided all the answers, for this was never the intention. Through the various activities and resources, you will have found an opportunity to explore and question the way that rehabilitation is provided and make comparisons with those services that you are familiar with.

Now reflect back on your experiences and try to answer one final question. Just what is meant by rehabilitation, and what more do you need to know?

References

Borrie, M. J., Campbell, A. J., Caradoc-Davies, T. H. (1986) Urinary incontinence after stroke: a prospective study. *Age and Ageing* 15, pp. 177.

Brunning, H., Huffington, C. (1985) Altered images *Nursing Times* 81 (31), pp. 24–7.

Carr, E. K., Kenney, F. D. (1992) Positioning of the stroke patient: a review of the literature. *International Journal of Nursing Studies* 29 (4), pp. 355–69.

Davis, S., O'Connor, S. E. (1999). *Rehabilitation Nursing: Foundations for Practice.* London: Ballière Tindall.

Department of Health (1992) *The Health of the Nation.* London: HMSO.

Ebrahim, S., Nouri, F., Barer, D. (1985) Measuring disability after stroke. *Journal of Epidemiology and Community Health* 39, pp. 86–9.

Forbes, E. J., Fitzsimons, V. (1993) Education: the key for holistic interdisciplinary collaboration. *Holistic Nursing Practice* 7 (4), pp. 1–10.

Fried, B. J., Leatt, P. (1986) Role perception among occupational groups in an ambulatory care setting. *Human Relations* 39 (12), pp. 1155–74.

Gibbon, B. (1991) Measuring stroke recovery. *Nursing Times* 87 (44), pp. 32–4.

Gibbon, B. (1993) Implications for nurses in approaches to the management of stroke rehabilitation. *International Journal of Nursing Studies* 30 (2), pp. 133–44.

Hamrin, E. (1982) Attitudes of nursing staff in general medical wards towards the activation of stroke patients. *Journal of Advanced Nursing* 7, pp. 33–42.

Kirkevold, M. (1997) The role of nursing in the rehabilitation of acute stroke patients: toward a unified theoretical perspective. *Advanced Nursing Science* 19 (4), pp. 55–64.

Kratz, C. R. (1978) *Care of the Long-Term Sick in the Community: Particularly Patients with Stroke.* Edinburgh: Churchill Livingstone.

Lincoln, N. B., Edmans, J. A. (1990) A re-evaluation of the Rivermead ADL Scale for elderly patients with stroke. *Age and Ageing* 19, pp. 19–24.

Mahoney, F. I., Barthel, D. W. (1965) Functional evaluation: the Barthel Index. *Maryland State Medical Journal* 14, pp. 61–5.

Mariano, C. (1989) The case for interdisciplinary collaboration. *Nursing Outlook* 37 (6), pp. 285–8.

McEwen, M. (1994) Promoting interdisciplinary collaboration. *Nursing and Health Care* 15 (6), pp. 304–07.

Mullins, L. L., Keller, J. R., Chaney, J. M. (1994) A systems and cognitive functioning approach to team functioning in physical rehabilitation settings. *Rehabilitation Psychology* 39 (3), pp. 161–78.

Myco, F. (1984) Stroke and its rehabilitation: the perceived role. *Journal of Advanced Nursing* 9, pp. 439–7.

Nolan, M., Nolan, J. (1998a) Stroke 2: expanding the nurse's role in stroke rehabilitation. *British Journal of Nursing* 7 (7), pp. 388–92.

Nolan, M., Nolan, J. (1998b) Stroke 1: a paradigm case in nursing rehabilitation. *British Journal of Nursing* 7 (6), pp. 316–22.

Nolan, M., Nolan, J. (1998c) Rehabilitation: scope for involvement in current practice. *British Journal of Nursing* 7 (9), pp. 522–6.

O'Connor, S. E. (1993) Nursing and rehabilitation: the interventions of nurses in stroke patient care. *Journal of Clinical Nursing* 2, pp. 29–34.

O'Connor, S. E. (1997) *An investigation to determine the nature of nursing in stroke units.* Unpublished PhD thesis. University of Southampton, Southampton.

Patrick, C. (1972) Forgotten patients on medical wards. *Canadian Nurse* 68, pp. 27–31.

Pearson, P. H. (1983) The interdisciplinary team process or the professional's Tower of Babel. *Developmental Medicine and Child Neurology* 25 (3), pp. 390–5.

Roper, N., Logan, W. W., Tierney, A. J. (1985) *The Elements of Nursing.* Edinburgh: Churchill Livingstone.

Rudd, A.G., Irwin, P., Rutledge, Z., Lowe, D., Morris, R., Pearson, M.G. (1999) The national sentinal audit of stroke: a tool for raising standards of care. *Journal of the Royal College of Physicians* 30, pp. 460–4.

Strasser, D. C., Falconer, J. A., Martino-Saltzmann, D. (1994) The rehabilitation team: staff perspectives of the hospital environment, and interprofessional relations. *Archives of Physical Medicine and Rehabilitation* 75, pp. 177–82.

Stroke Unit Trialists' Collaboration (1995) A systematic review of specialist multi-disciplinary team (stroke unit) care for stroke inpatients. The *Cochrane Database* of *Systematic Reviews* Issue 1.

Stockwell, F. (1972) *The Unpopular Patient.* London: RCN.

Wade, D. T. (1988) Measurement in rehabilitation. *Age and Ageing* 17 pp. 289–92.

Waters, K. (1991) *The role of the nurse in rehabilitation of elderly people in hospital.* Unpublished PhD thesis. University of Manchester, Manchester.

Waters, K. R., Luker, K. A. (1996) Staff perspectives on the role of the nurse in rehabilitation wards for elderly people. *Journal of Clinical Nursing* 5, pp. 105–14.

Whiting, S., Lincoln, N. (1980) An ADL assessment for stroke patients. *Occupational Therapy* February, pp. 44–6.

Wolfe, C., Rudd, A., Beech, L. (eds) (1996) *Stroke Services and Research: An Overview with Recommendations for Future Research.* London: Stroke Association.

World Health Organisation (1980) *International Classification of Impairments, Disabilities and Handicaps.* New York: WHO.

World Health Organisation (1999) ICIDH-2 *International Classification of Functioning and Disability: Beta 2 Draft.* New York: WHO.

Resources

📖 Further reading

Department of Health (2001) *National Service Framework for Older People.* London: HMSO.

Annotated bibliography

Anderson, R. (1992) *The Aftermath of Stroke.* Cambridge: Cambridge University Press.
   Stroke affects the personal, social, professional and family lives of patients and their carers. This book is based on a study in which 173 stroke patients and their family carers were followed from the time of the stroke for a period of 18 months. It tells of their experience of the illness and examines their patterns of coping, including physical, social, economic and emotional aspects. The book is written for all health care professionals involved with stroke patients and their carers, and directs attention to the practices which can improve the quality of life for people with chronic illness.

Barer, D. H. (1991) Stroke in Nottingham: provision of nursing care and possible implications for the future. *Clinical Rehabilitation* 5, pp. 103–10.
   Report of a cross-sectional survey to measure the extent of the burden of stroke on health service resources. A total of 822 patients were surveyed out of a population of 700,000: 232 were in hospital (28%) 221 were in nursing homes (27%) and 369 at home with district nurse support (45%). District nurses spend most time with the elderly, long-standing stroke patients. Increase in the proportion of elderly in the population and improvements in medical practice, which reduce fatalities in the early stages, are likely to increase the number of elderly disabled survivors.

Braithwaite, V., McGown, A. (1993) Caregivers' emotional well-being and their capacity to learn about stroke. *Journal of Advanced Nursing* 18, pp. 195–202.
   Study examining the effect of distress on the capacity of informal care givers of stroke patients to absorb information about stroke and care giving. Care givers were given information at a seminar and were pre-and post-tested. Knowledge after the seminar was best predicted by age and pre-seminar knowledge. Emotional state did not affect how much they learnt, although emotional carers may be too shocked at the time. The data suggests that, given time to accept the care giving role, emotional care givers are receptive to learning about stroke and stroke patients' needs.

Davies, S. M. (1994) An evaluation of nurse-led team care within a rehabilitation ward for elderly people. *Journal of Clinical Nursing* 3, pp. 25–33.
   Report of small quasi-experimental study considering the introduction of nurse-led team care against quality of care, job satisfaction, length of stay (LOS). Multi-method approach. Claims for nurse-led team care is based on time and presence with patient. Nurse-led team care improved quality, but had no effect on LOS or job satisfaction. It is still not clear how many members of a team can work effectively together nor what the mechanisms are for establishing appropriate team responsibilities and interprofessional boundaries.

Gibbon, B. (1993) Implications for nurses in approaches to the management of stroke rehabilitation: a review of the literature. *International Journal of Nursing Studies* 30 (2), pp. 133–41.

Literature review paper which contends that there is no generally agreed one best way to manage stroke patients. The three principle ways, that is principles of SRU in GMW and peripatetic stroke service, are considered in the light of the implications for nurses. The author contends that understating and undervaluing nursing leads to underuse of essential resource. The findings of this paper have now been superseded by the systematic review conducted by the Stroke Unit Trialist's Collaboration.

Hamrin, E. K. F., Lindmark, B. (1990) The effect of systematic care planning after acute stroke in general hospital medical wards. *Journal of Advanced Nursing* 15, pp. 1146–53.

An experimental research project sought to determine the effect of systematic care planning on the functional outcome of stroke patients. Whilst empirical evidence of greater satisfaction for both nurses and patients was reported, no statistically significant improvement could be found. It is noteworthy that the care plans were devised by a member of the research project group rather than the ward-based nurses.

McLean, J., Roper-Hall, A., Mayer, P., Main, A. (1991) Service needs of stroke survivors and their informal carers: a pilot study. *Journal of Advanced Nursing* 16, pp 559–64.

Pilot study which sought to determine the needs of stroke patients and its survivors. Information was obtained about psychological, physical, social and service needs together with the feelings of stroke survivors and their informal carers. Methodology was by interview of patient and carers separately in their own homes. Research tools were refined and demonstrated several unmet needs in the psychosocial domain. Main finding was for more information about stroke and for counselling in relation to care problems arising out of the disability.

O'Connor, S. E. (1993) Nursing and rehabilitation: the interventions of nurses in stroke patient care. *Journal of Clinical Nursing* 2, pp. 29–34.

This paper explores the therapeutic intervention of nurses given that it has been at the centre of debate for some time. It reviews existing (English-language) literature and concludes that the role of the nurse is still vague and that if nurses fail to define it, then others will.

Bibliography

Baker, J. (1996) Shared record keeping in the multidisciplinary team. *Elderly Care* 10.(26), pp. 39–41.

Donnan, G. A. (1992) Investigation of patients with stroke and transient ischaemic attacks *The Lancet* 339, pp. 473–7.

Grenville, J., Lyne, P. (1995) Patient-centred evaluation and rehabilitative care. *Journal of Advanced Nursing* 22, pp. 965–72.

Kalra, L., Yu, G., Wilson, K., Roots, P. (1995) Medical complications during stroke rehabilitation. *Stroke* 26, pp. 990–4.

Kirkevold, M. (1990) Caring for stroke patients: heavy or exciting? *Image: Journal of Nursing Scholarship* 22 (2), pp. 79–83.

Marmot, M. G., Poulter, N. R. (1992) Primary prevention in stroke. *The Lancet* 339, pp. 344–7.

Redfern, S., Ross, M. (1999) *Nursing Older People.* 3rd Edition. Edinburgh: Churchill Livingstone.

Smith, M. (1999) *Rehabilitation in Adult Nursing Practice.* Edinburgh: Churchill Livingstone.

@ Web pages

Stroke Forum: **www.strokeforum.com**

National Rehabilitation Information Centre: **www.naric.com**

Cornucopia of rehabilitation information: **www.codi.buffalo.edu.com**

Archive of disability research:
   www.mailbox.ac.uk/lists-a-e/disability-research/archive.com

Association of Rehabilitation Nurses: **www.rehabnurse.org/index.com**

International Classification of Impairments, Activity and Participation:
   www.who.int/msa/mnh/ems/icidh/icidh.com National Service Framework for Older People: **www.doh.gov.uk/nsf/olderpeople.htm**

Essence of Care: patient-focused benchmarking for health care practitioners.
   www.doh.gov.uk/essenceofcare.htm

Useful addresses

The Stroke Association is the only UK charitable organisation solely concerned with combating stroke. It was launched in November 1991 when the Chest, Heart and Stroke Association (CHSA) handed its work in chest and heart disease to other national charities enabling it to concentrate on stroke.

The Stroke Association sponsors programmes of research, health education and community services. The association produces a wide range of publications and cassettes in clear every-day language to help patients and carers to understand stroke and its effects.

The Stroke Association can be contacted at CHSA House, Whitecross Street, London, EC1Y 8JJ.

13

Insights into Pain Management

Eileen Mann

Introduction

The aim of this chapter is to study the nursing care of patients experiencing pain. Pain is multi-dimensional, highly complex and individual to the sufferer. To add to pain's complexity, it can be acute, such as the pain associated with trauma or surgery. Pain can become chronic and long term, perhaps involving nerve damage following trauma or a virus. Pain can sometimes be present in the absence of obvious pathology, or it can be experienced as an acute exacerbation of some chronically painful condition. This may often be the case with a progressive non-malignant degenerative disease such as arthritis, or pain may be termed malignant and be associated with cancer.

Learning outcomes

The aims of this chapter are to enable the student to:

- Describe the physiology of pain.
- Explain the multi-dimensional nature of pain, exploring the reasons why it is such an individual experience.
- Evaluate a selection of methods for assessing pain in a variety of clinical settings.
- Identify what makes acute pain different to chronic pain, and why chronic pain so often defies effective treatment.
- Discuss the pharmacological and non-pharmacological strategies that can be used to manage pain effectively.
- Analyse some of the barriers to good pain management.
- Use appropriate referral channels for pain management outside the individual sphere of practice.
- Use relevant literature and research to inform practice.

Concepts

- The patient
- Chronic pain
- Acute pain
- Multidisciplinary teams
- Psychosocial influences
- Neurophysiology
- Pharmacological strategies

- Non-pharmacological strategies
- Information giving
- Empowerment
- Pain assessment
- Evidence based practice
- Clinical governance
- Interdisciplinary collaboration

As pain is a multi-dimensional phenomenon the following scenario looks at a family's experiences of pain. The experiences of the Johnson family, both past and present, will be used to explore many of the factors that make pain such a complex and challenging health care issue.

Studying a family's individual experiences of pain provides us with the opportunity to explore a wide range of scenarios. By understanding the context in which each scenario takes place, we shall be able to define the complexities, analyse

> ### Activity 13.1
>
> The complexity of pain is quite difficult to understand and if you come across any words or phrases and you are unsure of their meaning, make sure you refer to a dictionary.

the issues, and describe the challenges that each scenario poses. As nurses, more than any other health care professional, encounter patients in pain on a daily basis, it is vital that you feel confident to care for patients suffering from a vast range of painful conditions. Pain and nursing are inextricably linked, but there is evidence to show that nurses do not always fulfil the function of assessment and management of pain and some nurses are not always familiar with the methods of effective pain control (Akinsanya 1985). All pain presents health care professionals with a challenge, but acute pain is now far better understood. The last decade or so has seen great technological change in the management of acute pain. As a result, it is acute pain that will be explored in greatest depth within the following chapter.

> ## Scenario *Introducing Mary Johnson and her family*
>
> The Johnson family is currently having a particularly stressful time. Mary Johnson, who is 42 years old, is in hospital having just undergone major bowel surgery. She is anxiously awaiting the results of pathology tests following the removal of a tumour from her ascending colon. Her husband, who is 47 years old, is having to take time off work to visit and support his wife, and to look after their three children, Martin who is 13 years old, Amy who is 10 years old and Phillip who is 5 years old. Mark is also supporting his elderly parents Clive and Phyllis Johnson, who are both in their

seventies and becoming increasingly immobile. Phyllis Johnson suffers from a range of disabling conditions, including rheumatoid arthritis and osteoporosis. Clive Johnson is now experiencing increasing problems associated with his diabetes, and has recently undergone surgery for cancer of the prostate.

Mary's experience
Although Mary's postoperative pain is being reasonably well controlled via the thoracic epidural she has placed in her back, it is taking a large hourly volume of epidural solution to achieve this. Mary is still very tense and finds moving and getting comfortable difficult. Factors other than the physical painful stimulation arising from the tissue damage of surgery could explain why Mary's pain is proving more difficult to control.

Activity 13.2

Think back to a time you were in pain. Did other factors, such as fear that the pain might signify a serious injury, or boredom, make a difference to how much pain you felt?

Mary has many other stressful factors in her life that could potentially make pain more difficult to control:

- She is anxious about the pathology results as there is a chance that the tumour is malignant.
- Mary is also finding it difficult to relax. She is not sleeping particularly well and worries about how the family is coping without her.

However, before looking at some of the psychosocial factors that can impact on the successful management of pain, we need to know something of the neurophysiology of pain, as we currently understand it.

We have all experienced pain, although there are a small group of children with a very rare and usually fatal condition where they lack pain conducting nerve fibres (Melzack and Wall 1988). For the rest of us, we all have a 'pain history'. It might be that in the past our pain has been transient and short-lived. For

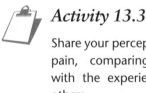

Activity 13.3

Share your perceptions of pain, comparing these with the experiences of others.

others less fortunate, it may have been experienced as a lifetime of pain which is unremitting and intractable, that is resistant to therapy. However, when we try to actually define what pain is, it puzzles and confounds a universally accepted definition. In

1986 the International Association for the Study of Pain (IASP), a group of international leaders in the field, got together and came up with an all encompassing definition:

> Pain is an unpleasant sensory and emotional experience associated with actual or potential tissue damage.

This definition at least helps to illustrate pain as a multi-factorial phenomenon, different for each individual regardless of the cause, and even different for each individual depending on the time of day, what else is going on around them, and how they are actually feeling at the time. But McCaffery (1972) put it very simply; recognising that only the individual in pain could really know what it was like, therefore she describes: 'Pain is whatever the person says it is and exists whenever he says it does.'

? **The meaning of pain – why is it that each individual's experiences of pain may differ so widely from another's?**

Despite being the same age, gender, weight and having experienced similar painful stimuli, individuals may display entirely differing degrees of pain tolerance. Some will experience intense suffering and distress while others will appear almost indifferent. Many factors can influence how much pain we feel and whether the pain causes suffering or is dismissed as being almost trivial. The following factors may be significant:

- The meaning of the pain is important, do we know its cause?
- Were we expecting it and prepared for it?
- Could it signify serious or even life-threatening disease?
- Are we from a cultural or family background that openly displays 'pain behaviour' such as crying and groaning loudly, or has our background instilled into us that it is important to maintain a 'stiff upper lip'?
- Spiritual faith may be an important factor, a strong belief that it is 'God's will' enables some people to endure hours of pain and discomfort with serenity.

So many factors seem to influence how we respond to pain. Buddhism is a philosophy specifically designed to come to terms with human suffering and fakirs or 'holy men' will walk on nails, hold a difficult posture for hours, or fast for weeks. These men practise what William James discovered in the early part of this century: 'that human beings, by changing the inner attitudes of their minds, can change the

> *Activity 13.4*
>
> Try identifying some other factors which might influence the way individuals experience pain. How much of this is culturally determined?

outer aspects of their lives' (cited in Brand and Yancey 1993). These and many more factors can contribute to the pain we feel and how we may try to control pain using various strategies and coping mechanisms (see Chapter 3 on child and family health).

Activity 13.5

A If you wish to read more on this subject, then read either of these useful chapters: Chapter 4 in Hawthorne and Redmond (1998); or Chapter 3 in Fordham and Dunn (1994).

B Access the up to date information on pain research, relief and control which can be located on the Internet (see the section on Web Pages).

The peripheral nervous system

In order for the nurse to help Mary manage her pain it is necessary to have an appreciation of the physiology of pain. If you are unfamiliar with the anatomy and physiology of the nervous system, it may be useful to access a basic introductory text before working through this chapter.

The peripheral nervous system is made up of nerve endings which have receptors embedded into them. These nerve endings join up like the roots of a tree to form larger branches. The branches then enter the central nervous system as either spinal nerves entering the spinal cord or cranial nerves that enter directly into the brain. Once part of the central nervous system, the nerves relay information to the brain where the meanings of these messages are perceived and responded to.

The nerve endings that are associated with transmitting pain are termed nociceptors and can be found extensively on skin, periosteum and joint surfaces, and within arterial walls, subcutaneous tissues, muscle fascia and viscera. There are two types of nerve fibres that specifically transmit painful stimuli, *a* delta fibres which transmit very fast signals and act as a rapid protective mechanism, and the slower *c* fibres that continue to remind us damage has occurred.

> **Think about a personal experience of pain; for example, have you ever burnt yourself? What was it like? What did you do to try and lessen the pain and why did you do that?**

If you put your hand on a hot plate, you whip it away quickly, even before you become fully conscious of what you have done. This is because your *a* delta fibres have responded very rapidly, informing your brain of an intense burning sensation. The pain is sharp, easy to locate and your muscles respond almost before you are aware of what you have done. These fibres are protecting you by making you take rapid evasive action before more damage occurs. Once the damage has occurred though, the dull diffused throbbing pain that comes with redness, swelling and inflammation continues, to tell you that some tissue is damaged. These are your slower *c* fibres busy sending off continuous signals. These signals are hard to ignore and almost demand you rest your hand to allow for healing to take place, and to prevent further damage. To lessen the pain, putting your hand under running water helps. By doing this, not only are you cooling the area, but other nerve fibres that normally transmit touch, coolness and warmth are stimulated, and this helps to modulate or override the pain that is felt.

The response of damaged tissues

Traumatised tissue releases breakdown products, which ultimately form chemical cascades. Prostaglandin *e* is a potent pain-producing by-product of one of these cascades. Using non-steroidal anti-inflammatory drugs (NSAIDS) may block some of its unpleasant effects. Trauma also affects the blood vessels causing spasm, oedema and liberation of platelets that break down into another potent pain producing neuropeptide called 'substance P'. Other pain stimulating substances are liberated from traumatised tissue and blood vessels. These substances set up a chain reaction of inflammation, swelling, redness, increased sensitivity and more pain. Being able to cool traumatised tissue such as a bruise or sprain with an ice pack causes vasoconstriction. This may help to reduce some of the immediate inflammatory response.

The production of kinins and other substances continues to irritate the nerve endings, causing pain. These pain stimulated nerve endings will send a message to the brain of any noxious, or potentially tissue damaging event such as burning, freezing, crushing, bruising, or the cutting of the skin with a sharp instrument.

When mentioning what happens when you burn your hand, we described how there are a mass of nerve fibres located on the skin that transmit sensations that do not signify damage or potential damage, and may even be quite pleasurable. These are the *a* beta fibres that transmit sensations of gentle heat, coolness, touch and vibration. Stimulation of these nerve fibres can promote well-being such as the sensation we experience on a warm summer's day with the sun on our bodies, or a covered hot-water bottle soothing an aching stomach. Or alternatively, the relief of a cool poultice applied to an inflamed area, or even the pleasurable sensation of a massage on aching muscles. They are significant to pain perception as we shall explain.

Gate Control Theory

This groundbreaking theory was the result of the collaborative work of the British professor of anatomy and physiology Patrick Wall and the Canadian psychologist Ronald Melzack, first published in 1965 (Melzack and Wall 1965). When you think about it, our knowledge of pain pathways is really very recent. The 1960s saw a period of intense progress within other fields of medicine, particularly surgery with the early human organ transplants, but at that time we were only just starting to understand some of the puzzles of pain. It is therefore not so surprising that until recently pain was so ineffectively managed. Our lack of knowledge, widespread misconceptions and, historically, a lack of scientific interest, meant that for the majority of patients, pain was an

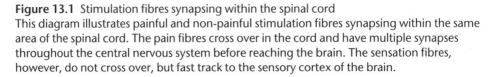

Activity 13.6

For more in-depth text on acute pain neurophysiology, refer to the discussion of acute and post-operative pain in either Wall and Melzack (1965) or Melzack and Wall (1996).

inevitable part of their post-trauma and post-operative experience.

The discovery of the three different nerve fibres helped us to understand the first principles of the Gate Control Theory. The pain or nociceptive transmitting *a* delta and *c* fibres, and the sensations transmitted by *a* beta fibres, synapse in a specific area of the spinal cord's grey matter called the *substantia gelatinosa*. Melzack and Wall's Gate Control Theory proposed that it was in this area that a principal pain modulating or regulating mechanism took place, able to act as a sort of gate. The gate was either opened by the stimulation of nociceptors enabling pain signals to reach the brain, or closed by modulating factors such as other competing non-painful sensations that inhibit this process. As there was a finite capacity for transmitting any sensation up the central nervous system to the brain, it was possible to bombard the substantia gelatinosa with so much stimulation, it limited the number of pain signals that could effectively reach the brain at any one time. As the stimulation transmitted by the *a* beta fibres reached

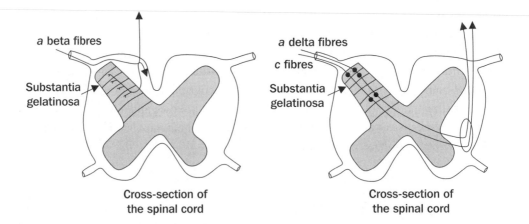

Figure 13.1 Stimulation fibres synapsing within the spinal cord
This diagram illustrates painful and non-painful stimulation fibres synapsing within the same area of the spinal cord. The pain fibres cross over in the cord and have multiple synapses throughout the central nervous system before reaching the brain. The sensation fibres, however, do not cross over, but fast track to the sensory cortex of the brain.

the brain faster and via fewer synapses, it took precedence over all but major painful sensation.

This helps to explain why the application of a cool or a warm poultice and the other similar practical physical pain relieving remedies such as rubbing a bruise can actually be effective.

? Using the information you have about Mary, consider how psychosocial factors might impact on her perception of pain?

So far the Gate Control Theory has helped to explain why stimulating the skin with a non-painful sensation can help to reduce pain. However, the theory goes on to shed more light on how it is possible for the brain and body to further regulate how much pain we perceive at any one time.

We have talked about the substantia gelatinosa appearing to have a gating mechanism within it, this ability to 'gate' pain sensation would seem to be a feature of other areas of the central nervous system, where similar gates can also be opened or closed depending on types of stimulation. Apart from sensation at the periphery, chemicals produced within the brain and the body can also activate these gates. This helps to explain just how multi-factorial the sensation and perception of pain can become – a truly bio-psychosocial event that depends on other factors far more than on straightforward painful stimulation. This understanding is important as it also helps to shed a little light on some of the other puzzles of pain.

? Thinking about what we have discussed above, can you now come up with more reasons why Mary's pain is proving difficult to relieve.

It may be useful to consider why:

- Pain may be resistant to the usual pain relieving drugs
- Other factors can be very influential
- Non-pharmacological strategies may help

Exploring Mary's recent experience of surgery enables us to track the physiological response of acute pain, as well as explain the impact of some psychosocial influences. Not only has Mary experienced extensive tissue damage that resulted when her skin and muscles were cut with the surgeon's scalpel, she also experienced intermittent visceral pain prior to her surgery.

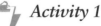

Activity 13.7

Talk to a practitioner who has experienced difficulty helping an individual manage their pain despite the use of strong analgesia. What reasons did they give for this?

> ## Mary's experience of pain
>
> Although the bowel does not transmit painful sensations if it is cut or burnt, the sensations when the bowel is stretched can be very intense. Mary is complaining about the intensity of abdominal pain, due to the tumour causing an intermittent blockage of her large bowel. Once the blockage had been removed, Mary experienced a different kind of pain, now due to gut distension caused by gas build up within the intestine as it gradually returns to normal function. Despite Mary having had effective analgesia to cover the pain of surgery, only a dense nerve block or rendering Mary semi-comatose would completely remove the visceral pain of abdominal distension. This pain provides the body with a potent warning sign that something may be wrong. Despite a well-placed epidural, Mary's pain is not responding to pharmacological strategies (pain relief) as well as was hoped. She is tense and anxious, which is causing a release of stress hormones, resulting in further muscle tension and discomfort.

The addition of non-pharmacological and other comfort strategies to her care could help to improve her pain relief. A care plan devised with Mary prior to surgery identified the ways in which Mary had coped with pain in the past and these strategies proved useful following her operation. Often, being in hospital isolates people from their own coping mechanisms and prevents them from using the simple strategies that they would use at home.

Non-pharmacological strategies

More and more nurses are developing an interest in non-pharmacological strategies for pain management. Often they are frustrated because some patients – even when given a strong cocktail of various drugs – sometimes fail to achieve adequate pain relief. Whilst some health care professionals can withdraw when a patient's pain is proving to be a challenge, the nurses have no such option.

Professional conversation

Marion, staff nurse caring for Mary

Information giving

'As the staff nurse caring for Mary post-operatively, I was able to reassure Mary that the periodic cramping pains that she was experiencing were a positive sign that gut function was beginning to return to normal. In the case of wind pain, early ambulation, peppermint water and reassurance that the pain will only be transient is often all that is needed. For

Mary, prior knowledge helped remove the fear of any new cramping pain which ensured that, once she was over the immediate post-operative period, she was hardly troubled by the sensation.'

Other useful non-pharmacological strategies which are gaining in popularity may include:

- Simple massage
- A hot-water bottle
- Listening to music
- Transcutaneous nerve stimulation (TENS) – traditionally used to help control labour pains, muscular pain and some chronic pains

> ## Activity 13.8
>
> Look at an introductory text on nursing models and frameworks and find out how pain management strategies such as information giving could be incorporated into Mary's care plan.

It is helpful to consider the reasons why pain might be relieved by non-pharmacological strategies. The following diagram (Figure 13.2) helps to illustrate the circular pathways between the sensory cortex, or thinking part of the brain, the midbrain, thalamus and the area of spinal nerve input within the spinal cord.

? How can distracting attention away from the focus of the pain inflence the way that it is perceived?

> ## Activity 13.9
>
> **A** Knowledge of non-pharmacological strategies can provide nurses with a repertoire of therapies to enhance analgesia. See a text on aromatherapy and refer to Stevenson (1995); and Carroll (1997) discussed in the bibliography. Alternatively, several books on pain have good sections on non-pharmacological strategies to manage pain such as Fordham and Dunn (1994, pp. 102–24); Hawthorn and Redmond (1998, pp. 204–18); McCaffery and Beebe (1994, pp. 161–95); Carroll and Bowsher (1993, pp. 136–45, and also pp. 146–65 on physiotherapy for the relief of pain which provides an overview of how another discipline can play a significant part in the management of pain).
>
> **B** Ask a physiotherapist about their experiences of using TENS in post-operative pain management. Read either McQuay and Moore on the use of TENS in acute postoperative pain (1998, pp. 172–9); or you may want to read a book on TENS in which case read Walsh (1997).

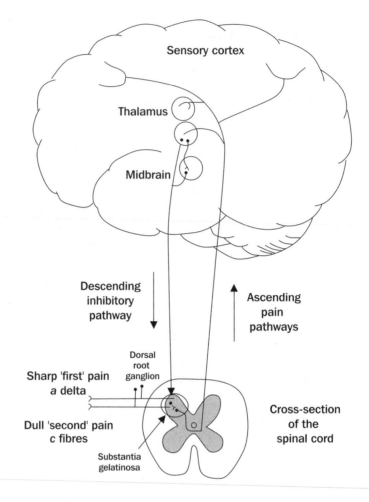

Figure 13.2 Neural pathways between brain and spinal cord
(Reproduced from Eileen Mann and Eloise Carr (2000), Pain: Creative Approaches to Effective Management. Basingstoke: Palgrave Macmillan.)

Professional conversation

Alan, Mary's named nurse

Pre-operative assessment

'As Mary's named nurse I tried to ensure that Mary felt both as comfortable and relaxed as possible. I believe it is important to find sufficient time to answer queries and address any concerns either as part of the assessment or separately. Listening to patients builds trust and confidence and enables rapport to develop. Having pain ignored or disbelieved can render even quite forceful personalities vulnerable and anxious. Mary was certainly eager to have her questions answered, which we tried to do confidently and sensitively. She wanted to know all about her surgery and what was going to happen. Shade (1992) argues that being familiar with the ward routines and what to expect can improve the outcome for patients. Mary was introduced to other patients and this helped her to feel more relaxed in her strange surroundings. The anaesthetist also came to see her and explained how the epidural analgesia would help to control the pain that she would experience. He assured her that with this technique, the post-operative pain would usually be well controlled without the ghastly sickness and head spinning that she had experienced in the past.'

Mary's pre-operative care was documented in her care plan so that everyone was aware what had been explained to Mary, how she was coping, and how well she was orientated to her new surroundings. Mary read, watched television and listened to her tape-player before opting for some night sedation which ensured a good night's sleep. An early morning cup of tea, several hours before her surgery, came as a pleasant surprise.

Evidence-based practice

Post-operative nausea and vomiting

Not all patients need to go without clear fluids for many hours prior to surgery. New studies are showing that for most patients, consuming a small volume of clear fluid up to two hours before surgery is not only safe, but has also been shown to reduce post-operative nausea (Chapman 1996; Shevde and Triveldi 1991).

Pre-operative care

Although Mary had previously experienced periods of partial bowel obstruction, on admission to hospital her gut function was normal.

Mary received three drugs with her pre-medication. She was given a non-steroidal anti-inflammatory drug (NSAID) as pre-emptive analgesia, a drug to reduce the risk of sickness following surgery (an anti-emetic), and a sedating drug to make her feel sleepy and relaxed.

These strategies and interventions helped Mary to feel physically and mentally better prepared for her journey to the operating theatre. Other patients sitting in the beds around her told her not to worry and were very reassuring. The lady in the bed opposite had also previously experienced an epidural and told Mary how delighted she had been when the following day after surgery she had been able to sit out of bed and take a few steps without any significant discomfort at all.

Epidural analgesia

During Mary's operation, tissue was inevitably cut and damaged, resulting in the chemical inflammatory soup that causes the nociceptors to transmit pain. However, a light anaesthetic kept Mary asleep so she was not aware of this process.

An epidural catheter sited prior to surgery was used to instil bolus doses of two different drugs into the tissue around Mary's spinal cord where the pain messages would normally enter. One of these drugs was a local anaesthetic, and the other was a powerful opioid analgesic. As a result of these drugs, Mary was able to regain consciousness in the recovery room following her surgery, initially with no pain at all, and only mild pain when she tried to roll on to her side.

> ### Pain control during Mary's operation
>
> During the operation, the anaesthetist closely monitored Mary's physiological response to pain, carefully recording her blood pressure and pulse. The epidural space was injected before surgery commenced with a bolus dose of opioid, in this case diamorphine, and local anaesthetic, bupivicaine. Then periodically, Mary's epidural was topped up with further doses of bupivicaine. Once the operation was over, a 500ml bag of normal saline solution containing very dilute concentrations of local anaesthetic and the opioid fentanyl was commenced at a rate of 5ml per hour in the recovery room.

The following diagram (Figure 13.3) shows a cross-section through the spine to illustrate the location of the epidural space and the site of the needle through which a catheter can be threaded to achieve continuous post-operative pain relief.

The illustration in Figure 13.4 shows how local anaesthetic, for example bupivicaine, was able to control Mary's pain. You may find it helpful to refer to a general anatomy and physiology textbook for more detailed explanation of these complex physiological and biochemical processes.

This blocking of the chemical pathways on the nerve membrane effectively stops the transmission of pain.

How opioids work

The opioids (e.g. diamorphine, morphine and fentanyl) prescribed for Mary were able to halt painful transmissions by binding tightly to opioid receptors located on nerve membranes and within the central nervous system. Opioids are the principal drugs for potent intra-operative and post-operative pain relief. They have the advantage of being able to have their actions chemically reversed with the antagonist drug naloxone should a patient shows signs of overdose.

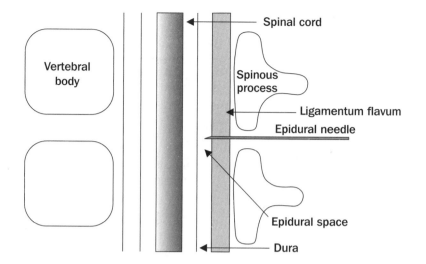

Figure 13.3 The epidural space.
(Reproduced from Eileen Mann (????))

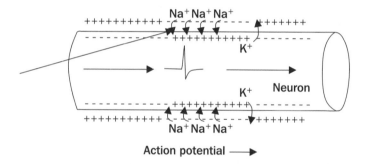

Figure 13.4 Local anaesthetic acts on the cell membrane
(Reproduced from Eileen Mann and Eloise Carr (2000), Pain: Creative Approaches to Effective Management. Basingstoke: Palgrave Macmillan.)

 Activity 13.10

Before you look at the next diagram look up the terms agonist and antagonist in a medical dictionary.

Activity 13.11

Within your own clinical area make a list of other pharmacological agents regularly used to control pain.

For further information on post-operative pain relief you may wish to refer to Alexander and Gardner (1994 pp. 1–24).

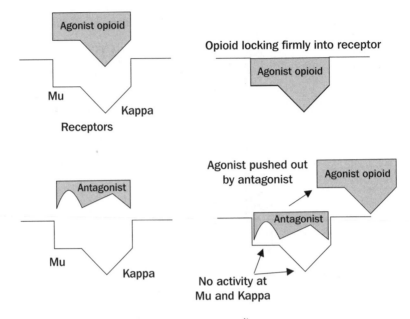

Figure 13.5 Opioids lock into receptors on nerve endings
Showing how opioids such as morphine lock into receptors located on nerve membranes and
how opioid antagonist naloxone can block the action of opioids.
(Reproduced from Eileen Mann and Eloise Carr (2000), Pain: Creative Approaches to Effective Management. Basingstoke:
Palgrave Macmillan.)

Mary's experience in the immediate post-operative period.

In the recovery room Mary awoke virtually pain free. The recovery staff showed her
the chart they would be using to assess her pain and how this would be continued by
the ward staff. The family came to see her on the ward later that first evening.
Despite Mark's concerns about Mary's diagnosis, the stress of coping with the children, and the demands of his elderly parents, his good humour and the chattering of
the children were able to act as a short-term distraction. In truth Mary felt quite
exhausted and was quite pleased when they left. She found the position in which she
was most comfortable, and this enabled her to see the television, which also acted as
a distraction. A little later she was invited to use some essential oils which were prepared by one of the nurses who was also an aromatherapist. This combined use of a
number of pain relieving strategies enabled Mary to fall asleep.

Feelings of well-being, the use of distraction, and the use of humour can increase the
body's own ability to close the pain gates and keep them closed. However, by day two,
with Mary waiting to hear the results of her pathology, pain had become more of a
problem. Evidence suggests that both fear and anxiety are implicated in winding pain
up and making it harder to control. Although the surgeon explained that his initial

examination of the tumour suggested it may be benign, Mary was anxious and generally found it difficult to relax.

A good rapport between a patient and the nurse is important if specific needs are going to be effectively anticipated and met. Knowing the impact that fear and anxiety may have on Mary's experience of pain and her overall recovery, it was essential that nursing time was set aside to address this.

Professional conversation

Alan, Mary's named nurse

Pain, fear and anxiety

'I have come to know Mary quite well and although she outwardly appears stoical and in control, I also know that during the past few days she has been consumed with anxiety that the tumour in her bowel may prove malignant and that she could soon die from cancer. Mary wants to see her children grow up and is frightened that they will not manage without her. In her notes I have written that during the ward round, Mary's surgeon explained to her that although he couldn't be sure, he felt it was unlikely that the tumour he removed was malignant. I have also taken some time to explain to Mary that certain bowel tumours treated early enough can usually result in a complete cure. She has expressed a wish to know the pathology results immediately they are received, and to be kept informed of all her options should the tumour prove to be malignant. Mary wants to be fully informed with her husband present if the news is not good, and I have documented this in her notes. I found time to just sit with Mary tonight, she wanted nothing more than to hold someone's hand.'

The amount and type of pain experienced by Mary needed to be assessed throughout the post-operative period in order to ensure that pain control was having maximum effect. Mary had earlier been shown the chart when she had asked about pain control. This had been used in the recovery area and was now in use back on the ward.

 How would you assess Mary's pain? Which types of pain assessment tools exist within your own clinical area?

 Evidence-based practice

The assessment of pain

In order for nursing and medical staff to manage pain effectively, they must have a means of assessing pain and the effects of any treatment that is offered. The best way of assessing acute pain is to use a simple, but validated pain assessment tool that ideally relies on a patient's verbal response. In

Mary's case, staff need to be able to regularly assess the location, intensity and impact on well-being of any pain experienced. The quality or description of her pain also helps to signify whether it is resulting from an ineffective epidural or whether it is perhaps the odd spasm of the gut caused by trapped wind as it begins to function normally again. A simple verbal or numerical rating system is ideal for assessing the intensity of any pain. In an acute situation it is quick and easy to perform. For further information on pain assessment refer to Schofield (1995) and Briggs (1995) discussed in the bibliography at the end of this chapter.

Examples of some of the more commonly used pain assessment tools include:

Table 13.1 Pain assessment tools

Visual analogue score

No pain _____ **worst pain**

Simple verbal rating

No pain   Mild pain   Moderate pain   Severe pain

Numerical rating

1 2 3 4 5 6 7 8 9 10

For small children and for people with a learning disability using a 'faces chart' may be easier for them to understand.

Figure 13.6 A 'faces' chart for children
(Reproduced from Eileen Mann and Eloise Carr (2000), Pain: Creative Approaches to Effective Management. Basingstoke: Palgrave Macmillan.)

 Question: Which of these tools would you select to assess Mary's pain and why?

The use of a simple pain assessment tool combined with questions about Mary's general wellbeing is all that is needed. An open question asking how she is feeling and then getting her to score her pain intensity was more effective than just asking 'have you any pain'? A numerical check on a 1 to 10 scale (1 = no pain and 10 = the worst pain ever)

will ascertain the severity of any discomfort present. This scoring system, when used again after Mary has been asked to move and cough effectively, will give an indication of whether the epidural is doing its job adequately or needs adjustment or supplementing with other therapy.

Simple verbal numerical rating

Mary's perceived level of pain at 22.00 hrs on the second post-operative day was:

1 2 3 4 5 6 7 **8** 9 10

The vocabulary of pain is also important and can give a powerful indicator of what the cause of the pain may be. We talked earlier of the sharp spasm-type pain that comes when wind is trapped in the gut. Tissue trauma pain tends to be of a dull and diffused nature. Nerve damage pain is often referred to as having a burning sensation; these descriptors can act as a powerful diagnostic tool to experienced clinicians.

However, with technological methods of pain control, such as epidural analgesia, other assessments have to be made:

- Is the amount of opioid causing sedation?
- Does the patient feel excessively itchy and nauseous?
- Is the local anaesthetic in the infusion exacerbating any post-operative hypotension?
- Does the patient have normal sensation?
- Is the patient suffering from motor loss?
- Is urine output satisfactory?

? **Why is it that all these factors, not only any pain that may be experienced, have to be assessed on a regular basis and any problems encountered acted upon immediately?**

Poor analgesia, hazardous or unpleasant side-effects would indicate that an immediate review of the current strategy is required. There is a need to establish whether Mary's epidural is still in the right place, and the infusion rate high enough to provide adequate analgesia without resulting in unwanted side effects. Could analgesia be improved by giving Mary another drug, such as regular paracetamol or a non-steroidal anti-inflammatory drug? If other remedies prescribed to control potential side-effects such as nausea, itching or constipation are becoming ineffective, then these medications will also need adjustment.

Pain assessment is not just 'have you any pain? It needs to ascertain far more than that and each clinical area will probably need to devise its own assessment tool, appropriate for the analgesia regimes that are currently used.

> ### Activity 13.12
>
> For further information regarding the management and monitoring of patients with an epidural, see King and Jacob (1993, pp. 211–18) or McCaffery and Beebe (1994, pp. 101–8).

Post-operative analgesia

It is often beneficial to combine several pain relieving drugs that have different modes of action. We have already discussed how Mary's epidural infusion combined a local anaesthetic with an opioid drug. If the epidural fails to provide optimum analgesia, administering additional drugs, such as paracetamol and or one of the non-steroidal anti-inflammatory drugs (NSAIDs), may result in improved analgesia. Should Mary be particularly worried about the removal of drains or of having short procedures carried out that cause pain, the use of entonox may be useful as a way of administering very short-acting pain relief.

Entonox is unfortunately often overlooked as a short-term treatment for acute pain. This is despite the fact that it is extremely safe and can be very effective in providing brief additional analgesia. It is particularly useful to use when a patient is waiting for an oral pain killer to work, or is having a painful and unpleasant procedure performed that is only going to take a few minutes.

Entonox is a 50 per cent mixture of oxygen and nitrous oxide, which has a very rapid onset of action and is excreted almost as rapidly. Entonox comes in a portable cylinder and has been used for many years to help control labour pain in childbirth, by ambulance crews and in Accident and Emergency departments. Entonox is contraindicated for very few people although some may feel a little drowsy, dizzy or sick. (See also the use of Entonox in childbirth in Chapter 2 on maternal health.)

> ### Activity 13.13
>
> A For further information on Entonox, read Lawler (1995, pp. 19–21); and Toulson (1990, pp. 23–6).
>
> B The following includes a list of commonly used analgesic preparations. You may like to find out their mode of action, normal dose, contra-indications and side-effects by reference to a pharmacology textbook.

Analgesic drugs

There are several ways of classifying analgesic drugs, but usually they are grouped into the strong opioids, weak opioids and non-opioid drugs.

Strong opioids

- Morphine
- Diamorphine
- Fentanyl
- Pethidine

Weak opioids

- Codeine
- Dihydrocodeine
- Dextropropoxyphene (often combined with paracetamol to give Co-proxamol)
- Tramadol

Non-opioid drugs

- Aspirin
- Paracetamol
- Non-steroidal anti-inflammatory drugs (NSAIDS)

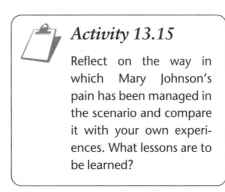

Activity 13.14

For further information on pharmacological strategies, refer to Hawthorn and Redmond (1998, pp. 145–203). Or, if you have a special interest in emergency medicine, then there is good text on pain control in Illingworth and Simpson (1994, pp. 267–302). For a compilation of results on the efficacy of various analgesic therapy, refer to McQuay and Moore (1998).

? Have you seen other pharmacological strategies used to control acute pain? Look up the term adjuvant medication.

Although acute pain is less complex than chronic pain, sometimes even acute pain can prove difficult to control with analgesic drugs alone. When this is the case, a more in-depth pain assessment can help elicit other causes. Finding the cause of a pain that is not responding to the therapies so far mentioned means that different drugs – called adjuvant therapies and often used in chronic pain, or the pain experienced with terminal disease –

Activity 13.15

Reflect on the way in which Mary Johnson's pain has been managed in the scenario and compare it with your own experiences. What lessons are to be learned?

can sometimes be helpful. An example would be the use of buscopan when gut spasm is particularly troublesome, or using an anxiolytic agent such as midazolam or diazepam when anxiety is a major feature.

Each member of the Johnson family can recount their own experiences of pain, even the youngest member Phillip. How the family responded at the time helps to shape how children grow up to view pain either as something to be dreaded and feared, or as a normal part of life, for the most part endurable and not overwhelming. Our upbringing and culture help to formulate this response. We all know of some children who will become terrified and distressed at what appears to be a mildly painful stimulus, but conversely we often see those stoical little souls who barely squirm, often during quite unpleasant painful procedures. Even in small children, we are able to measure the degree of stimulation occurring in nerve fibres. Although this may have a bearing on the amount of pain perceived, it cannot identify the degree of distress caused. If children pick up the signals from their parents that pain is always to be feared and avoided at all cost they will rapidly become distressed by any painful stimuli. This is all part of our central processing of pain. Once the painful stimulation has reached our brains, then it is our brains that dictate just how much the pain will trouble and distress us as a result.

The Johnson family's experiences of pain

Martin's worst memory of pain was experienced when he broke a leg falling out of a tree. The pain was initially severe, but once the leg was splinted and immobile the pain reduced substantially. Whilst in hospital Martin received good analgesia. He was given a small dose of oral immediate-release morphine syrup. In order that Martin's leg could be examined he was encouraged to use Entonox. When he went home, his mother was given several days supply of the NSAID diclofenac and advised to give Martin this drug regularly with paracetamol in addition for any breakthrough pain that may occur. For Martin, his first experience of severe pain was not an unduly negative one; his pain was recognised, believed and acted upon promptly. This experience has ensured Martin does not view hospitals with fear and anxiety and he has confidence in the ability of health care professionals to manage pain competently.

Amy's worst experience was following an accident when her fingers were trapped in a car door. The pain was excruciating, sickening and frightening. She had one of her fingernails removed in hospital without adequate analgesia and she was then sent home. The occasional paracetamol given by her mother once she left casualty had been insufficient to control the dull throbbing pain that seemed to be with her for days. For Amy, hospitals are uncaring, frightening places, and she dreads going there again.

Phillip's only real memory of pain is the occasional earache he has experienced following a cold. Never really severe pain but none the less he remembers the pain as being horrible. For Phillip a dose of paracetamol, lots of cuddles from his mother and a course of antibiotics quickly solved the problem. Getting the infection under control is the key to treating Phillip's pain.

? What was your worst childhood experience? Has this left you with any problems such as a fear of needles, or going to the dentist? You may wish to access further information on the perception of pain in an introductory psychology textbook and also consider the sociology of pain in an introductory sociology text.

Mark Johnson's intense pain experience

Mark Johnson has a vivid memory of renal colic. Again the pain was intense, but this time not because of tissue damage, but because an area of viscera, insensitive to being cut or bruised, responded dramatically and painfully to being distended by a trapped stone. Mark's renal colic pain responded effectively to his general practitioner giving him an injection of 100mg pethidine and 50mg of diclofenac orally.

? Have you seen pethidine used in the past? In what way is pethidine different from morphine?

Although pethidine is a short-acting opioid, and therefore of limited use for most pain control, the fact that it is reputed to cause less smooth muscle spasm means it is often given for renal and biliary colic. However, the use of pethidine is now being questioned especially because its duration of action is often so short. For Mark's father and mother though, it has been a different story. Their advanced years have brought with them a variety of chronically painful conditions that, for the most part, defy totally effective treatment and prove far more of a challenge to effective control.

? Both morphine and pethidine are controlled drugs. What special arrangements are required of the nurse for the safe storage and administration of such medication?

Clive Johnson's pain experiences

Clive Johnson's pain experiences have been gained during a lifetime of activity and illness. In his youth he experienced severe and inadequately controlled acute pain following injuries sustained during the Korean War. Unfortunately, he also now experiences chronic pain in his left foot as a result of nerve damage that has occurred with his late onset-diabetes. Not only does Clive experience neuropathic (nerve damage) pain, he has developed a large ulcer above his ankle. Despite the best efforts of his GP and community health team, no single drug therapy provides long-term, complete pain relief and the pain is with Clive most of the time.

? Why is chronic pain so different? Talk to someone who regularly experiences episodes of recurrent periodic pain, such as migraine, or pain which is present on a more or less permanent basis. Find out how they cope with and manage their pain.

Acute pain is usually related to a specific event or injury which results in immediate pain being experienced. It is accompanied by a response within the autonomic nervous system which will initially leave the sufferer with visible signs such as pallor, sweating, tachycardia and alterations in blood pressure. Acute pain nearly always responds to analgesia and treatment of the cause of the pain. For instance, pain following the tissue damage of surgery or trauma will usually respond well to psychological preparation, adequate doses of analgesia (Foley 1993), sleep and effective comfort strategies. Because the pain has resulted from an event, it is self-limiting. Once the event is over or the tissue healing, the pain naturally subsides.

In many ways, chronic pain is far more complex and is not just an extension of acute pain. Chronic pain is usually defined as pain that lasts for more than three months. It can be associated with a chronic pathological process that ensures pain is ongoing. It can be as a result of changes in the central nervous system that make chronic pain quite different from just a 'long-lasting' acute pain. Or pain may be present in the absence of any obvious cause, presenting an extremely complex picture with the psychosocial implications of not being believed. Patients with chronic pain do not exhibit the autonomic response seen with early acute pain as their system has adapted; this sometimes leads to inexperienced staff doubting the existence of the pain. The experiences of the senior members of the Johnson family enable us now to explore some of these issues in greater depth.

Professional conversation

Carol, practice nurse

Pain and wound management

'I have been dressing Clive's leg ulcer on and off, at the Practice for the last three months. He has been having serious problems with hardly any healing taking place, and we became quite worried as Clive has diabetes. During a recent stay in hospital, the tissue viability specialist nurse examined his leg ulcer and dressed it on a few occasions. Clive found dressing changes very painful. The nurse recommended that Clive take some combination analgesia one hour before she arranged to visit him which helped considerably, and she also got him to use Entonox whilst she was dressing the wound. Since Clive has been back with us, he has suffered little pain as the combination analgesia does work well, and we have introduced this more widely across the practice.'

Why might Clive's pain have been less severe when dressings were changed at the Practice rather than in the hospital? Why is Clive's diabetes a worry to the practice nurses? (For further information, see Casey (1998, pp. 49–54.)

Clive has had neuropathic pain for many years. Part of his foot has no sensation, but on the other side he feels pain all the time. Accepting this as part of his diabetes, he has never really sought further treatment. All the 'painkillers', he has taken in the past for his foot pain have either had no effect whatsoever, or left him feeling lethargic and constipated.

 What strategies may be useful in controlling Clive's neuropathic pain?

Evidence-based practice

Pain and disability in diabetes

Whilst patients are in hospital with a chronic condition, specialist care may be able to stabilise chronic conditions with drug adjustments. Diabetes may be better controlled and neuropathic pain may respond to a trial of a low dose tricyclic antidepressant such as amitriptyline. Patients need to be assured that these drugs are not being used because staff think the pain is not real and just the result of depression. The drug has a particular action, not fully understood, that in small doses can be effective in treating painful diabetic neuropathy (McQuay and Moore 1998). One of the side-effects of amitriptyline is sedation. By having the drug at night, a better sleep pattern may be established enabling patients to cope better with pain.

A well-evaluated trial of oral morphine might possibly be useful when pain is particularly troublesome, but should be combined with therapy to control side-effects such as constipation. Unfortunately, many patients with neuropathic pain fail to respond to opioids at doses that medical staff are comfortable with. There are still concerns about addiction even when the evidence does not support this risk (Ferrell et a, 1992). However, effective doses of opioids for chronic pain may lead to intolerable or unmanageable side-effects even when attempts are made at controlling these. Furthermore, if pain is a feature of a numb area, there is always less confidence that opioids would necessarily provide pain relief (Jadad et al 1992). Sometimes nerve membrane stabilising drugs, usually used to treat epilepsy, may prove useful. (See Backonja et al 1998, pp. 1831–6.)

Neuropathic pain often fails to respond to analgesia as the mechanism of pain may be due to a malfunction in the peripheral or central nervous system *and not from* the nerve terminal stimulation that happens with an acute tissue damage, inflammatory response, or chronic inflammatory condition such as arthritis. Understanding some of the theories of chronic pain mechanism enables potentially more effective treatment to be tried.

Not all chronic pain has an identifiable cause like a painful diabetic neuropathy. For some unfortunate patients, severe pain is present in the absence of any discernible pathology. Neuropathic pain is often described as having a burning sensation with intermittent shock-like sensations. Although not fully understood, it is thought the pain can arise from a malfunction or hyperexcitability at the periphery. This means that nerves transmitting pain may be so excitable that they fire following a range of physical, chemical and metabolic changes. Changes may also occur in the central nervous system following nerve damage, with hyperexcitability extending into the dorsal horn of the spinal cord and a loss of some of the modulating pathways.

Chronic pain can also be maintained when psychological factors are contributing. We all seem to equate pain with damage and the fact that this may not be the case frequently needs reinforcing. The fear of masking damage will often lead to patients not taking analgesia, or developing avoidance and disability. This fear can be more disabling than pain itself (Crombez et al 1999). In addition, the majority of people trying to find an end to their pain could well be suffering from depression, anxiety and dependence on pharmacological strategies. The psychology of pain is a fascinating subject covered in Skevington (1995).

? **If you were looking after a patient who complained of uncontrolled chronic pain, who would you ask for advice?**

Interdisciplinary collaboration

Whilst in hospital, some patients may benefit from advice by a specialist nurse or health care professional. Although interdisciplinary advice may also be arranged in the community, it is often in hospital that a first contact is made with one, or combinations of the following professionals:

- A pain specialist or pain team for assessment, information and a possible trial of therapy.
- A specialist who deals with particular chronic conditions such as diabetes or Parkinson's disease.
- A dietician for advice on diet. Obesity can lead to immobility and this can exacerbate pain, isolate sufferers and reduce social interaction.
- An occupational therapist can help with mobility and independence in the home.
- A physiotherapist can be an invaluable resource, especially when mobility and muscle spasm are the major problems.
- A social worker might help those families struggling to manage on their own.
- Voluntary, charitable and self-help organisations may be particularly helpful in providing specialist support and information.

Effective interprofessional working combines the expertise of several specialities. Good quality pain management is not just about drugs and therapies. Interprofessional collaboration may often improve the quality of outcome for patients, especially those struggling with chronically painful conditions for which no cure can be found. An early referral to a chronic pain or rheumatology clinic may be appropriate.

> Phyllis experiences chronic pain from rheumatoid arthritis and back pain, following frequent crush damage in her osteoporotic spine.

Phyllis Johnson's experience enables us to study something of the processes of chronic inflammatory pain, as well as ongoing musculo-skeletal pain.

? **Who would be best placed to advice Phyllis on her treatment and pain control?**

Phyllis's analgesia is predominantly:

- An NSAID, which she takes with a drug to help protect her stomach from the ulceration that can be a factor with long-term NSAID use.
- Additional paracetamol.
- Low-dose oral morphine for moderately severe flare-ups help her to maintain her mobility.
- When her condition has a very severe flare-up, she has had local anaesthetic with a corticosteroid injected directly into her affected joint. Sometimes she has to increase her dose of systemic steroids to control the inflammatory response.

> Phyllis is currently attending the multi-disciplinary rheumatology clinic. At the clinic the effects of the prescribed drugs and treatments that help to keep her chronic inflammatory condition under control and relieve her pain are evaluated and adjusted.

Musculo-skeletal pain

Phyllis's osteoporosis means it is vital that she keeps active for as long as possible. With her bones already demineralised and prone to fracture, the less mobility she has, the weaker they become. However, she is now finding it harder to get about and has quite severe damage to her spinal vertebrae. Opioids and adjuvant drugs are of only limited benefit and for the most part, she stoically endures her pain, determined to still find enjoyment in life. She keeps her mind occupied, reading books, watching television, playing cards with her friends and trying to remain cheerful, and these serve her reasonably well as coping strategies. She is well supported by her family, and maintaining her social interactions helps to ensure that she does not become completely overwhelmed by her pain.

You can see by the scenarios of Clive and Phyllis that their pain is far more complex. Firstly, pharmacological strategies often prove quite disappointing and for sufferers, there is often no foreseeable end in sight for their pain. It becomes something they have learnt to live with and many have suffered in silence, despite recent and ongoing scientific attempts to find effective treatments. The effect of chronic pain on the family unit is also an important issue that is often overlooked (Snelling 1994). Fortunately, both Clive and Phyllis have had some reasonably early access to multi-disciplinary health care, which has helped to educate them and to control some of the symptoms that trigger their pain. Other chronic pain syndromes are even more complex and less understood. Considerable numbers of patients are left feeling abandoned, frustrated and helpless by the so far lack of scientific explanation and the seeming lack of success in treating many of their conditions.

 What sort of pain assessment tool would be suitable for use with chronic pain sufferers like Phyllis and Clive?

Assessing chronic pain

Many patients with chronic pain never get to have their pain fully assessed or evaluated. Unlike acute pain, where an assessment can be very brief in order to initiate and evaluate treatment, a comprehensive chronic pain assessment can be a lengthy affair. Once this has been carried out, for many patients assessing their pain on a four-hourly basis can be counterproductive. This is particularly the case when they have been suffering for many years and use distraction as a coping strategy. Regular assessment for these people just keeps refocusing their minds on their pain.

 Evidence-based practice

Pain questionnaires

Most assessment of chronic pain takes the form of questionnaires. One of the best known questionnaires which produces a multi-dimensional scale is the McGill Pain Questionnaire (MGPQ). This was first devised by Ronald Melzack (Melzack 1975) and is especially valuable as a research tool or for use by specialist pain clinics. Words that are commonly used to describe pain are grouped together into several categories: sensory, affective and evaluative. Patients are given the questionnaire, which can take up to 20 minutes to complete, and asked to select one word from each subcategory that is most appropriate to describe their pain. For example, one category has the following words: dull, sore, hurting, aching and heavy. This particular subcategory describes a sensory aspect of pain. Within each group, the individual words are graded numerically according to increasing intensity, for instance hurting would score a higher figure than sore. When all the numbers are added up, you get an overall score or pain-rating index. The chart is combined with a body map to mark the location of pain and can include a visual analogue score for pain intensity.

Pain diaries can be very helpful, but patients need to feel motivated to use them and they can be unsuitable for the elderly or cognitively impaired patient. The Oxford Pain Chart (McQuay 1990) is an example of how categorical scales have been incorporated into a pain dairy.

Personality and depression measures are also used as assessment tools in chronic pain management. It is suggested that patients with chronic pain tend to score more highly on hypochondriasis, hysteria and depression scales, although this is controversial (Dolin et al 1996) and most of the time, we have no way of knowing what came first, the pain or the depression.

? How can the effectiveness of both pain assessment and pain management be evaluated?

Using clinical effectiveness and evidence-based research to improve the quality of pain relief

Over the past 20 years the relief of pain has attracted a much higher profile than was the case in the 1960s, 1970s and even early 1980s. Pain has been selected as the target for clinical guidelines by many of the major pain organisations established over the past two decades. The evolution of the science of pain, and the development of protocols and guidelines are beginning to provide us with a 'standard of care' for which health care professionals and organisations could well be held accountable. The gradual introduction of a culture of pain assessment using reliable, validated assessment tools provides us with a numerical measure that can be used to evaluate quality initiatives. Regular audit is invaluable as a way of evaluating the effectiveness of what we are doing at the moment, deciding whether we are satisfied, and if not, devising a standard to aim for in order to improve outcomes in the future. Measuring the quality of care for audit purposes depends on making explicit the quality of practice to be expected. Prior to the development of pain assessment tools, which are still in need of improvement, we lacked a reliable form of measurement and this probably accounted for why quality pain relieving initiatives were slow to take off.

Once an effective system is established to measure the quality of the pain relief, you then have a structure in place that can be adapted to measure the effectiveness of other interventions. The findings of any evaluation provide evidence of the suitability, or otherwise, of the use of such an intervention. This contributes to evidence-based practice.

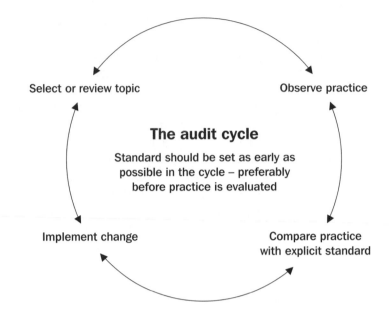

Figure 13.7 The audit cycle
Introducing systematic review and regular evaluation of what you are trying to achieve can help improve the quality of pain relief for patients.
(Reproduced from Eileen Mann and Eloise Carr (2000), Pain: Creative Approaches to Effective Management. Basingstoke: Palgrave Macmillan.)

A current definition of evidence-based practice is, 'that it is the conscientious, explicit, and judicious use of current best evidence in making decisions about the care of individual patients' (Sackett et al 1996, p. 2). This would seem fairly straightforward, but applying the principles to good pain management can sometimes prove very frustrating.

> Can you think of reasons why we have been slow to realise the value of good pain management and sometimes ineffective in implementing good practice?

Barriers to effective pain relief

- There can be many barriers to good pain relief; some subtle, others not so subtle.
- Patients can inhibit good analgesia with low expectations about pain relief or feelings that pain is inevitable (Carr 1997).
- Patients may be reluctant to take analgesia for fear of masking pain and therefore damage (Crombez et al 1999).
- Patients and staff may harbour concerns about perceived untreatable or intolerable side-effects of analgesia.
- Unfounded concerns about addiction and tolerance (Ferrell et al 1992).
- Access to education in pain management for health care professionals has been patchy and haphazard (Griepp 1992; Marcer and Deighton 1988).

- The incorporation of regular pain assessment and evaluation of analgesia into mainstream patient assessment and monitoring has been slow. Without good assessment and documentation, the needs of the patient cannot be adequately communicated to all those responsible for the patient's care.

Professional conversation

Theo Greaves, clinical nurse specialist, pain team

Organisational barriers to pain management

'Organisations also create barriers to effective pain management when dated guidelines are incorporated into hospital policy with little if any review (Carr and Mann 1998). For example, two nurses checking a controlled drug will often lead to lengthy delays responding to patients' requests for strong analgesia. The two-nurse check policy was a guideline of the Duthie Report (1988) and not a legal requirement as is often assumed. Questioning what you do and why can often stimulate lively debate and open up previously unidentified issues. Hospitals have traditionally been slow to change, but pressure to review this culture is now widespread. In 1846, the first anaesthetic provided pain-free surgery – 150 years later patients should not have to endure unrelieved pain anywhere in hospital (McQuay and Moore 1998).'

 ### What may the future hold?

Nurses have been pivotal in many of the developments in pain management. They can continue to influence pain management by improving knowledge, and looking to change practice when outcomes fall short of those desired or expected. Pain management is part of the very essence of nursing; incredibly frustrating and stressful when it is poor, but exhilarating for all concerned when it is effective. Exciting developments in drug therapies could well be on the horizon, but in the meantime an improved knowledge of current pharmacological and non-pharmacological strategies could mean nursing having a more active role in pain management.

Extending nursing practice can contribute further to the developments of the last decade. The introduction of clinical guidelines under which certain drugs may be administered under protocol without a doctor's prescription is already with us (DOH 1989). The future may hold all sorts of possibilities for the further development of nursing expertise in the field of pain management. Nurse prescribing has extended practice way beyond that

> ### Activity 13.16
> Look around your clinical area and see if you can identify any changes that could contribute to improved pain management. How could they be implemented?

previously undertaken by nurses (DOH 1999, 2002). The NHS Plan (DOH 2000) suggests that by 2004, a majority of nurses should be able to prescribe medicines independently or supply medicines under Patient Group Directions, which will enable some nurses to supply 'prescriptions only medicines' under the general direction of a doctor.

Conclusion

In this chapter we have endeavoured to introduce pain management using a family-based scenario. The scenario incorporated acute post-operative pain, exploring both the physiological and psychological components that help to influence the success, or failure, of pain management strategies. We touched on the pharmacology of some of the most commonly prescribed pain relieving drugs, and the assessment strategies that need to be in place if pain management therapies are to be evaluated effectively. We looked at how some non-pharmacological strategies can be utilised to help reduce post-operative pain and how coping strategies may increase pain tolerance. We also looked briefly at how interdisciplinary working may enhance patient care and what the barriers may be that inhibit a timely or effective response to a patient's plea for pain relief.

Education into pain management has always been one of the major stumbling blocks to establishing good analgesia. This is now changing and pain management is becoming firmly established within both pre-registration and post-registration curricula. Easy access to ongoing education for all health care professionals is essential. The development of guidelines based on up-to-date evidence, combined with efforts to improve the way we manage pain must continue to be a major nursing priority. The stress that poor analgesia can cause both patients and staff alike should not be underestimated. It is hoped this chapter has helped to introduce this fascinating subject and the further reading section should provide a guide to where more in-depth text may be obtained.

References

Akinsanya, C. Y. (1985) The use of knowledge in the management of a patient's pain: the nurses' role. *Nurse Education Today* 5, pp. 41–6.

Alexander, J. I., Gardner, F. V. (1994) Prevention and management of postoperative pain. In: Gibson, H. B. (ed.) *Psychology, Pain and Anaesthesia.* London: Chapman and Hall.

Baillie, L. (1993) A review of pain assessment tools. *Nursing Standard* 7 (23), pp. 2529.

Brand, P., Yancey, P. (1993) *Pain: The Gift Nobody Wants: A Surgeon's Journey of Discovery.* London: Marshal Pickering/HarperCollins.

Briggs, M. (1995) Principles of acute pain assessment. *Nursing Standard* Feb. 9 (19), pp. 23–7.

Carr, E. C. J. (1997) Overcoming barriers to effective pain control. *Professional Nurse* 12 (6), pp. 412–16.

Carr, E. C. J., Mann, E. M. (1998) *Partnering Patients to Manage Pain after Surgery: A Teaching and Learning Guide.* Bournemouth: IHCS Bournemouth University.

Carr, E. C. J., Mann, E. M. (2000) *Pain: Creative Approaches to Effective Management.* Basingstoke; Palgrave, Macmillan.

Chapman, A. (1996) Current theory and practice: a study of preoperative fasting. *Nursing Standard* Jan 20, 10 (18), pp. 33–7.

Crombez, G., Vlaeyen, J. M. S., Heuts, P. H. T. G., Lysens, R. (1999) Pain-related fear is more disabling than pain itself. *Pain* 80, pp. 329–39.

Department of Health (1989) *Report of the Advisory Group on Nurse Prescribing.* 1st Crown Report. London: HMSO.

Department of Health (1999) *Review of the Prescribing, Supply and Administration of Medicines.* 2nd Crown Report. London: HMSO.

Department of Health (2000) *The NHS Plan.* London: HMSO.

Department of Health (2002) *Extending Independent Nurse Prescribing within the NHS in England: A Guide to Implementation.* London: DOH.

Dolin, S. L., Padfield, N. L., Pateman, L. A. (1996) *Pain Clinic Manual.* Oxford: Butterworth Heinemann.

Duthie, Prof. R. B. (1988) *DOH Guidelines for the Safe and Secure Handling of Medicines.* A Report to the Secretary of State for Social Services. London: HMSO.

Ferrell, B. R., McCaffery, M., Rhiner, M. (1992) Pain and addiction: an urgent need for change in nurse education. *Journal of Pain and Symptom Management* 7 (2), pp. 117–24.

Foley, K. M. (1993) Pain assessment and cancer pain syndromes. In: Doyle, D., Hanks, G. W. C., MacDonald, N. (eds) *Oxford Textbook of Palliative Medicine.* Oxford: Oxford Medical Publications, ch. 4.2.2, pp. 148–65.

Griepp, M. E., (1992) Under medication for pain: an ethical model. *Advances in Nursing Science* 15 (1), pp. 44–53.

International Association for the Study of Pain (IASP) (1986) Classification of chronic pain. Descriptions of chronic pain syndromes and definitions of pain terms. *Pain.* Supplement 3.

Jadad, A. R., Carroll, D., Glynn, C. L, Moore, R. A., McQuay, H. J. (1992) Morphine responsiveness of chronic pain: double-blind randomised crossover study with patient controlled analgesia. *Lancet* 6 June, 339 (8806), pp. 1367–71.

Marcer, D., Deighton, S. (1988) Intractable pain: a neglected area of medical education in the UK. *Journal of the Royal Society of Medicine* 81, pp. 698–700.

McCaffery, M. (1972) *Nursing Management of the Patient with Pain.* Philadelphia, PA: J. B. Lippincott.

McQuay, H. (1990) Assessment of pain, and effectiveness of treatment. In: Hopkins, A., Costain, D. (eds) *Measuring the Outcomes of Medical Care.* London: Royal College of Physicians, Kings Fund Centre for Health Services Development.

Melzack, R., Wall, P. D. (1965) Pain mechanisms: a new theory. *Science* 150, pp. 971–9.

Melzack, R. (1975) The McGill pain questionnaire: major properties and scoring methods. *Pain,* pp. 1277–99.

Sackett, D., Richardson, W. S., Rosenburg, W., Haynes, B. (1996) *Evidence-Based Medicine.* London: Churchill Livingstone.

Schofield, P. (1995) Using assessment tools to help patients in pain. *Professional Nurse.* August 10 (11), pp. 703–6.

Shade, P. (1992) PCA: Can client education improve outcomes? *Journal of Advanced Nursing* 17, pp. 408–13.

Shevde, K., Triveldi, N. (1991) Effects of clear fluids on gastric volume and ph in health volunteers. *Anaesthesia Analgesia* 72, pp. 528–31.

Skevington, S. (1995) *Psychology of Pain.* Chichester: J. Wiley and Sons.

Snelling, J. (1994) The effect of chronic pain on the family unit. *Journal of Advanced Nursing* 19, pp. 543–51.

Toulson, S. (1990) More than a lot of hot air. *Nursing* 11–24 Jan, 4 (2) pp. 23–6.

Resources

📖 Further reading

Backonja, M., Beydoun, A., Edwards, K. et al (1998) Gabapentin for the symptomatic treatment of painful neuropathy in patients with diabetes mellitus: a randomised controlled trial. *JAMA* 280, pp. 1831–6.

Casey, G. (1998) The management of pain in wound care. *Nursing Standard* 13 (12), pp. 49–54.

Carr, E. C. J. (1992) Overcoming barriers to effective pain control. *Professional Nurse* 15 (1), pp. 89–100.

Carroll, D. (1997) A non-pharmacological approach to chronic pain. *Professional Nurse Study Supplement* Oct. 13 (1), S12–S14.

Carroll, D., Bowsher, D. (1993) *Pain Management and Nursing Care.* Oxford: Butterworth Heinemann.

Fordham, M., Dunn, V. (1994) *Alongside the Person in Pain: Holistic Care and Nursing Practice.* London: Baillière Tindall.

Hawthorn, J., Redmond, K. (1998) *Pain Causes and Management.* Oxford: Blackwell Science.

Illingworth, K. A., Simpson, K. H. (1994) *Anaesthesia and Analgesia in Emergency Medicine.* Oxford: Oxford University Press.

King, V., Jacob, P. (1993) Special procedures. In: Carroll, D., Bowsher, D. (eds) *Pain Management and Nursing Care.* Oxford: Butterworth Heinemann, ch. 15.

Lawler, K. (1995) Entonox: too useful to be limited to childbirth. *Professional Care of Mother and Child* 5 (1), pp. 19–21.

Lawler, K. (1997) Pain assessment. *Professional Nurse* 13 (1), Study Supplement – Pain Control, S5–S8.

McCaffery, M., Beebe, A. (1994) *Pain: Clinical Manual for Nursing Practice.* London: Mosby.

McQuay, H., Moore, A. (1998) *An Evidence-Based Resource for Pain Relief.* Oxford: Oxford University Press.

Melzack, R., Wall, P. D. (1996) *The Challenge of Pain.* 3rd Edition. London: Penguin Books.

Park, G., Fulton, B. (1992) *The Management of Acute Pain.* Oxford: Oxford University Press.

Stevenson, C. (1995) Non-pharmacological aspects of acute pain management. *Complementary Therapies in Nursing and Midwifery* 1, pp. 77–84.

Thomas, V. J. (ed.) (1997) *Pain: Its Nature and Management.* London: Baillière Tindall.

Toulson, S. (1990) More than a lot of hot air, *Nursing* 11–24 Jan., I 4 (2), pp. 23–6.

Wall, P. D., Melzack, R., (eds) *Textbook of Pain.* 3rd Edition. Edinburgh: Churchill Livingstone.

Walsh, D. (1997) *TENS – Clinical Applications and Related Theory.* Edinburgh: Churchill Livingstone.

Welchew, E. (1995) *Patient Controlled Analgesia.* London: British Medical Journal Publishing Group.

Annotated bibliography

Alexander, J. I., Gardner, F. V. (1994) Prevention and management of postoperative pain. In: Gibson, H. B. (ed.) *Psychology, Pain and Anaesthesia.* London: Chapman & Hall.

This chapter explores various strategies that could improve pain management for patients following surgery. It looks at various pharmacological techniques as well as pre-operative preparation for both children and adults.

Baillie, L. (1993) A review of pain assessment tools. *Nursing Standard* 7 (23), pp. 25–9.

A useful and comprehensive review of pain assessment tools currently in use.

Briggs, M. (1995) Principles of acute pain assessment. *Nursing Standard* 9 Feb. (19), pp. 23-7.

This article looks less at pain assessment tools and more at the various factors which influence and direct acute pain assessment. Particularly useful in highlighting the importance of a positive nurse–patient relationship.

Carr, E. C. I (1992) Overcoming barriers to effective pain control. *Professional Nurse* 15 (1), pp. 89–100.

A thought provoking article that discusses the barriers patients put up that can inhibit good pain management. It also discusses the professional, institutional and organisational barriers that can also influence the quality of the pain management patients' experience.

Carroll, D., Bowsher, D. (1993) *Pain Management and Nursing Care.* Oxford: Butterworth Heinemann.

This book adopts a nursing approach to provide essential and relevant information on many aspects of pain management. Chapters including acute, chronic and cancer pain, as well as sections on the management of pain in the elderly and children.

Carroll, D. (1997) A non-pharmacological approach to chronic pain. *Professional Nurse, Study Supplement,* Oct. 13 (1), pp. S12–S14.

This article reviews some of the evidence, or lack of it so far, to support the use of a range of non-pharmacological strategies. The article critiques some of the work published so far that unfortunately, in many cases, has proved inconclusive, usually due to methodoligical problems. The text is useful to help support an evidence-based approach to pain management and emphasises the need for further study.

Casey, G. (1998) The management of pain in wound care. *Nursing Standard* 13 (12), pp. 49–54.

To my knowledge, the only article entirely devoted to the often ignored problem of invoked pain during the care of acute or chronic wounds.

Fordham, M., Dunn, V. (1994) *Alongside the Person in Pain: Holistic Care and Nursing Practice*. London: Baillière Tindall.

Again very much a nursing perspective that makes this book an interesting and informative read.

Hawthorn, J., Redmond, K. (1998) *Pain: Causes and Management*. Oxford: Blackwell Science.

A book that considers physiological, spiritual, psychological and social components of pain, covering pharmacological and non-pharmacological strategies. Also, there is a useful section that explores some of the barriers that have inhibited good pain management in the past.

Illingworth, K. A., Simpson, K. H., (1994) *Anaesthesia and Analgesia in Emergency Medicine*. Oxford: Oxford University Press.

This book covers all aspects of analgesia with a particular focus on what can be used in an emergency situation. Although written primarily for medical staff, it is also very useful for nursing staff and students who wish to know more about analgesia for specific situations, or who want more information about the use of local anaesthesia.

Johnson, M. I., Ashton, C. H., Thompson J. W. (1991) An in-depth study of long term users of transcutaneous electrical nerve stimulation (TENS): Implications for clinical use of TENS. *Pain* 44, pp. 221–9.

Useful article for those with a particular interest in TENS.

Lawler, K. (1995) Entonox: too useful to be limited to childbirth. *Professional Care of Mother and Child* 5 (1), pp. 19–21.

Article giving advice about the various situations where Entonox can provide useful analgesia. Also provides some explanations as to why Entonox is under-used at present.

Lawler, K. (1997) Pain assessment. *Professional Nurse* 13A, Study Supplement – Pain Control, S5–S8.

Text for those wishing more information on pain assessment.

McCaffery, M., Beebe, A. (1994) *Pain: Clinical Manual for Nursing Practice*. London: Mosby.

Although both the authors are American, this version has been extensively edited by Jane Latham to make it more appropriate for a British nursing audience. The book describes in detail how pain affects children and the elderly, as well as the rest of the general population. There are extensive nursing care guidelines, and suggested care plans that help to organise a patient's care and to facilitate communication between health care professionals.

McQuay, H., Moore, H. (1998) *An Evidence-Based Resource for Pain Relief*. Oxford: Pain Research Unit, University of Oxford.

This is the first book of its kind to bring together the reviews of drug and therapy trials. It is very helpful for those wanting information on how to assess the evidence and to be able to judge the value of that evidence. The book is divided into evidence for acute pain and chronic pain management and although it concentrates heavily on drug trials, it does include some other therapies as well.

Melzack, R., Wall, P. D. (1988) *The Challenge of Pain*. 2nd Edition. London: Penguin Books.
Vital book for anyone wanting to know far more about pain perception, why it is such a complex phenomenon and why it can prove such a challenge to treat. Despite the authors being the originators of the Gate Control Theory, their text is always clear and fascinating to read.

Park, G., Fulton, B. (1992) *The Management of Acute Pain*. Oxford: Oxford University Press.
This forms part of a series of books by Oxford Medical Publications that are comprehensive yet straightforward guides to caring for patients in pain. *The Management of Acute Pain* explains the mechanisms involved in pain perception and how the commonly used pharmacological therapies work to control pain.

Schofield, P. (1995) Using assessment tools to help patients in pain. *Professional Nurse*. August 10 (11), pp. 703–6.
Some straightforward information explaining the basic principles of pain assessment and why it is such a vital component of good pain management.

Skevington, S. (1995) *Psychology of Pain*. Chichester: J. Wiley and Sons.
This book is not a particularly easy read, but is especially useful for those with an interest in the psychological and emotional aspects of pain.

Stevenson, C. (1995) Non-pharmacological aspects of acute pain management. *Complementary Therapies in Nursing and Midwifery* 1, pp. 77–84.
Much of the research so far into complementary therapies or non-pharmacological aspects of pain management have concentrated on how they may be useful in helping to control chronic pain. This article looks at psychological approaches and physical therapies that may be of value in helping to control acute pain.

Thomas, V. A. (ed.) (1997) *Pain: Its Nature and Management*. London: Baillière Tindall.
An up-to-date book written by educators and clinicians who deal with pain management.

Toulson, S. (1990) More than a lot of hot air, *Nursing* 11–24 Jan., 4 (2), pp. 23–6.
Text extolling the virtues of using Entonox, especially within an accident and emergency department. Often this useful analgesic is overlooked by nursing staff, and yet its use can be not only effective but very safe as well.

Walsh, D. (1997) *TENS – Clinical Applications and Related Theory*. Edinburgh: Churchill Livingstone.
A book that goes into some depth on the physiology underpinning the use of TENS and advises on how to apply TENS in practice.

Welchew, E. (1995) *Patient Controlled Analgesia*. London: British Medical Journal Publishing Group.
A book especially for the student who has a particular interest in the development, application and management of patients receiving patient controlled analgesia.

@ Web pages

llwww.bournemouth.ac.uk/acad-depts; email: emann@bournemouth.ac.uk
Database of systematic reviews of pain relief: **www.jr2.ox.ac.uk/Bandolier**

Doctor's Guide to the Internet: Pain Management Information and Resources:
www.pslgroup.com/PAINMGT.HTM

Evidence-based/research

Agency for Health Care Policy and Research USA: **www.ahcpr.gov/**
Database of systematic reviews and research into pain relief: **www.ebando.com/**
Evidence-Based Healthcare Resources (with links to other sites):
www.grilib.demon.co.uk/ebm.htm
Health education systematic review discussion list:
www.mailbase.ac.uk/lists/sys-review/
Health Technology Assessment, NHS Research and Development Programme, providing
reviews of services for chronic pain control: **www.soton.ac.uk/-hta**
NHS Centre for Reviews and Dissemination, University of York:
www.york.ac.uk/inst/crd/welcome.htm
US National Institutes of Health – Pain Research: **http://www.nih.go**

Cancer and palliative care

Cochrane Cancer Network: **www.canet.demon.co.uk/**
King's College London, Department of Palliative Care and Policy:
www.kcl.ac.uk/kis/schools/kcsmd/palliative/top.htm
Sheffield Palliative Care Studies Group:
www.shef.ac.uk/uni/academic/D-H/dsas/spcsg/publicat.htm
VMO Programme on Cancer Control: **http://who-pcc.iarc.fr/**

Pain management

Pain Management Online: **www.painmngt.com/pi-0001.html** links to the following
organisations:
American Academy of Pain Management
American Pain Society
Chronic Pain Outreach
International Spinal Injection Society
National Headache Foundation
Neuro Modulation Society National
Roxanne Pain Institute
European Federation of IASP Chapters: **http:\\users.skynet.be/efic**
International Association for the Study of Pain: **http://www.halcyon.com/iasp**
The Pain Society: **www.ncl.ac.uk/-nrjh/painsoe/html**

Paediatric pain

Paediatric pain discussion list: **is.da..ca/-pedpain/ppmlist.html**
Science helping children: **is.dal.ca./~pedpain/pedpain.html**

💻 Video

Partnering Patients to Manage Pain after Surgery. I1ICS Bournemouth University, Royal
London House, Christchurch Road, Bournemouth, Dorset BH1 3LT.
A video and booklet that challenges some of the traditional practices surrounding post-
operative pain management and offers some solutions.

✉ Useful addresses

European Federation of IASP Chapters, EFIC Scientific Secretariat, Mrs C. de Lusignan,
Place Carnoy 11, Box 110, B 1200-Brussels, Belgium.
International Association for the Study of Pain (IASP), 909NE, 43' Street, Suite 306, Seattle,
WA 98105, USA.
Pain Society (UK Chapter IASP), 9 Bedford Square, London, WC1B 3RA.
RCN Pain Forum, Royal College of Nursing, 20 Cavendish Square, London, WIM OAB.

14 Insights into Palliative Care Nursing

Lynda Rogers and Pauline Turner

Introduction

This chapter focuses on the effects of caring for a person with a life-threatening illness. Joan has advanced breast cancer. This chapter will follow the experiences of Joan and her family. It will also explore the professional and personal issues for Helen and Gerald, two student nurses both of whom have had professional contact with Joan and her family. Helen worked with the multi-professional team who cared for Joan whilst she was an in-patient at the local hospice. She was also involved when the multi-professional team at the hospice arranged for Joan to return home as she had requested. Gerald had contact with Joan when he was working on the oncology unit in the acute hospital trust.

Aim

The aim of this chapter is that students will gain an insight and understanding of aspects of loss, grief and bereavement, with a focus on palliative care

---

Learning outcomes

The students will have an understanding of:

- The recognition of how the disease may have an effect on the physical, psycho-social and spiritual well-being of a person.
- The family as the unit of care.
- The importance of self-awareness in relation to aspects of loss, grief and bereavement.
- The principles of effective communication with the client/patient, their family and members of the health care team.
- The identification of the principles of palliative care, which includes considering the quality of life and the needs of the family as the unit of care.
- An awareness of the involvement and dynamics of the multi-disciplinary team and its contribution to effective patient care.

Concepts

- Cancer and palliative care
- Terminal illness
- Self-awareness
- Loss, grief and bereavement
- Quality of life
- Specialist services

- The multi-disciplinary team
- Reflective practice
- Whole person care
- The family as the unit of care
- Spirituality
- Death and dying

> ### Activity 14.1
>
> There may be other concepts that you have already decided you would like to explore. Ensure you have noted these down. As you work through the text yet more may arise.

Nurses will meet people with cancer and other life-threatening illnesses in many different settings. These include:

- Inpatient mental health units
- Paediatric wards
- Outpatient departments
- General medical and surgical wards
- Specialist units such as oncology, radiotherapy and haematology wards.

They will also meet people in the community setting who are receiving treatment in their own home or at the health centre or GP clinic. Also, nurses become involved through services for people with learning disability.

Practice tip

Check out the function and activities of any departments that are newly brought to your attention. This promotes improved communication between departments and between patients and staff.

The importance of a holistic approach is vital in cancer care. Holistic care takes into account the physical, psychological, social and spiritual implications of the disease as well as the individual's own needs. For this reason, it is important that nurses who are dealing with people facing a diagnosis of serious illness, death or aspects of loss, grief and bereavement have good communication and assessment skills. It is also important that

> ### Activity 14.2
>
> Write your own definition of holistic care before reading on.

health care professionals develop a high level of self-awareness which will enable them to give and receive support. These various aspects will be looked at in the chapter. It will focus on the knowledge and skills needed by nurses to care for patients who are experiencing a serious illness which can result in death. This review will also consider the nursing skills needed to support a patient and their family during the stages of the cancer journey. Her story enables other group members to reflect on their own beliefs and experiences in relation to caring for a person who has a diagnosis of cancer, as well as considering the needs of the patient's/client's family.

Scenario *Meet the students*

Helen Shape, 20 years old. Born in Surrey, England, Helen has been educated in local schools and has progressed to sixth form education in her local sixth form college. She commenced her nursing programme 11 months ago and is currently completing her common foundation programme.

Her parents are both well and Helen lives with them and her two sisters aged 22 years and 15 years when she is not at university. Helen has a varied social life and has always enjoyed helping people. She has been a member of the local St John Ambulance Brigade since she was 11 years old. She thinks this may have influenced her choice of career, although this was not the only influence. Helen also attended Brownies and Guides from the age of 7. She gained the Baden Powell Award when she was 14 years old. She also achieved badges for swimming and athletics.

Her parents used to encourage her to attend the local Church of England church when she lived at home but she has not made regular attendance in recent years. Since Helen commenced her nursing career, she has become interested in other faiths.

During her sixth form period of education she gained a part-time job as a waitress in a local restaurant and worked Saturday and Sunday evenings. She feels this job has enabled her to meet a variety of people and get to understand their different moods (especially when their food was not to their liking). She considers that she has learnt to communicate in different ways with people.

Gerald O'Keefe, 20 years old. Born in Ireland, Gerald has been educated in a Catholic boarding school and received further education at a local college where he gained his 'A' levels. He commenced his nursing programme 11 months ago and is currently completing his common foundation programme.

Gerald's parents are alive and well. They both come from Ireland, but the family moved to England in 1986 because of his father's job. The family home is now in Hampshire. Gerald lives with his parents and sister aged 18 when he is not at university. His sister commenced university studies this year, but had to return home for a short period as she had a serious kidney infection. She will return to university in the spring. Gerald is very fond of his sister and he felt quite concerned when she was ill and he could not go home to visit her during term time. Gerald feels the experience of concern for his sister when she was ill has made him aware of how patients'/clients' families may feel when their relatives are ill. Like Helen, Gerald enjoys a varied and active social life. He enjoys sport and has always played football and cricket in season. He also plays badminton and has joined the university badminton club. Gerald says that 'like all good students', he enjoys a few drinks at the local 'pub' or university social club with his friends.

Gerald is a practising Catholic and attended the local Catholic church with his family whilst in Ireland. He still attends the local Catholic church when he is at home with his parents.

Whilst studying for 'A' levels, he worked in a local store. When he gained his full driving licence, he changed his job to work as a care assistant in a local nursing home. He feels this work has helped him to gain experience before he applied for his nursing course.

Enquiry-based learning

Helen and Gerald, along with the other members of their cohort, have just completed the third clinical placement of their common foundation programme (CFP) in nursing. They are now in school for a theory component of their programme. The school uses enquiry-based learning as its method of learning. Every week they meet in their learning group, which enables the students to explore with each other and their facilitator aspects of their theoretical and clinical learning. As this is the first time the group have met for a number of weeks, they have chosen to share some of their clinical experiences with each other and to reflect on the learning they have gained from these experiences.

Helen shares her experience of working with a patient who she has helped care for both in the hospice setting and in the patient's own home.

This reflection also enables the group to consider their own needs in relation to caring for people who are experiencing aspects of loss, grief and bereavement or who are dying. The group use a tool which they have adapted, with their facilitator's help, from the Gibbs (1988) cycle of reflection (see Chapter 1) and from Schon's (1983) principles of reflection to enable them to clarify the process and their thoughts.

Adapted reflective tool

These are the stages that the students work through:

1 Telling the story – reflection 'on', describing the event.
2 Examining your feelings in relation to the story – did I feel sad, happy, angry, afraid, ignorant, stupid?

3 Evaluation – what have I learnt? Analysis, picking out the major points from the event.

4 Developing and learning – how will the previous three stages help to enhance my practice or actions/behaviour in the future?

Helen's reflective story

Joan, aged 53, was admitted to the hospice. Her past medical history showed that she had a diagnosis of breast cancer three years ago. She had previously been admitted to the oncology unit for radiotherapy and chemotherapy treatment after having had a partial mastectomy. More recently she was admitted to a medical ward with severe breathlessness.

Activity 14.3

Check out your understanding of terminology that may be unfamiliar. For example, review your understanding of the following:

- Radiotherapy
- Chemotherapy
- Partial mastectomy

You may like to review the assessment of breathing in Chapter 5 on nursing adults.

Helen explains to the group the admission process used at the hospice. This process is one which assesses the holistic needs of both the patient and their family. Helen also explains to the group how everyone in the multi-disciplinary team becomes involved with Joan's care.

Activity 14.4

If you have the opportunity, try to negotiate a visit to a local hospice.

Helen continues relating Joan's story

Joan was well for a couple of years, but over the last six months she has been feeling increasingly tired and unwell. A couple of months ago she noticed she was becoming breathless on climbing stairs, but this has become much worse and she is now breathless all the time. A chest X-ray shows that she has a pleural effusion as a result of lung metastases. The first line of medical treatment will be to perform a chest aspiration to drain the fluid from her lung.

When Helen had completed the first part of her story the group formulated a set of questions related to Joan and her care and nursing needs.

> ### Activity 14.5
> Check out your understanding of pleural effusion.

> ### Activity 14.6
> Before reading on, write down the questions that you would like to explore further if you were a member of this group. (To find out more about the nature of cancer and its treatments, read a specific text such as *Cancer Care: Prevention Treatment and Palliation*, edited by David 1995.)

Set out below are some of the questions or aspects of Joan's care which the group identified that they needed to explore further in order to enhance their knowledge and understanding:

 What members of the multi-disciplinary team and the multi-agency team would be found at a hospice? What are their key roles?

 Why does pleural effusion cause breathlessness?

 What other symptoms might Joan experience in relation to the pleural effusion?

How can these be relieved?

What are metastases? How do they occur? How would you explain 'lung metastases' to a junior colleague?

Some important points about breathlessness

Breathlessness is a common and very distressing symptom in patients with advanced cancer and is most associated with lung, colorectal, breast and prostate cancers (Reuben and Mor 1986; Heyse-Moore et al 1991). It is an unpleasant sensation of being unable to breathe easily. While Joan is waiting for the chest aspiration to be carried out, nursing management of her breathlessness is extremely important. Like pain, there is an emotional component to breathlessness so it is vital that the nurse spends time with Joan, reassuring her and providing measures that will reduce her anxiety. Breathlessness is extremely frightening as many patients fear that they will suffocate or choke to death during a breathless attack.

Activity 14.7

Before reading on compile a list of nursing actions which you think may help to alleviate Joan's distress. You may like to review the section on assessment of breathing in Chapter 5 on nursing adults.

Measures which will help include:

- Upright positioning in bed, using firm pillows which are piled one on top of the other (not the 'armchair' arrangement).
- Use of cool air – a fan or open windows.
- Encourage diaphragmatic breathing – patients often breathe only from the top part of their chest.
- Sitting with the patient and the family giving reassurance.
- Administering opioids; for example, morphine helps to reduce the sensation of breathlessness.

Joan's family

Joan has a husband, Robert, two sons and a daughter. The two sons live away but Ellie, aged 15, is still at school. Robert is a long-distance lorry driver and he has found Joan's deteriorating health very worrying over the last few months. Ellie does not talk about her mother's illness and spends a lot of her time upstairs in her bedroom or out with her friends.

Working with the whole family

'Cancer can affect a family in much the same way as it affects a body', writes Murray-Parkes (cited by Monroe in Saunders and Sykes 1993), 'causing deterioration if left untreated.' Working with the whole family is therefore important and individual family member's needs will have to be ascertained, and where possible addressed.

Evidence-based practice

Glasper and Lowson (1998) argue that family-centred care is not just about enabling the family to have knowledge and understanding of the diagnosis and treatments and health care interventions, but about being enabled to *participate* in the care. The participation should be encompassed within a holistic approach to the patient's/client's health care needs and interventions.

A genogram can be a useful way of alerting the professional team to the needs of the family. A genogram is a diagrammatic representation of a family, like a family tree, which provides important information about the family and its support networks. (Giossi 1997). Gathering information for a genogram can be initiated by the nurse or doctor

Activity 14.8

Think about Robert and Ellie's needs. What are the important issues for them? What about Joan and Robert's two sons?

in their assessment interview and can be built up gradually. Or Joan could be asked to draw this herself. Some patients like doing this as it gives them control over what information they are prepared to share. It can also be a way for them to identify who, in their circle of friends and family, is able to provide support and who may need support themselves. For some people, however, sharing such information might be painful and can only emerge over time in a trusting relationship (Sheldon 1993). (Refer to Figures 4.1 and 7.1 in Chapters 4 and 7 on adolescent health and learning disabilities for examples of family genograms.

Joan's genogram gives information about her family which can be used sensitively and appropriately by members of her own family, as well as the multi-disciplinary team. From Joan's genogram it is possible to see that her mother died with breast cancer. This immediately raises the issue about possible hereditary factors, and indicates that Ellie will need to be offered follow-up and screening in the future as her risk of developing breast cancer is increased (McPherson et al 1995). Since this is the case, it is even more important that Ellie gets the right sort of information about her mother's illness and has the opportunity to ask questions.

The genogram also demonstrates that Joan has a very supportive sister, although she may have anxieties of her own about breast cancer. Robert's parents live locally and are fit and well. Family support therefore may be good, which is an important factor since

Activity 14.9

Before reading on identify what should be included in a family assessment.

Robert's work takes him away from home for many hours at a time.

However, assessment of the family's needs will change over time. At the moment, for example, Joan is still mobile and able to carry out her own personal care, as well as some household tasks. By asking both Joan and Robert the question, 'What is most worrying for you at the moment?', the nurse will be able to focus on aspects which are of immediate concern (Monroe 1993).

A checklist of areas to enquire about is provided below.

Family assessment should include enquiry about the following areas:

- Psychological and emotional needs.
- Information needs – about the disease and treatment, about the services available at home and how to access them.
- Individual family member's – in this case, Ellie's – needs.
- Support networks – family, friends, neighbours.
- Finances or financial support.

Communication

One of the points raised by various members of the group is the importance of positive communication. Quite a number of the group describe how they have observed members of the multi-disciplinary team in their last placement talking with clients/patients and their families. They also highlight the importance of good intercommunication between team members.

Evidence-based practice

The importance of good nurse–patient communication in the care of cancer patients

Much has been written about the importance of good communication when caring for patients with cancer and their families. The challenge is to enter into open and honest dialogue in a way that enables them to express their anxieties and fears. This requires the development of good communication skills, which will mean paying attention to our non-verbal messages (body language) and the use of verbal skills such as:

- Active listening
- Open questioning
- Reflecting back to the patient our understanding of what they have said.

This requires courage, sensitivity, and a high level of self awareness. Practice this skill whenever you feel comfortable to try. Wilkinson (1991) suggests that nurses may facilitate or 'block' communication with patients. 'Blocking' may occur as a way of distancing ourselves from the uncomfortable or painful expression of emotions. Faulkner and Maguire (1994) describe some of these 'distancing techniques', and suggest that we need to recognise them and ask ourselves why we are using them. Examples of 'blocking' or 'distancing' include:

- Ignoring cues
- Selective attention to cues
- Inappropriate encouragement
- Premature reassurance
- False reassurance
- Switching the topic
- Premature problem solving
- Passing the buck
- Avoiding
  (Faulkner and Maguire 1994)

Activity 14.10

Think about 'blocking' and 'distancing'. Clarify what is meant by each of these terms, checking your understanding with others. Consider in what ways you may have personally 'blocked' or 'distanced' yourself from patients or others, or have observed others using these devices.

Reflective accounts by two students in the group

Student C

'I know that I have "blocked" effective communication with a patient. I asked a patient how he was feeling yesterday and he replied, "Rough". Without thinking, I continued, "But that pain in your leg is a lot better today isn't it?" He muttered his agreement and went back to reading his paper. I was doing something else at the time and was relieved not to have to continue the conversation with him. But later when I thought about this incident, I realised that I had switched the focus from an emotional one (how he was feeling) to a physical one (his pain) and had effectively "blocked" further conversation with him on this matter.'

Student D

'I know what you mean, said another student in the group. I was talking to a patient who was waiting to have a fairly unpleasant procedure performed. She told me she was feeling very anxious about it and I said something to the effect that it was "fairly normal to feel like that". When I read Wilkinson's study, I realised that I had used "blocking" tactics by reassuring the patient that it was normal for her to feel like that, but without hearing her out as to what her anxieties really were. I hope that by reflecting on incidents like this I will be more aware of my own communication with patients and will listen more attentively to what they are really saying.'

Activity 14.11

See also Chapter 6 (on mental health) and texts such as: MacLeod-Clark (1983); Buckman (1992); Sheldon (1993); Faulkner and Maguire (1994); and Egan (1990).

Helen is encouraged to continue with Joan's story

Joan's condition had steadily worsened since her last admission to hospital. She had had regular check-ups at the outpatient breast clinic and a recent bone scan showed that she had bone metastases in her ribs and in her lumbar and thoracic spine. Despite this, Joan still managed to be reasonably independent. However, one morning as she was walking to the telephone, she slipped and fell, fracturing her femur. Her GP admitted her to hospital, and she subsequently had surgery to pin her femur. The operation was successful, but Joan's mobility was now much reduced and she was in a lot of pain. The orthopaedic team referred her to the hospital palliative care team, who discussed pain control with the ward staff and arranged for her to be transferred to a palliative care unit for rehabilitation and symptom management.

Activity 14.12

Find out if there is a palliative care team identified in the area where you work. What is the role of individual members of the team? How is the team contacted?

Later in your programme you may find it very useful to negotiate to spend some time with individuals in the team.

Before reading on, consider the client groups that a palliative care team may support.

Palliative care teams

Specialist palliative care services provide care for people whose disease is not responsive to curative treatment. Some of these teams deal only with cancer patients, but many others offer a service to people who are dying from non-malignant diseases such as motor neurone disease and HIV and Aids.

The key principles of palliative care include:

- Emphasis on quality of life, including good symptom control.
- Autonomy and choice.
- A holistic approach.

- The dying person and those who matter to that person as the unit of care.
- Open and sensitive communication with patients, their informal carers and professional colleagues (National Hospice Council 1995).

The palliative care unit

Joan was admitted to the palliative care unit for rehabilitation. She was keen to go home and a team approach was adopted to enable Joan's wish to be achieved. Whilst in the hospice, Joan's needs were assessed. This included her physical needs such as pain control. The assessment was based on a holistic approach and encompassed her psychological, social and spiritual needs.

During Joan's admission it became clear that her cancer was advancing fairly rapidly and her condition deteriorating. She rarely referred to her illness. Instead, her predominant attitude seemed to be one of 'keeping cheerful'. She talked often about her plans for the future, including where the family would take their holidays next year. She also mentioned returning to work. She was a secretary and worked for years with a firm of solicitors until about 18 months ago when she was made redundant. Some of the ward staff had said that she was 'in denial' and wanted to challenge some of her statements. It felt uncomfortable for them that she had not 'accepted it'.

 ## Activity 14.13

From your practice experience you may like to reflect on patients that you have cared for. In what ways have you noticed that people react to the knowledge that they are not getting better, or how might people react?

Evidence-based practice

Psychological responses to dying

There are several theoretical frameworks which have been described over the last 30 years as a way of understanding the process through which people who are facing death pass. It is important to remember that they are only frameworks, in other words they are meant to act as a guide to help others understand people's responses at such a time. They cannot be a true representation of how an individual is feeling – only he or she can know that, and each person will have a different set of values, beliefs and perspective about what is happening. Kubler Ross (1969) is one of the most well known theorists and her description of the 'stages of dying' has influenced many people's thinking. These stages are:

- Denial
- Anger

- Bargaining
- Depression
- Acceptance

For a wider reading of the issues around the 'stage theories of dying', please refer to other further reading such as the texts by Buckman (1992); and Clark and Seymour (1999).

Other writers have proposed a three-stage model of the grieving process. However, a closer look at theories about coping mechanisms (Lazarus 1984) would suggest that denial is a way of coping with stress and provided that it is not detrimental to the patient and family, it serves its purpose well. Buckman (1992) suggests that professionals should assess denial in patients to see if it is working for or against them.

One thing that needs to be borne in mind, however, is the effect that Joan's denial might be having on Ellie and the rest of the family and their need to prepare psychologically for the future. Even so, Joan's denial may not need to be challenged as long as Robert is aware that Joan is not going to get better and is able to talk with Ellie about this. A useful way of gently introducing this topic with Robert, if he has not directly asked about Joan's prognosis, is the 'what if' question; for example, 'what if Joan's condition is progressing more rapidly than we had expected?' Another approach is 'planning for the worst and hoping for the best' (Sheldon 1993). By this Sheldon suggests that, although the family and health care professionals should not deny the future, the condition or illness is becoming worse or that there will be no improvement, the patient/client and their family should focus on 'today'. This 'hoping for the best' approach can enable people to focus on how they feel or are coping today. This is sometimes referred to as 'living for today'.

Religious or spiritual considerations

Religious beliefs and systems can provide a sense of peace and well-being for a person or group of people who have a particular faith. Health care professionals have a responsibility to respect other beliefs and faiths and, where possible, to provide for their religious needs. Acute hospitals normally have a chaplaincy that can provide religious, spiritual and social support for both the patient/client and their family.

Activity 14.14

Your clients and patients will come from a wide range of cultural backgrounds and will hold many different and varying beliefs. If your client is a Sikh, a Muslim or perhaps Jewish, would you know what formalities or wishes should be taken into account? Find out in your next practice visit what information is available on the full range of faiths.

Preparing for Joan's return to home

There are a wide range of issues in discharge planning or transferring care. The primary health care team will need some information to be prepared to take on their roles. The community palliative nursing team will also be involved.

To ensure that Joan would be able to return home, a network of care provision is set in place. Her GP and the primary care team would be informed, and a discharge plan would be sent to them to ensure that all Joan's current health care needs are known and understood by the health care professionals who will continue to provide for her needs. The specialist palliative care team may also continue to visit Joan at home. Knowing precisely what information is helpful is important for continuity of care.

Activity 14.15

Whenever you can, take the opportunity to arrange to work with colleagues in the community. Find out the details of their roles and what hospital-based nurses should pass on for effective communication to facilitate seamless care. Try to become involved in discharge planning to consolidate and put into practise the new information gained.

Dying at home – the facts

Most people, if given the choice, would prefer to die at home. The majority will spend most of the last year of their life at home, although a large percentage of people still die in acute hospital environments (Clarke 1997, cited in Clark and Seymour 1999). The main people involved in care are the relatives or close friends, so their needs too must be taken into account. Others include the GP, district nursing team and, if required, occupational therapist. It may be that other specialist practitioners, such as the community psychiatric nursing team, can be of help to either the client and/or family members.

Despite death becoming less of a taboo subject, many people will not have seen a death and would need information and support about what to expect during the last stage of living.

Evidence-based practice

Stress and anxiety experienced by students
Lazarus (1984) defines stress as a condition which can occur when a situation leads an individual to perceive a discrepancy between demands of the situation and their personal biological, psychological and sociological ability to cope with the issue. Stress can be positive, enabling the individual to overcome a situation such as moving faster in the morning to ensure that you

arrive in time to catch a bus; however, too many stressors can result in negative stress effect and anxiety.

In interviews with student nurses Rogers (1992 and 2002) found that those who were unprepared to cope with patients who were experiencing aspects of loss, grief and bereavement suffered stress and anxiety. Students who had opportunities to explore aspects of loss, grief and bereavement in the early stages of their nurse education programmes said that, although they still needed support in the clinical environment, they felt more able to cope when clients/patients and relatives were given 'bad news'.

Helen explained that Joan went back home where her care needs were looked after by her family and members of the primary health care team. Joan died as she had wished, in her own home with her family around her.

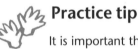

Practice tip

It is important that not only family and friends of the client/patient are able to express themselves but also all members of the health care team as well.

Reflecting and sharing with the group

After Helen has shared her story she used the reflective cycle to explore her own feelings. She was also able to consider what she had learnt from this experience and what could help her future practice. One of the things she said she had learnt was the importance of communication, not only how to actively listen to patients and clients, but to feel comfortable with silence. She said she realised that just being with someone, sitting quietly with them, perhaps holding their hand, seemed so helpful.

The group spent time sharing their own experiences about caring for someone who is experiencing aspects of loss, grief and bereavement.

Gerald explained that there were times when he felt very vulnerable whilst working on the oncology unit. 'The staff were very nice to me; everyone understood that because I was a psychiatric student undertaking my 'adult placement', I had very little experience of dealing with people who had acute physical needs'. I wanted to help at times but felt so useless. I was glad that my assessor (mentor) gave me time to explore my feelings. Whenever possible we would sit down and talk about what I had done. Sometimes I was able to question treatment and nursing care. But at other times, we would just talk about my feelings. It made me feel part of the team and not just a visitor. It helped me learn about oncology treatment, but also to understand that not everyone responded well to treatment. I also realised how useful my psychi-atric nursing skills were.'

Other group members also shared their own feelings of insecurity regarding this aspect of care. Some talked about not knowing what to say to patients or relatives; feeling guilty for smiling, being seemingly unable to control facial expressions; over-sensitivity in listening out for cues from the patient and wondering what meaning to attribute to them; being unsure of what to pass on to more senior colleagues and what is a confidential, as opposed to a casual, remark. This sharing seemed to help the group to feel less insecure and to realise that others in the group felt the same as they did.

However, the group also reflected on sessions they had attended at the beginning of their course. These small group sessions enabled them to explore in safety their own values and beliefs related to death and dying. They were also able to express their own concerns about practice. Some group members remembered asking what it would be like looking after someone who was dying; what did a dead person look like. At the same time, other students reiterated how they had shared their own previous experi-ences related to loss, grief and bereavement. Gerald reflected again on his experiences whilst working in a nursing home before he started his nursing programme. 'You know we had a lot of theory about loss, grief and bereavement and were told what it could be like to care for people who are dying. But it's not until you care for someone who is dying that you start to think about what it must be like to have your life cut short by a terminal illness.' 'I understand what you are saying', replied Helen quietly. They both sat staring in front of them, seemingly lost in their own thoughts.

Evidence-based practice

Learning to demonstrate caring attitudes

Field (1996) and Clark (1993) both suggest that many people in Western societies still have a limited experience and awareness of death and dying, or of aspects of loss, grief and bereavement.

However, health care professionals have come a long way since Elizabeth Kubler-Ross gave her opinion in 1969. She suggested that because many people had such little knowledge of death and found the experience fright-ening, many doctors and nurses were not able to provide a peaceful death despite their efforts to provide for their physical needs. This resulted in a 'gruesome, lonely, mechanical and dehumanised death' (1969, p. 7).

Corless (1990) argues that a nurse's behaviour towards a patient who is dying is determined by personal attitudes. Further, it is argued that if a nurse feels uncomfortable or has a limited understanding of the needs of the dying person and their family's needs, they are more likely to demonstrate avoid-ance behaviour and less likely to demonstrate appropriate caring attitudes to their patient/client group.

Loss, grief and bereavement

Gerry and Helen had had an opportunity to start to explore their own beliefs about loss, grief and bereavement when they first started their nursing course. They had spent some time in a small group, talking with a teacher about their fears and feelings in relation to starting to work with people who were sick and vulnerable. Some people in their group had commented that they had not seen anyone who was dead. Another person had expressed fears about being asked questions by relatives which they would feel unable to answer, such as what was wrong with a patient or how long the patient had to live.

Activity 14.16

A You may find it helpful to identify any fears you may have about caring for people who have a terminal disease. Perhaps you could work with a friend or colleague with whom you feel comfortable in sharing your feelings. You may find you have similar worries or they might be quite different.

B Consider what you would say to a patient who was experiencing a life-threatening illness if you had to admit them onto your ward or visit them in their home.

C Consider how you think you could have helped to support Joan, her husband and her children, in both acute and community settings.

Practice tip

Taking the time to rehearse such potentially stressful situations is often helpful in developing your practice skills. Some students create the opportunity to use role-play to practise, seek feedback and share ideas to enhance their understanding.

Evidence-based practice

Considerations for change to the preparation of pre-registration students in relation to loss, grief and bereavement and care of the terminally ill

A lack of adequate training and preparation within nurse education in relation to this aspect of care has been found to lead to difficulties when communicating with dying people and those suffering aspects of loss, grief and bereavement. This was more recently supported by Kelsey's study (1992) when she mooted that education and training were inadequate to deal with this area of care. However, Rogers's current research (2002) has found that if student nurses have exposure to this aspect of professional health care early in their course, then they are better prepared and more able to accept the needs of both the patient who is suffering loss and bereavement as well as the family's demands on them, the health care professionals. She also found that by enabling students to talk about their fears and concerns about working with very sick patients of all age groups, they started to explore for themselves their own vulnerability and mortality.

'Do you remember the session we had, talking with patients and relatives who may have fears and anxieties about diagnosis?'

'Yes I do. I wasn't sure what to expect . . . it was about ways in which we could use communication skills.'

'It focused on ways in which we could be part of the multi-professional team helping to 'break bad news'.'

'I found learning about active listening and the use and benefit of silence when a patient is trying to express themselves very helpful.'

(Extracts from PhD student transcripts 1995 and 1996, Rogers 2002)

Irving (1993) stresses the importance of nurses (and other health care professionals) learning effective communication skills. If these professionals feel unable to speak honestly and openly with their patients in a way which is appropriate to their patient's age, educational and language ability, then they could well develop a 'conspiracy of care'. They appear to avoid appropriate communication with the patients and their relatives because they do not know what to say or do when they are confronted with awkward questions. They may even use 'blocking' techniques (Faulkner and Maguire 1994).

Kigers's study (1994) found that students often felt confused and unable to deal with experiences of death and aspects of loss, grief and bereavement, commenting that the 'system does not provide for support needs in relation to coping with the experience of death . . .' (p. 685).

Sneddon and Eagle (1991) argue that specific teaching in relation to these subjects can improve confidence and reduce anxiety and

> ### Activity 14.17
>
> Consider your own communication skills. Would you feel comfortable sitting quietly with a patient or relative whilst they find the words to tell you how they feel?

stress. This is further supported by Reisetter and Thomas (cited in Nebaeur 1996), who state that improvements in students' study programmes, focusing holistically on this area of care, can reduce stress and improve client contact and care.

Rogers (2002) has found that a programme of study which starts to examine aspects of loss, grief and bereavement early on in the curriculum can not only reduce stress and anxiety in the students, but can enhance and improve the quality of intervention that these same students feel they can provide whilst working within the multi-disciplinary professional health care team.

Carl Rogers (1983) argues that we need to become self-aware. By examining our own beliefs and attitudes we can begin to know ourselves, and in doing so enhance the care we give to our patients/clients. It will also enhance our own professional and personal self-esteem.

The end of the group session

At the end of their session, the group recognised how much they had learnt from listening to each other's experiences. They also realised how much information they had gathered which would be carried forward and used as they progress and examine other concepts. All the members of the group agreed. This exploration was not the end of this experience, but a stage in a long trajectory of life-long learning. They recognised that individually and as a group, they could use some of the information and knowledge gained during this session to develop their practice skills, as well as to enhance their knowledge base.

Conclusion

While working through this chapter, many issues will have arisen for you about caring for a person with a life-threatening illness. Although this example relates to a person with breast cancer, you will already have met many individuals affected by a variety of different forms of cancer or other life-threatening situations. All have particular nursing needs and the same principles of holistic care must be considered, whether the person is in hospital, in a hospice or is being nursed at home, to ensure the best quality of life is attained for each individual.

Joan and her family have specific needs and the importance of communication with the patient, family and between members of the health care team has been emphasised. There are many excellent examples of multi-disciplinary team work in palliative care practice. These are as a result of reflective practice where the needs of patient and family are at the centre.

Loss, grief and bereavement raise professional and personal issues for all members of the health care team who need to support each other as well as the patient and family. Perhaps you have been able to relate to the two student nurses and reflected on your experiences to date of caring for people experiencing a great loss, for example, loss of a limb, or coping with a terminal illness. You may wish to consider your own deficits in knowledge and understanding, and plan how you can access both information and support. Using a reflective tool may help you to review your own practice and highlight possible areas to further develop self-awareness to most effectively care for people in such challenging situations.

References

Buckman, R. (1992) *How to Break Bad News: A Guide for Health Care Professionals.* Basingstoke: Papermac.

Clark, D. (ed.) (1993) *The Future for Palliative Care: Issues of Policy and Practice.* Buckingham: Open University Press.

Clark, D., Seymour, J. (1997) What is qualitative research and what can it contribute to palliative care? *Palliative Medicine* 11, pp. 159–66.

Clark, D., Seymour, J. (1999) *Reflections on Palliative Care.* Buckingham: Open University Press.

Corless, I. B. (1990) Attitudes, subjective norms and behavioural intentions of nurses towards dying patients and their families: a critique of the study by N. L. Waltman. *Oncology Nursing Forum* 17 (3) supplement, pp. 55–60.

David, J. (ed.) (1995) *Prevention, Treatment and Palliation.* London: Chapman Hall.

Egan, G. (1990) *The Skilled Helper.* New York: Brooks Press.

Field, D. (1996) Awareness and modern dying. *Mortality* 1 (3), pp. 255–65.

Faulkner, A., Maguire, P. (1994) *Talking to Cancer Patients and Their Relatives.* Oxford: Oxford University Press.

Giossi, C. (1997) The use of the genogram in palliative care. *Palliative Medicine* 11, pp. 455–61.

Glasper, E. A., Lowson, S. (eds) (1998) *Innovations in Paediatric Ambulatory Care: A Nursing Perspective.* Basingstoke: Macmillan – now Palgrave Macillan.

Gibbs G. (1988) cited in Burns and Bulman (eds) *Learning by doing: A Guide to Teaching and Learning Methods.* Oxford: Further Education Unit, Oxford Brooks

Heyse-Moore, L. H., Ross, V., Mullee, M. (1991) How much of a problem is dyspnoea in advanced cancer? *Palliative Medicine* (5), pp. 20–6.

Irvin, B.M. (1993) Teaching palliative nursing to students. *Nursing Standard* September, 7 (50), pp. 37–9.

Kelsey, S. (1992) Can we care in the end: do nurses have the skills for terminal care? *Professional Nurse* January, pp. 216–19.

Kiger, A. M. (1994) Student nurses involvement with death: the image and the experience. *Journal of Advanced Nursing* 20 (4), pp. 686–97.

Kubler-Ross, E. (1969) *On Death and Dying.* London: Routledge Press.

Lazarus, R. S. (1984) *Stress, Appraisal and Coping.* New York: Springer Veriag Press

Macleod-Clark, J. (1983) Nurse patient communication. In: Barnett, S. (ed.) *Nursing Research: Ten Studies in Patient Care.* Chichester: Wiley Press.

McPherson, K., Steel, C., Dixon, J., Cancer – Epidemiology, risk factors and genetics. In: Dixon, J. M.(ed.) (1995) *ABC of Breast Diseases.* London: BMJ Publishing Group.

Monroe, B. (1993) Psychosocial dimensions of palliation. In: Saunders, C., Sykes, N. (eds) *The Management of Terminal Malignant Disease*. 3rd Edition. London: Edward Arnold.

Murray-Parkes, C. cited in Monroe, B. (1993) Psychosocial dimensions of palliation. In: Saunders and Sykes *The Management of Terminal Malignant Disease*.

National Hospice Council (1995) *Guidelines on Research in Palliative Care: Getting Good: Practice into Practice*. London: NHC.

Reisetter, K., Thomas, B. (1986) Cited in Nebaeur, M., Prior, D., et al (1996) Nurses perception of palliative care nursing. *International Journal of Palliative Nursing* (1).

Reuben D. B., Mor, M. (1986) Dsyspnea in terminal cancer patients. *Chest* 89, pp. 234–6.

Rogers, C. (1983) *Freedom to Learn for the 80's*/New York: Merrill Press.

Rogers, L. (1992) *Unpublished MA dissertation*, University of Southampton.

Rogers, L. (*extracts from student transcripts during field study 1995 and 1996*) for PhD thesis: presented for award June 2002.

Schon, D. (1983) *The Reflective Practitioner*. London: Jossey-Boss.

Sheldon, F. (1993) Communication. In: Saunders and Sykes *The Management of Malignant Terminal Disease*.

Sneddon, M., Eagle, P. (1991) Educational support in palliative care. *Nursing Standard* 5 (12), pp. 38–9.

Wilkinson, S. (1991) Factors which influence how nurses communicate with cancer patients. *Journal of Advanced Nursing* 16, pp. 677–88.

Resources

📖 Further reading

Buckman, R. (1992) *How to Break Bad News: A Guides for Health Care Professionals*. Basingstoke: Papermac.

David, J. (ed.) (1995) *Prevention, Treatment and Palliation*. London: Chapman Hall.

Faulker, A., Maguire, P. (1994) *Talking to Cancer Patients and Their Relatives*. Oxford: Oxford University Press.

Sheldon, F. (1993) Communication. In: Saunders and Sykes *The Management of Malignant Terminal Disease*.

Index